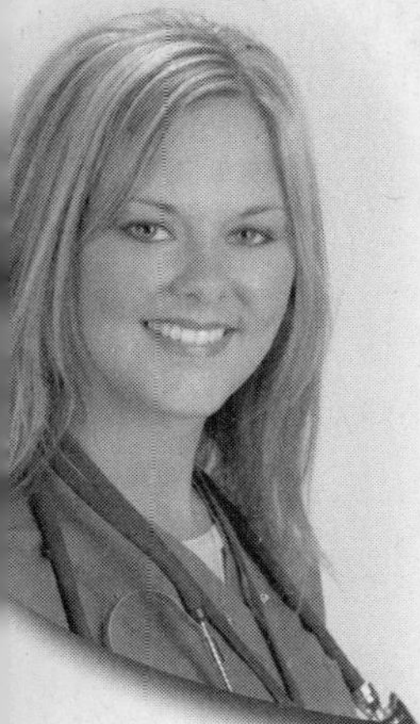

“The review modules are so he[illegible] give me bulleted highlights and concise, [illegible] information…
To top it off, you also get critical thinking exercises!
These books are fantastic! They have undoubtedly been the greatest review item I have found.”

Kimberly Montgomery
Nursing student

Terim Richards *Nursing student*

“I immediately went to my nurse manager after I failed the NCLEX® and she referred me to ATI. I was able to discover the areas I was weak in, and focused on those areas in the review modules and online assessments. I was much more prepared the second time around!”

Molly Obetz *Nursing student*

“The ATI review books were very helpful in preparing me for the NCLEX®. I really utilized the review summaries and the critical thinking exercises at the end of each chapter. It was nice to review the key points in the areas I was weak in and not have to read the entire book.”

Lindsey Koeble *Nursing student*

“I attribute my success totally to ATI. That is the one thing I used between my first and second attempt at the NCLEX®....with ATI I passed!”

Danielle Platt *Nurse Manager • Children’s Mercy Hospital • Kansas City, MO*

“The year our hospital did not use the ATI program, we experienced a 15% decrease in the NCLEX® pass rates. We reinstated the ATI program the following year and had a 90% success rate.”

“As a manager, I have witnessed graduate nurses fail the NCLEX® and the devastating effects it has on their morale. Once the nurses started using ATI, it was amazing to see the confidence they had in themselves and their ability to go forward and take the NCLEX® exam.”

Mary Moss *Associate Dean of Nursing and Health Programs • Mid-State Technical College • Rapids, WI*

“I like that ATI lets students know what to expect from the NCLEX®, helps them plan their study time and tells them what to do in the days and weeks before the exam. It is different from most of the NCLEX® review books on the market.”

Pharmacology For Nursing Practice
Review Module Edition 3.0

Contributors

Viola G. Benavente, RN, MSN, CNS
Assistant Professor
Department of Acute Nursing Care
School of Nursing
University of Texas Health Science Center
San Antonio, Texas

Jennifer Clausen, PharmD
Saint Luke's Hospital South
Overland Park, Kansas

Margaret S. Grinslade, RN, PhD
Department of Chronic Nursing Care
School of Nursing
University of Texas Health Science Center
San Antonio, Texas

Karen Hill, RN, PhD, MSN
Assistant Professor of Nursing
Southeastern Louisiana University
Hammond, Louisiana
Textbook Author

Sue Kilgore, RN, BSN
Park University
Parkville, Missouri
Shawnee Mission Medical Center
Shawnee Mission, Kansas

Judith Klinefelter, RN, DEd
Associate Professor of Nursing
Dean of the College of Nursing
Pennsylvania State University
University Park, Pennsylvania

Adrianne Linton, RN, PhD, MSN
Associate Professor of Nursing
University of Texas—Austin
Austin, Texas
Textbook Author

Joan Luckmann, RN, MA

University of Washington
Seattle, Washington
Textbook Author

Laura R. Sprinkle, PharmD, MSN

Clinical Specialist
Saint Joseph Health Center
Kansas City, Missouri

Melissa Thomas, RN, MSN

Clinical Nurse Specialist
Saint Luke's Hospital
Kansas City, Missouri

Patricia Van Tine, RN, MA

Clinical Professor
Santa Ana College
Santa Ana, California

Carolyn Wyss, RN, MSN

Associate Professor of Nursing
Walters State University
Morristown, Tennessee
Textbook Author

Editor-in-Chief

Leslie Schaaf Treas, RN, PhD(c), MSN, CNNP

Director of Research and Development
Assessment Technologies Institute™, LLC
Overland Park, Kansas

Editor

Jim Hauschildt, RN, EdD, MA

Director of Product Development
Assessment Technologies Institute™, LLC
Overland Park, Kansas

Copyright Notice

Important Notice to the Reader of this Publication

Assessment Technologies Institute™, LLC is the publisher of this publication. The publisher reserves the right to modify, change, or update the content of this publication at any time. The content of this publication, such as text, graphics, images, information obtained from the publisher's licensors, and other material contained in this publication are for informational purposes only. The content is not providing medical advice, and is not intended to be a substitute for professional medical advice, diagnosis, or treatment. Always seek the advice of your primary care provider or other qualified health provider with any questions you may have regarding a medical condition. Never disregard professional medical advice or delay in seeking it because of something you have read in this publication. If you think you may have a medical emergency, call your primary care provider or 911 immediately.

The publisher does not recommend or endorse any specific tests, primary care providers, products, procedures, processes, opinions, or other information that may be mentioned in this publication. Reliance on any information provided by the publisher, the publisher's employees, or others contributing to the content at the invitation of the publisher, is solely at your own risk. Healthcare professionals need to use their own clinical judgment in interpreting the content of this publication, and details such as medications, dosages or laboratory tests and results should always be confirmed with other resources.†

This publication may contain health or medical-related materials that are sexually explicit. If you find these materials offensive, you may not want to use this publication.

The publishers, editors, advisors, and reviewers make no representations or warranties of any kind or nature, including, but not limited to, the accuracy, reliability, completeness, currentness, timeliness, or the warranties of fitness for a particular purpose or merchantability, nor are any such representations implied with respect to the content herein (with such content to include text and graphics), and the publishers, editors, advisors, and reviewers take no responsibility with respect to such content. The publishers, editors, advisors, and reviewers shall not be liable for any actual, incidental, special, consequential, punitive or exemplary damages (or any other type of damages) resulting, in whole or in part, from the reader's use of, or reliance upon, such content.

Introduction to Assessment-Driven Review

To prepare candidates for the licensure exam, many different methods have been used. Assessment Technologies Institute™, LLC, (ATI) offers Assessment–Driven Review™ (ADR), a newer approach for customized board review based on candidate performance on a series of content-based assessments.

The ADR method is a four-part process that serves as a type of competency-assessment for preparation for the NCLEX-RN®. The goal is to increase preparedness and subsequent pass rate on the licensure exam. Used as a comprehensive program, the ADR is designed to help learners focus their review and remediation efforts, thereby increasing their confidence and familiarity with the NCLEX-RN® content. This type of program identifies learners at risk for failure in the early stages of nursing education and provides a path for prescriptive learning prior to the licensure examination.

The ADR approach may be preferable to a traditional "crash course" style of review for a variety of reasons. Time restriction is a fundamental barrier to comprehensive review. Because of the difficulty in keeping up with the expansiveness of information available today, a more efficient and directed approach is needed. Individualized review that starts with the areas of deficit helps the learner narrow the focus and begin customized remediation instead of a blanket A-to-Z approach. Additionally, review that occurs sequentially over time may be preferable to after-the-fact efforts after completion of a program when faculty are no longer available to assist with remediation.

Early identification of content weaknesses may prove advantageous to progressive program success. "Smaller bites" for content achievement and a shortened lapse of time between the introduction of course content and remediation efforts is likely to be more effective in catching the struggling learner before it is too late. Regular feedback keeps learners "on track" and reduce attrition rate by identifying the learner who is "slipping." This approach provides the opportunity to tutor or implement intensified instruction before the learner reaches a point of no return and drops out of the program.

Step I: Proctored Assessment

The ADR program is a method using a prescriptive learning strategy that begins with a proctored, diagnostic assessment of the learner's mastery of nursing content. The topics covered within the ADR program are based on the current NCLEX-RN® Test Plan. Proctored assessments are administered in paper-pencil and online formats. Scores are reported instantly with Internet testing or within 24 hours for paper-pencil testing. Individual performance profiles list areas of deficiencies and guide the learner's review and remediation of the missed topics. This road map serves as a starting point for self-directed study for NCLEX® success. Learners receive a cumulative Report Card showing scores from all assessments taken throughout the program—beginning to end. Like reading a transcript, the learner and educator can monitor the sequential progress, step-by-step, an assessment at a time.

Step II: Modular Reviews

A good test is one that supports teaching and learning. The score report identifies areas of content mastery as well as a means for correction and improvement of weak content areas. Eight review modules contain concise summaries of topics with a clinical overview, therapeutic nursing management, and client teaching. Key concepts are provided to streamline the study process. The ATI modules are not intended to serve as a primary teaching source. Instead, they are designed to summarize the material relevant to the licensure exam and entry-level practice.

Learners are taught to integrate holistic care with a critical thinking approach into the review material to promote clinical application of course content. The learner constructs responses to open-ended questions to stimulate higher-order thinking. The learner may provide rationales for actions in various clinical scenarios and generate explanations of why the solution may be effective in similar clinical situations. These exercises serve as the venue to shift from traditional didactic memorization of facts toward the use of analytical and evaluative reason in a client-related situation. The clinical application scenarios involve the learner actively in the problem-solving process and stimulate an attitude of inquiry.

These exercises are designed to provoke creative problem solving for the individual learner as well as collaborative dialogue for groups of learners in the classroom. Through group discussion, learners discover the technique of elaboration. Learners use group dialogue to increase their understanding of nursing content. In study groups, they may pose questions to their peers or explain various topics in their own words, adding personal experiences with clients and examples from previously acquired knowledge of the topic. Together they learn to reframe problems and assemble evidence to support conclusions. Through the integration of multiple perspectives and the synergy involved in the exchange of ideas, this approach may also facilitate the development of effective working relationships and patterns for lifelong learning. Critical thinking exercises for each topic area situate instruction into a problem-solving environment that can capture learners' attention, increase motivation to learn, and frame the content into an application context. Additionally, the group involvement can model the process for effective team interaction.

Step III: Non-Proctored Assessments

The third step is the use of online assessments that allow users to test from any site with an Internet connection. This online battery identifies specific areas of content weakness for further directed study. The interactive style provides the learner with immediate feedback on all response options. Rationales provide additional information about the correctness of an answer to supplement learners' understanding of the concept. Detailed explanations are provided for each incorrect response to clarify topics that learners often confuse, misunderstand, or fail to remember. Readiness to learn is often peaked when errors are uncovered; thus, immediate feedback is provided when learners are most motivated to find the answer. A Performance Profile summarizes learners' mastery of content. Question descriptors for each missed item are used to stimulate inquiry and further exploration of the topic. The online assessment is intended to extend the learners' preparation for NCLEX® in a way that is personally suited to their deficiencies.

Step IV: ATI-PLAN™ DVD Series

This multi-disk set contains more than 28 hours of nursing review material. The DVD content is designed to complement ATI's Content Mastery Series™ review modules and online assessments. Using the ATI-PLAN™ navigational points, learners can easily find the content areas they want to review.

Recognizing that individuals process information in a variety of ways, ATI developed the ATI-PLAN™ DVD series to offer nursing review in a way that simulates the classroom. However, individuals viewing the ATI-PLAN™ DVDs can navigate through more than 28 hours of material to their topics of choice. Nursing review is available at the convenience of the learner and can be replayed as often as necessary to ensure mastery of content.

The regulation of personal learning goals and the ability to plan and pursue academic intentions are the keys to successful learning. The expert teacher is the one who can determine individual learning needs and appropriate strategies to master learning. The ADR program is an efficient method of helping students prepare for the nursing licensure exam using frequent and systematic content review directed by the identified areas of content weakness. The interactive approach for mastery of nursing content focused in the areas of greatest need is likely to increase student success on the licensure exam.

ATI's ADR method parallels the nursing process in concept and in design. Both provide a framework for solving actual and potential problems purposefully and methodically. Assessment ADR-style is accomplished with ATI's battery of proctored assessments. Diagnosis is facilitated by the individual and group score reports the proctored assessments generate. Planning for improving performance in identified areas of weakness incorporates ATI's modular review system. Implementation begins with modular review and culminates in use of ATI's online assessments to validate improvement. Evaluation is reflected in the score reports, and performance can then be strengthened or further improved with the ATI-PLAN™ DVD series. Just like the nursing process, ATI's ADR prescriptive learning method often leads to specific, measurable results and highly desirable outcomes.

Table of Contents

CHAPTER 1

Basic Pharmacologic Principles

Key Points

- Pharmacokinetics include processes that affect a drug from the time it enters the body until it leaves the body:

  Absorption: Passage of medication from administrative site to entry into the blood stream.

  Distribution: Transport of medication to target tissue, including binding to plasma protein albumin.

  Metabolism/biotransformation: Degradation of medication preparation for excretion.

  Excretion: Elimination of medication from the body.
- Age, gender, genetic/ethnic characteristics, pathologic alterations, and body size are important variables affecting drug actions.
  - Systemic metabolic differences at the age extremes can produce pronounced drug effects different from those in young and middle-aged adults.
- **Therapeutic Index** (margin of safety) is a serum drug concentration within the therapeutic range (i.e., dosage sufficient to be effective, but a peak serum concentration below the level of toxicity).
- Tolerance occurs when the body becomes accustomed to a drug and larger doses are needed to achieve the same effects.
- All drugs in a particular classification generally have the same use, similar modes of action, and similar side effects.
  - Once key information about a drug classification is known, the nurse will have a great deal of information when identifying a specific medication with a known classification, even though the specific drug may be unfamiliar.
- **Noncompliance** (client's failure to follow prescribed medication therapy) is a major treatment problem.
  - Many factors contribute to noncompliance, such as:
    - Experience of adverse effects
    - Lack of understanding about disease process or drug
    - Lack of financial resources
    - Physical limitations
    - Psychological limitations
- Teaching the public, as well as individual clients, how to take medication accurately and safely is a major nursing responsibility.
- **Drug interactions** can be beneficial or detrimental. When two or more drugs are given at the same time, they frequently interact in some way.

Pharmacokinetics

Factors Affecting Absorption

- Route of administration and conditions at absorptive site influence rate of absorption:
  - Injectables are absorbed more rapidly than oral drugs; intramuscular (IM) is faster than subcutaneous (SC) due to richer blood supply.
  - Intravenous (IV) drugs are instantly absorbed.
- Drug form:
  - Special tablet coatings or additives are meant to delay absorption.
  - Liquid form of oral medication is absorbed faster because no dissolution is required.
  - Some injectable and topical medications have substances added to prolong their absorption times.
- Gastric emptying time and gastrointestinal motility
- Timing: Presence of food or other drugs in stomach, especially antacids

Factors Affecting Distribution

- Circulation, cardiac output, and blood supply to site of drug action
- Binding of drug to plasma protein albumin and tissue binding
- Level of plasma protein albumin
- For oral drugs, amount of drug metabolized in liver before reaching systemic circulation ("first-pass phenomenon")
- Blood-brain barrier prevents many drugs from entering central nervous system (CNS)

Factors Affecting Metabolism/Biotransformation

- Condition of the liver—since most drugs are degraded (detoxified) by liver enzymes
- "First-pass" through the liver accounts for the reason that many drugs are given in larger doses by mouth (PO) than by injection.
- Chemicals or drugs that stimulate production of transforming enzymes will speed metabolism of other drugs, possibly decreasing their effects.
- Chemicals or drugs that decrease production of transforming enzymes will slow metabolism of other drugs, causing drug accumulation and increasing adverse effects.

Factors Affecting Excretion

- Condition of the kidneys, since most drugs are excreted in urine
- Chemicals, foods, or other drugs that alter the pH of the urine

Drug Half-Life

- Amount of time required for serum concentration of a drug to decrease by 50%
- Dependent on rate of drug excretion
- Determines frequency of administration
- Not dependent on dose

Drug Interactions

Interactions occur when the pharmacokinetics or action of one drug are modified by another drug or food.

Drug-Drug Interactions

Additive effects:

- Two drugs with similar mechanisms of actions sum their effects
    - 1+1 = 2 (alcohol and sedatives cause increased sedation).

Synergism or potentiation:

- Two drugs with different mechanisms of action produce greater effects
    - 1+1 = 3 (codeine and aspirin together produce greatly increased pain relief).

Interference:

- One drug accelerates or slows the metabolism or excretion of another (barbiturates, warfarin [Coumadin], and cimetidine [Tagamet] affect the metabolism of many other drugs; probenecid [Benemid] slows the renal excretion of penicillin).

Displacement:

- Two drugs compete for drug binding sites on albumin.

Antagonism:

- Effects of two drugs that cancel each other
    - 1+1 = 0; may be due to competition for binding sites on cell membranes (e.g., naloxone [Narcan] prevents opiates from binding to receptor sites in CNS).
- Basis for specific antidotes given to antagonize the toxic effects of another drug or chemical

Incompatibility:

- Physical interaction of two drugs that interfere with the effect of at least one of the drugs (magnesium in antacids inactivates tetracycline if in the stomach at the same time).
- Pharmacist or another qualified resource should be consulted before mixing drugs in IV solution or syringe.
- Basis for administration of drugs to bind or inactivate a toxic drug or chemical in the gastrointestinal tract.

Drug-Food Interactions

- Food slows absorption of most drugs, but usually does not affect drug's action with important exceptions. Interaction between:
    - Tyramine-containing foods (beer, wine, aged cheeses, chicken livers) and monoamine oxidase (MAO) inhibitor drugs such as phenelzine (Nardil) can cause severe hypertension and intracranial hemorrhage.
    - Foods containing vitamin K (green leafy vegetables, broccoli, bananas, fish) antagonize the action of the oral anticoagulant warfarin (Coumadin).
    - Dairy products and tetracycline form an insoluble nonabsorbable compound.

- Grapefruit juice inhibits the metabolism of several drugs, including calcium channel blockers, which can result in increased drug levels, possibly to the point of toxicity.
- Acidic foods and iron increase absorption of iron.

- Many food supplements and herbs can potentiate or interfere with drug actions.

Adverse Drug Effects

Allergy (hypersensitivity): Immune (antigen-antibody) response to a drug to which the client was previously exposed and sensitized

Carcinogenicity: Ability of some drugs and chemicals to alter body cells and cause a variety of cancers

Dependence: Craving for a drug that may or may not be accompanied by physiologic dependency; most often involving drugs that alter CNS function

Gastrointestinal effects: Most medications can cause nausea, vomiting, and diarrhea. Giving the medication with food, if not contraindicated, will often lessen these unpleasant effects; however, absorption may be affected.

Hematologic effects: Some drugs, especially those to treat cancers, cause bone marrow depression, making clients susceptible to infection, anemia, and abnormal bleeding.

Hepatotoxicity: Ability of many drugs to damage the liver, especially since the liver metabolizes most drugs (as well as alcohol)

Idiosyncrasy: Unusual, unexpected response to medication; may be based on individual's genetic makeup

Nephrotoxicity: Ability of some drugs, such as aminoglycoside antibiotics, to damage the renal tubule, causing renal insufficiency or failure

Teratogeneticity:

- Ability of a drug to cause abnormalities in a developing fetus when taken by the mother
- The U.S. Food and Drug Administration (FDA) Pregnancy Risk Categories classify drugs according to the risk they impose on the developing fetus. Category X drugs should not be given to pregnant women or women who may become pregnant.

Medication Administration

Client Rights

- Clients have the right to participate in planning their care and to participate in decision-making about their health care.
- The nurse has a role as a client advocate and can give clients the tools they need to be informed, active participants by teaching them how to prevent or avoid medical problems. These may include education about their disorders, about the drugs and other medical therapy measures prescribed, and by counseling them about available resources to encourage health maintenance and compliance.
- Clients always have the right to refuse treatment.

Medication Order Interpretation

- The nurse must be familiar with:
  - Drug names (generic and trade)
  - Systems of measurement (metric, household and apothecary)
  - Medical terminology
- Abbreviations used in medical charting and prescriptions in order to interpret and follow medication orders accurately. *(See following table).*

With the tremendous emphasis on client safety today, health care organizations are attempting to eliminate certain abbreviations that may not be interpreted as intended. The Institute for Safe Medication Practices (ISMP) Council publishes a list of abbreviations ("ISMP List of Error-Prone Abbreviations, Symbols and Dose Designations") that are often misunderstood and have led to client injury and death. It is available at http://www.ismp.org/PDF/ErrorProne.pdf. In 2003, the Joint Commission on Accreditation of Healthcare Organizations (JCAHO) along with the ISMP began requiring health care organizations to eliminate the use of five of the dangerous abbreviations. The abbreviations to avoid in the health care setting include: U (units) and IU (international units); QD (every day), QOD (every other day); MSO4 and MS (morphine sulfate); MgSO4 (magnesium sulfate); trailing a zero (2.0 mg), and lack of leading zero (.2 mg).

Table 1: ISMP List of Error-Prone Abbreviations, Symbols, and Dose Designations

Abbreviation	Intended Meaning	Misinterpretation	Correction
μ g	microgram	Mistaken as "mg"	Use "mcg"
AD, AS, AU	Right ear, left ear, each ear	Mistaken as OD, OS, OU (right eye, left eye, each eye)	Use "right ear," "left ear," or "each ear"
OD, OS, OU	Right eye, left eye, each eye	Mistaken as AD, AS, AU (right ear, left ear, each ear)	Use "right eye," "left eye," or "each eye"
BT	Bedtime	Misinterpreted as "BID" (twice daily)	Use "bedtime"
cc	Cubic centimeters	Mistaken as "u" (units)	Use "mL"
D/C	Discharge or discontinue	Premature discontinuation of mediations if D/C (intended to mean "discharge"_ has been misinterpreted as "discontinued" when followed by a list of discharge medications	Use "discharge" and "discontinue"
IJ	Injection	Mistaken as "IV" or "intrajugular"	Use "injection"
IN	Intranasal	Mistaken as "IM" or "IV"	Use "intranasal" or "NAS"
HS	Half-strength	Mistaken at bedtime	Use "half-strength" or "bedtime"
hs	At bedtime, hours of sleep	Mistaken as half-strength	Use "half-strength" or "bedtime"

Abbreviation	Intended Meaning	Misinterpretation	Correction
IU**	international unit	Misread as IV (intravenous) or 10 (ten)	Use "units"
o.d. or OD	Once daily	Mistaken as "right eye" (OD-oculus dexter), leading to oral liquid medications administered to the eye	Use "daily"
OJ	Orange juice	Mistaken as OD or OS (right or left eye); drugs meant to be diluted in orange juice may be given in the eye	Use "orange juice"
Per os	By mouth, orally	The "os" can be mistaken as "left eye" (OS-oculus sinister)	Use "PO," by "mouth," or orally
q.d. or QD**	Every day	Mistaken as q.i.d., especially if the period after the "q" or the tail of the "q" is misunderstood as an "i"	Use "daily"
qhs	At bedtime	Mistaken as "qhr" or every hour	Use "at bedtime"
qn	Nightly	Mistaken as "qh" (every hour)	Use "nightly"
q.o.d. or QOD**	Every other day	Mistaken as "q.d" (daily) or "q.i.d." (four times daily) if the "o" is poorly written	Use "every other day"
q1d	Daily	Mistaken as q.i.d. (four times daily)	Use "daily"
q6PM, etc.	Every evening at 6 p.m.	Mistaken as every 6 hours	Use "6 PM" nightly" or "6 PM daily"
SC, SQ, sub q	Subcutaneous	SC mistaken as SL (sublingual); SQ mistaken as "5 every;" the "q" in "sub q" has been mistaken as "every" (e.g., a heparin dose ordered "sub q 2 hours before surgery" misunderstood as every 2 hours before surgery)	Use "subcut" or "subcutaneously"
ss	Sliding scale (insulin) or $^1/_2$ (apothecary)	Mistaken as "55"	Spell out "sliding scale," use "one-half" or "$^1/_2$"
SSRI	Sliding scale regular insulin	Mistaken as selective-serotonin reuptake inhibitor	Spell out "sliding scale (insulin)"
SSI	Sliding scale insulin	Mistaken as Strong Solution of Iodine (Lugol's)	Spell out "sliding scale (insulin)"
t/d	One daily	Mistaken as "tid"	Use "1 daily"
TIW or tiw	3 times a week	Mistaken as "3 times a day" or "twice in a week"	Use "3 times weekly"

Abbreviation	Intended Meaning	Misinterpretation	Correction
U or u**	Unit	Mistaken as the number 0 or 4, causing a 10-fold overdose or greater (e.g., 4U seen as "40" or 4u seen as "44"); mistaken as "cc" so dose given in volume instead of units (e.g., 4u seen as 4cc)	Use "unit"

Dose Designations and Other Information	Intended Meaning	Misinterpretation	Correction
Trailing zero after decimal point (e.g., 1.0 mg)**	1 mg	Mistaken as 10 mg is the decimal point is not seen	Do not use trailing zeros for doses expressed in whole numbers
No leading zero before a decimal dose (e.g.,.5 mg)**	0.5 mg	Mistaken as 5 mg if the decimal point is not seen	Use zero before a decimal point when the dose is less than a whole unit
Drug name and dose run together (especially problematic for drug names that end in "L" such as Inderal40 mg; Tegretol300 mg	Inderal 40 mg Tegretol 300 mg	Mistaken as Inderal 140 mg Mistaken as Tegretol 1300 mg	Place adequate space between the drug name, dose, and unit of measure
Numerical dose and unit of measure run together (e.g., 10mg, 100mL	10 mg 100 mL	The "m" is sometimes mistaken as a zero or two zeros, risking a 10- to 100-fold overdose	Place adequate space between the dose and unit of measure
Abbreviations such as mg. or mL. with a period following the abbreviation	mg mL	The period is unnecessary and could be mistaken as the number 1 if written poorly	Use mg, mL, etc. without a terminal period
Large doses without properly placed commas (e.g., 100000 units; 1000000 units)	100,000 units 1,000,000 units	10000 has been mistaken as 10,000 or 1,000,000; 1000000 has been mistaken as 100,000	Use commas for dosing units at or above 1,000, or use words such as 100 "thousand" or 1 "million" to improve readability

Drug Name Abbreviations	Intended Meaning	Misinterpretation	Correction
ARA A	vidaravine	Mistaken as cytarabine (ARA C)	Use complete drug name
AZT	zidovudine (Retrovir)	Mistaken as azathioprine or aztreonam	Use complete drug name
CPZ	Compazine (prochlorperazine)	Mistaken as chlorpromazine	Use complete drug name
DPT	Demerol- Penergan-Throazine	Mistaken as diphtheria-pertussis-tetanus (vaccine)	Use complete drug name
DTO	Diluted tincture of opium, or deodorized tincture of opium (Paregoric)	Mistaken as tincture of opium	Use complete drug name
HCI	Mistaken as hydrochloric acid or hydrochloride	Mistaken as potassium chloride (The "H" is misinterpreted as "K")	Use complete drug name unless expressed as a salt of a drug
HCTZ	hydrochlorothiazide	Mistaken as hydrocortisone (seen as HCT250 mg)	Use complete drug name
MgS04**	magnesium sulfate	Mistaken as morphine sulfate	Use complete drug name
MS, MS04**	morphine sulfate	Mistaken as magnesium sulfate	Use complete drug name
MTX	methotrexate	Mistaken as mitoxantrone	Use complete drug name
PCA	procainamide	Mistaken as Patient Controlled Analgesia	Use complete drug name
PTU	propylthiouracil	Mistaken as meraptopurine	Use complete drug name
T3	Tylenol with codeine No. 3	Mistaken as liothyronine	Use complete drug name
TAC	triamcinolone	Mistaken as tetracaine, Adrenaline, cocaine	Use complete drug name
TNK	TNKase	Mistaken as "TPA"	Use complete drug name
ZnS04	zinc sulfate	Mistaken as morphine sulfate	Use complete drug name

Stemmed Drug Names	Intended Meaning	Misinterpretation	Correction
“Nitro” drip	nitroglycerin infusion	Mistaken as sodium nitroprusside infusion	Use complete drug name
“Norflox”	norfloxacin	Mistaken as Norflex	Use complete drug name
“IV Vanc”	intravenous vancomycin	Mistaken as Invanz	Use complete drug name

Symbols	Intended Meaning	Misinterpretation	Correction
dr	Dram	Symbol for dram mistaken as “3”	Use metric system
	Minim	Symbol for minim mistaken as “mL”	
x3d	For three days	Mistaken as “3 doses”	Use “for three days”
> and <	Greater than and less than	Mistaken as opposite of intended; mistakenly used incorrect symbol; “<10” mistaken as “40”	Use “greater than” or “less than”
/ (slash mark)	Separates two doses or indicates “per”	Mistaken as the number 1 (e.g., “25 unit/ 10 units” misread as “25 units and 110” units	Use “per” rather than a slash mark to separate doses
@	At	Mistaken as “2”	Use “at”
&	And	Mistaken as “2”	Use “and”
+	Plus or and	Mistaken as “4”	Use “and”
°	Hour	Mistaken as zero (e.g., q2 seen as q 20)	Use “hr,” “h,” or “hour”

** Identified abbreviations in the table are also included on JCAHO’s “minimum list” of dangerous abbreviations, acronyms and symbols that must be included in an organization’s “Do Not Use” list, effective January 1, 2004.

Source: Institute for Safe Medication Practices. Accessed online January 30, 2005, at http://www.ismp.org/PDF/ErrorProne.pdf.

- Drug orders can be written using either the generic (e.g., acetaminophen) or brand/trade (e.g., Tylenol) name. Each drug has only one generic name, but may have many trade names. Trade (also called proprietary) names usually have an ® or ™ after them, are capitalized, and are owned by a particular manufacturer.
- Most drug dosages are now ordered in the metric system (mg, mL). Drugs to be taken at home may be ordered in terms of household measures (tsp, oz). The apothecary system measures (grain, dram) are now obsolete and rarely used.
- If an order is unclear for any reason, the nurse has the responsibility to consult with the prescriber for clarification before attempting to carry out the order.
- If the nurse is unfamiliar with a drug being prescribed, he/she should consult a resource to obtain the necessary information before attempting to administer the drug.

- If the dose of a drug is outside the usual range according to references, the nurse has a responsibility to consult with the prescriber before administering it.

Routes

Oral (PO or by mouth)

- Most convenient and least expensive route of administration
- Absorption is usually slowest and may be erratic
- Cannot be used for unconscious, dysphagic, confused clients, or those with gastric suction
- Clients that may have trouble swallowing whole capsules or tablets may need to have the medication crushed and mixed with food or put down the feeding tube. Not all tablets and capsules can be crushed. Medications that are slow release, long acting, or sustained release are coated to control the release of the drug. This coating must remain intact to prevent uncontrolled release, or "dumping," of the dose. (Tablets should not be crushed if they have been coated. Capsules generally can be opened, but the beads cannot be crushed because they are generally the part that have been coated to control release of the medication). The nurse should follow the manufacturers' guidelines with regard to crushing and administering the medications with food or via the tube.
- Many medications cannot be given PO because gastric secretions destroy them.

Sublingual (SL) or buccal

- Absorption directly into large blood vessels under tongue or in cheek
- SL medications should not be swallowed to avoid inactivation in stomach (e.g., nitroglycerin [NTG] tablet).

Topical

- Direct application of liquid, cream, lotion, ointment, or patch to skin surface
- Absorption may be slow-release for prolonged systemic effect (e.g., nitroglycerin [NTG] paste) or for local effect only (e.g., hydrocortisone cream for itching).
- Drugs may be inserted into a body cavity (rectum, vagina) usually for local effect (e.g., Dulcolax suppository, spermicidal cream), or systemic action (Tylenol).
- Drugs may be dissolved in solution for spraying onto nasal mucosa or throat for local effect (e.g., cromolyn sodium).
- Drops of drug solution may be instilled into lower conjunctival sac of eye or into ear canal for local effect (e.g., pilocarpine for glaucoma).

Inhalation

- Administration directly into respiratory tract via nasal or oral routes (nebulizer or metered dose inhalation)
- Rapid absorption
- Systemic or local effect

Parenteral

Subcutaneous (SQ)

- Below the skin layers but above the muscle
- Sites in upper arm, thigh, abdomen

Intradermal (ID)

- Just under the epidermis
- Sites: usually inner aspect of lower forearm

Intramuscular (IM)

- Into the muscle
- Sites include deltoid, vastus lateralis, ventrogluteal, dorsogluteal
- The client should be instructed to relax the area to be used for an intramuscular injection, and the nurse should assess for relaxation. A relaxed muscle decreases the pain of the intramuscular injection.

Intravenous (IV)

- Into a vein
- Sites: usually of the arm or hand

Other parenteral routes used by primary care providers may be:

- Intraosseous (into bone)
- Intra-arterial (into an artery)
- Epidural (into the epidural space around the spinal cord)
- Intra-articular (into a joint)

Intravenous (IV) Fluids

Purpose of IV infusion:

- Maintain fluid and electrolyte balance
- Replace lost water and electrolytes
- Provide nutrients and calories
- Act as a diluent for medications. Drug references or the pharmacist should be consulted when drugs are reconstituted and diluted for IV administration, to be certain of compatibility between drug and solution components.

Types of solutions:

- **Isotonic**: Solutions with approximately the same osmolarity (concentration) as plasma (250-300 mOsm/L); used to replace extracellular fluid losses or prevent them without causing fluid shifts between extra- and intracellular compartments. Some isotonic solutions are:
  - Normal saline (0.9% sodium chloride)
    - Isotonic saline is the usual solution for reconstitution and dilution of drugs for IV administration.
  - Lactated Ringer's (Ringer's Lactate, LR, or LRI)
  - Dextrose solution (5% dextrose in sterile water, also called: D5W).
    - Once inside the body, the carbohydrate dextrose (glucose) is used for energy, leaving only water.

        - D5W and the hypotonic solutions below are effective for hydrating clients.
- **Hypotonic**: Solutions with lower osmolarity than plasma (less than 250 mOsm/L); used to provide mostly water in cases of dehydration or sodium excess (saline 0.33% or 0.45%). Hypotonic fluids should not be administered to clients with cerebral edema nor should they be used to irrigate wound or body cavities.
- **Hypertonic**: Solutions with higher osmolarity than plasma (more than 350 mOsm/L); used to provide electrolytes, treat water intoxication, and provide calories and nutrients. Examples include:
    - Dextrose in saline (5% dextrose in 0.9% sodium chloride, D5NS)
    - Dextrose 5% in half-strength saline (D5$^1/_2$NS)
    - Dextrose 10% in water
    - Dextrose 5% in Lactated Ringer's (D5LR)
    - Total parenteral nutrition solutions (TPN)
        - Once inside the body, the carbohydrate dextrose (glucose) is used for energy, leaving only water.
- Electrolyte replacements, such as potassium chloride, can be added to any IV solution to replace deficiencies.
    - Potassium chloride must never be given IV push or intraveneous piggyback (IVPB). Such errors have caused cardiac arrest.
    - Potassium must always be diluted in large volumes of IV fluid and administered by slow drip.
- Glucose in the form of dextrose is often a component of various IV solutions to provide some carbohydrate source for calories needed by the body for energy. Five percent (5%) dextrose in a liter of solution provides approximately 170 calories.

Calculations

- Most drug dosages are ordered in the metric system (cc, mL, g, mg, mcg). (*See table.*)
- Some drugs (e.g., insulin, heparin) are measured in units; electrolytes are often in mEq (milliequivalents).
- The nurse must be able to convert measurements within the metric system (e.g., grams to mg, liters to mL) as well as between metric and household systems (e.g., mL to tsp, oz to mL).
- The nurse must be able to calculate IV flow rates for use with an electronic controller or pump (mL/hr) or manually (gtts/min).

Equivalents and Methods of Calculation

Volume								
1 mL or ml	=	1 milliliter	=	0.001	liter	=	1	cc[1]
1 cL or cl	=	1 centiliter	=	0.01	liter			
1 dL or dl	=	1 deciliter	=	0.1	liter			
1 L or l	=	1 liter	=	1	liter	=	1,000	mL

Volume								
1 daL or dal	=	1 decaliter	=	10	liters			
1 hL or hl	=	1 hectoliter	=	100	liters			
1 kL or kl	=	1 kiloliter	=	1,000	liters			
Mass								
1 mcg	=	1 microgram	=	0.000001	gram			
1 mg	=	1 milligram	=	0.001	gram	=	1,000	mcg
1 cg	=	1 centigram	=	0.01	gram			
1 dg	=	1 decigram	=	0.1	gram			
1 g or gm	=	1 gram	=	1	gram	=	1,000	mg
1 daG or dag	=	1 decagram	=	10	grams			
1 hG or hg	=	1 hectogram	=	100	grams			
1 kG or kg	=	1 kilogram	=	1,000	grams	≈	2.2	lbs
1 grain or gr	=	1 grain	=	0.06	gram	=	60	mg
Common U.S. Measurements								
1 lbs	=	1 pound						
1 tsp	=	1 teaspoon	=	1/3	tablespoon	≈	5	mL
1 Tbs	=	1 tablespoon	=	3	teaspoons	≈	15	mL
1 oz	=	1 ounce	=	2	tablespoons	≈	30	mL[2]

1. 1 mL = 1.0000028 cm^3 or approximately 1 cm^3. A cube with sides of 1 cm has a volume of approximately 1 mL. The abbreviation "cc" for "cubic centimeter" is no longer in regular use outside of the medical environment.

2. 1 ounce = 29.5735 mL or approximately 30 mL.

- The wavy "equals sign" ≈ means approximately equal, but not exactly equal.
- Many times aspirin is ordered in grains, thus the nurse should be familiar with this measurement and how to convert it to grams or milligrams. One grain equals 60 milligrams; 0.25 or 1/4 grain, therefore, is 15 milligrams.

Dosage Calculation Using Ratio and Proportion Method

Pharmaceuticals are manufactured and packaged in varying strengths or doses. A nurse needs to be able to convert an ordered dosage into an amount that can be dispensed and administered given the pre-packaged medications that are on hand. A nurse can begin by looking at this problem as a ratio. Stating something as a ratio, such as the ratio of A to B is written as either A:B or as a fraction like this: $\frac{A}{B}$. Here we want the ratio of the dose that is ordered to the quantity of the medication that is available. A dosage can be ordered in many different measurements, such as mcg, mg, g, or units. However, the actual medications on hand may be manufactured in measurements that are only available in pre-determined tablets, mL, or ounces. Let's look at an example.

Assume the medication ordered is 500 mg in a single dose. However, the medication is only immediately available in tablets of 250 mg each. How would you determine how many tablets to give the client?

Begin by writing down the equation representing 500 mg per dose and 250 mg per tablet:

Step 1 $\frac{500 \text{ mg}}{1 \text{ dose}} = \frac{250 \text{ mg}}{1 \text{ tablet}}$

Cross-multiply the numerator of one side of the equation with the denominator on the other side of the equation in order to get rid of the fractions on each side of the equation. The result:

Step 2 500 mg x 1 tablet = 250 mg x 1 dose

The goal is to end up with "1 dose" all by itself on one side of the equation, so divide both sides of the equation by 250 mg:

Step 3 $\frac{500 \text{ mg x } 1 \text{ tablet}}{250 \text{ mg}} = \frac{250 \text{ mg x } 1 \text{ dose}}{250 \text{ mg}}$

Step 4 2 x 1 tablet = 1 dose or 2 tablets = 1 dose

2 = number of tablets to give to the client.

Dosage Calculations Requiring Measurement Conversion

In the previous example, the dosage and tablets were both measured in mg. However, in practice it won't always be that easy. Here's an example of a measurement conversion to be made before giving a unit dose.

Medication Order: Ampicillin 0.5 g PO (by mouth) qid. Available drug is ampicillin (Principen) 250 mg per capsule. Begin by writing down the equation representing 0.5 g per dose and 250 mg per capsule:

Step 1 $\frac{0.5 \text{ g}}{1 \text{ dose}} = \frac{250 \text{ mg}}{1 \text{ capsule}}$

The dose desired and the dose administered must be in the same form of measurement, therefore convert the 0.5 g to mg: 1 gram = 1,000 mg, so move the decimal point 3 numeral positions to the right: $0.5_1 0_2 0_3$ to get: 500 mg. Rewrite the equation as follows:

Step 2 $\frac{500 \text{ mg}}{1 \text{ dose}} = \frac{250 \text{ mg}}{1 \text{ capsule}}$

Cross-multiply the numerator of one side of the equation with the denominator on the other side of the equation in order to get rid of the fractions on each side of the equation. The result:

Step 3 500 mg x 1 capsule = 250 x 1 dose

The goal is to end up with "1 dose" all by itself on one side of the equation, so divide both sides of the equation by 250 mg:

Step 4 Dividing both sides by 250 mg $\frac{\text{500 mg x 1 capsule}}{\text{250 mg}} = \frac{\text{250 mg x 1 dose}}{\text{250 mg}}$

Step 5 2x1 capsule = 1 dose or 2 capsules = 1 dose

2 = number of capsules to give to the client.

Dosage Calculation Based on Client Weight

Medications are frequently administered in liquid formulations. A nurse needs to be able to calculate an ordered dosage based on client weight and then determine the amount of liquid medication to administer.

Medication order: Ibuprofen 10 mg/Kg/dose PO (by mouth) q 8hours PRN (as needed for) temperature > 102.5°F. The client weighs 40 pounds and has a fever of 103°F. Ibuprofen is available as an oral suspension containing 100mg/5mL.

Step 1 40lbs x $\frac{\text{1Kg}}{\text{2.2lbs}}$ = 18.2 Kg

The client's weight must be converted from pounds to kilograms in order to calculate a dosage.

Step 2 18.2 Kg x $\frac{\text{10mg}}{\text{Kg}}$ = 182 mg

The desired dose is calculated by multiplying the client's weight in kilograms by the prescribed dose.

Step 3 182 mg x $\frac{\text{5 mL}}{\text{100 mg}}$ = 9.1 mL

The quantity of medication to administer is calculated by multiplying the desired dose by the concentration of the suspension.

The nurse should administer 9.1 mL of the ibuprofen suspension to the client.

IV Flow Calculation

To calculate mL/hr for infusion pump or controller:

$$\frac{\text{mL IV fluid to administer}}{\text{number of hours to run}} = \text{number of mL per hour}$$

Example: Ampicillin 0.5 g in 100 mL D5W IVPB q 6h. Administer over 30 min.

Begin by writing down the equation that represents 100 mL administered over 30 minutes (or one-half hour):

Step 1 $\frac{100 \text{ mL}}{0.5 \text{ hr}}$

Step 2: Divide the numerator and the denominator by 0.5 in order to make the denominator equal to 1.

$$\frac{200 \text{ mL}}{1 \text{ hour}} = 200 \text{ mL/hour}$$

Set the IV pump to infuse at the rate of 200 mL in 1 hour. Note the IV pump is set by "rate per hour," so setting the pump to infuse at 200 mL/hr works in this instance because the IV bag only contains 100 mL of fluid; therefore no more than 100 mL will be infused.

To calculate IV drip rate for manual control:

First determine the "Drop Factor" of the particular IV tubing which is to be attached to the IV bag. The box the tubing is in is marked with a numerical value to indicate the Drop Factor. The wider the diameter of the tubing, the faster the fluid will reach the client. There are generally two types of tubing:

Macrodrip tubing: 10-20 drops/mL or 10-20 gtts/mL

Microdrip tubing: 60 drops/mL or 60 gtts/mL

All IV tubing has a clear chamber at the end near the IV bag where you can see the fluid dripping out of the IV bag before it enters the tubing. This where you count the rate per minute of the falling drops (use the second hand or seconds counter on your watch).

Generally speaking, there are three drip rate formulas commonly used. They are as follows:

Formula 1: Based on the volume of fluid to be infused onver a set period of time.

$$\frac{\text{Volume to be infused measured in mL (or cc) x Drop Factor of the IV set}}{\text{Amount of time over which the infusion is to occur}} = \text{Drops/minutes or gtts/min}$$

Formula 2: Based on specific dosage to be infused per minute

$$\frac{\text{Dosage per minute to administered x Drop Factor of the IV set}}{\text{Concentration of medication per mL}}$$

Make sure the unit of measurement is the same for the dosage (in the numerator) and the concentration (in the denominator).

Formula 3: Based on specific dosage per kilogram of body weight per minute

$$\frac{\text{Dosage per minute x Body weight in kg x Drop Factor of the IV set}}{\text{Concentration of medication per mL}}$$

Make sure the unit of measurement is the same for the dosage (in the numerator) and the concentration (in the denominator).

Example

The primary care provider orders a continuous infusion of heparin: 1000 mL of solution containing 40,000 units of heparin to run at 25 mL/hr. Calculate the flow rate using microdrip tubing.

Use Formula 1: $\frac{\text{25 mL x 60 gtts/ mL}}{\text{60 minutes}} = \text{25 gtts/min}$

The strict math for the solution of this formula is as follows:

Step 1 Write the formula: $\frac{\text{25 mL x (60 gtts)/ (1 mL)}}{\text{60 min.}}$

Step 2 The two mL terms cancel each other, and $\frac{60}{1}$ simply = 60, to get this: $\frac{\text{25 x 60 gtts}}{\text{60 minutes}}$

Step 3 Then, the 60s in the numerator and denominator cancel each other out to get this:

$\frac{\text{25 gtts}}{\text{1 minute}} = \text{25 gtts/min}$

Note: 25 mL/hr is used, not 1000 mL

Note: Because the 60 gtts and 60 min cancel each other, when using a microdrip IV set, the gtts/min is always the same as the ordered mL/hr. Therefore this problem could be solved without any calculation. However, a nurse should always conduct a calculation, and then double-check that calculation.

Medication Errors

Nurses can avoid making medication errors through unfailing adherence to the "five rights" of medication administration:

- Administer:
  - Right dose
  - Right drug
  - Right time
  - Right route
  - Right client
- Many nurses would include additional rights:
  - Right documentation of the medication administered
  - Right to know side effects and potential complications
  - Right to refuse treatment

Errors in self-administration of medications are especially common in the elderly because they:

- Often take multiple medications
- May have sensory defects making accurate measurement difficult
- May have memory deficits

Unfortunately, medication errors in hospitalized clients do occur. This is often due to a breakdown in the medication administration system rather than to the error of just one person.

Nurses have "the last clear chance" to avoid errors since they are the ones actually giving the drug to the client. Nurses should be knowledgeable and meticulous enough to catch errors in dosage, incorrect medications, drugs that may be inappropriate, or incorrect dosage form or routes before the drug is given.

Legal Responsibilities

Federal and state regulation of drugs stems from the *Food, Drug, and Cosmetics Act of 1938* and its many amendments, which have been passed to protect the safety of the public. The Act regulates manufacturing, distribution, labeling, and advertising of substances used as drugs.

The *Controlled Substances Act of 1971* regulates distribution of narcotics and other drugs of potential abuse, and categorizes medications according to their abuse potential.

- Most of these drugs affect the central nervous system.
- Individual states may also have laws controlling use of potentially abused drugs.
- The drugs have been organized by "schedules" as shown in the following table.

Drug Classification System

Schedule I	• The drug or other substance has a high potential for abuse. • The drug or other substance has no currently accepted medical use in treatment in the United States. • There is a lack of accepted safety for use of the drug or other substance under medical supervision.
	Examples: LSD, MDMA, marijuana, DMT, peyote, psilocybin, mescaline, heroin. Authorized research is permitted
Schedule II	• The drug or other substance has a high potential for abuse. • The drug or other substance has a currently accepted medical use in treatment in the United States or a currently accepted medical use with severe restrictions. • Abuse of the drug or other substance may lead to severe psychological or physical dependence.
	Examples: cocaine, hydrocodone, morphine, opium, opiates, meperidine, methadone, amphetamine, PCP, codeine, secobarbital, oxycodone
Schedule III	• The drug or other substance has a potential for abuse less than the drugs or other substances in Schedules I and II. • The drug or other substance has a currently accepted medical use in treatment in the United States. • Abuse of the drug or other substance may lead to moderate or low physical dependence or high psychological dependence.
	Examples: anabolic steroids, dronabinol (synthetic THC), ketamine, LSA.
Schedule IV	• The drug or other substance has a low potential for abuse relative to the drugs or other substances in Schedule III. • The drug or other substance has a currently accepted medical use in treatment in the United States. • Abuse of the drug or other substance may lead to limited physical dependence or psychological dependence relative to the drugs or other substances in Schedule III.
	Examples: chloral hydrate, meprobamate, phenobarbital, diphenoxylate with atropine sulfate, chlordiazepoxide, diazepam, diethylpropion
Schedule V	• The drug or other substance has a low potential for abuse relative to the drugs or other substances in Schedule IV. • The drug or other substance has a currently accepted medical use in treatment in the United States. • Abuse of the drug or other substance may lead to limited physical dependence or psychological dependence relative to the drugs or other substances in Schedule IV.
	Examples: buprenorphine, pyrovalerone, prescription medications containing low quantities of codeine, diphenoxylate, narcotic cough syrups

Nurses are responsible for administering controlled substances according to institutional regulations and state and federal laws. Detailed records must be kept of drugs administered.

Drug abuse by nurses and other medical personnel is a serious problem. It jeopardizes the safety of clients, the health care system, the nurse's license to practice, the nurse's health and livelihood, and subjects the nurse to criminal prosecution.

Errors in medication administration are one of the most common reasons for professional negligence (malpractice) lawsuits against nurses and their employers.

- The nurse is expected to be knowledgeable about drugs, their therapeutic use, dosage, action, possible adverse effects, and correct administration techniques.
- Expected practice includes accurate and appropriate documentation.
- Failure to conform to the standard of care regarding medication administration exposes the nurse to the accusation of liability for malpractice if a client is injured.

Compliance

- Client's willingness to follow the drug therapy regimen
- Factors contributing to noncompliance include:
  - Multiple drugs
  - Complicated scheduling
  - Experience of adverse effects
  - Lack of understanding about disease process or drug
  - Lack of financial resources
  - Physical or psychological limitations that make obtaining, measuring, or taking the drugs difficult

Fluid and Electrolyte Homeostasis

Fluid volume and osmolality disorders:

- Isotonic fluids
  - Oral rehydration fluids (e.g., Pedialyte)
  - Isotonic intravenous fluid (e.g., 0.9% NaCl [sodium chloride] in sterile water)
- Hypertonic fluid volume contraction:
  - Hypotonic fluids
    - Plain drinking water
    - Intravenous 5% dextrose in water
- Hypotonic fluid volume contraction:
  - 0.9% NaCl for mild hyponatremia with normal kidney function
  - Hypertonic fluids (3% NaCl) for severe hyponatremia
- Fluid volume expansion:
  - Diuretics and inotropics

Acid-base imbalances:

- Respiratory alkalosis
  - Non-pharmacologic treatment is preferred
  - A sedative such as diazepam (Valium) may be given to suppress hysteria.
- Respiratory acidosis
  - Initial efforts focus on correcting the cause.
  - Sodium bicarbonate may be needed for severe acidosis.

- Metabolic alkalosis
  - IV infusion of solution containing sodium chloride and potassium chloride
  - Severe alkalosis may be treated with dilute hydrochloric acid (HCl) infused through a central venous catheter, or by administering ammonium chloride.
- Metabolic acidosis
  - Initial efforts focus on correcting the cause.
  - Severe acidosis may be treated with oral or intravenous sodium bicarbonate.

Potassium imbalances:

- Hypokalemia
  - Potassium chloride (PO, IV)
  - Potassium phosphate
  - Potassium acetate
- Hyperkalemia
  - Calcium gluconate
  - Glucose and insulin
  - Sodium bicarbonate
  - Sodium polystyrene sulfonate (Kayexalate)

Magnesium imbalances:

- Hypomagnesemia:
  - Prevention: PO (by mouth) magnesium gluconate or magnesium hydroxide
  - Treatment: Parenteral magnesium sulfate
- Hypermagnesemia: Intravenous calcium gluconate

Nursing Intervention

- Give only normal saline (NS) with administration of blood products.
- Avoid NS infusion in persons with sodium restriction (e.g., cardiac rehabilitation).
- Use D5W in client with diabetes who have low blood sugar and are not hyperglycemic.
- Isotonic and hypertonic fluids increase the intravascular fluid volume, so the client must be monitored for fluid volume excess (tachycardia, increased blood pressure from baseline, polyuria, and tachypnea).
- Sodium bicarbonate is reserved for severe acidosis because it may elevate the pH too rapidly, causing alkalosis. The sodium can cause fluid volume excess.
- Potassium supplements can produce hyperkalemia leading to potentially fatal dysrhythmias.
- Clients with impaired renal function are at special risk for fluid volume excess and hyperkalemia.
- Oral potassium supplements can cause gastrointestinal irritation and ulceration.

- Potassium supplements are contraindicated with:
  - Hyperkalemia
  - Severe renal impairment
  - Potassium sparing diuretics
  - Hypoaldosteronism
- Monitor urine output before and during the infusion of potassium supplements. Stop the infusion immediately if renal failure develops.
- Potassium supplements must be diluted before administration. Concentrated solutions of potassium can have fatal effects due to cardiac dysrhythmias.
- When clients are receiving parenteral magnesium sulfate, always have injectable calcium gluconate available to counter the effects of hypermagnesemia.
- Parenteral magnesium sulfate can cause neuromuscular blockade leading to respiratory paralysis and heart block.

Client Education

- The nurse has a responsibility to teach clients about their medications so they can self- administer their prescribed drugs safely and accurately to obtain the maximum benefit from them.
- Failure to tell client about potential adverse effects and appropriate action to take should an adverse event occur can make the nurse vulnerable for liability should the client be injured.
- Nurses also have a responsibility to counsel clients and the public about appropriate use of medications (prescription as well as over-the-counter medications), dietary and herbal supplements, and the potential dangers of drug interactions.
- Nurses should instruct clients to take oral supplements as directed to prevent gastric irritation:
  - Do not chew enteric-coated tablets.
  - Dilute liquids as directed.
  - If you miss a dose, do not double the next dose.
  - Do not use salt substitutes; they contain potassium.
  - Notify your primary care provider of dark or bloody stools or abdominal pain.
- Instruct clients to keep appointments for laboratory work to monitor potassium level.
- Instruct clients to advise the primary care provider if they notice changes in the rhythm of their heartbeat.

Special Dosing Considerations

Drug Administration During Pregnancy and Lactation

- FDA Pregnancy Risk Categories serve to classify drugs according to the risk they impose on the developing fetus.
  - Category X drugs (e.g. estrogens, warfarin, several benzodiazepines, and "statin" antilipidemics) create clear fetal risk and their use is

contraindicated in pregnancy.
    - Category A drugs are generally considered safe during pregnancy.
- While some drugs are clearly identified as teratogens (substances that can damage rapidly growing cells of the fetus), many others remain unidentified.
    - To avoid possible harm, pregnant women should only use medications when there is a real necessity.
    - All medications should be avoided during the first trimester if possible. Use the smallest dose for the shortest time possible.
    - Avoid combination drugs.
- The nurse should counsel all pregnant women not to take any medication without approval from their obstetrician or health care provider.
- Mother and fetus should be monitored closely for adverse effects.
    - Most drugs taken by the mother are passed into breast milk to some degree.
        - For some, the amount is so small it causes no significant effect.
        - For others, the effects on the nursing infant are unknown or potentially harmful.
    - Drugs should be given only in the lowest effective doses for the shortest possible time, and only when the benefits outweigh potential harm.
    - If a drug is necessary, the mother should take it after nursing and 3-4 hours before the next feeding or pumping.
        - To maintain milk supply, continued nursing or pumping is necessary.
        - Advise the client to discard the milk if drug ingestion occurs during the lactation period.

Drug Administration

To children:

- Responses to medications often occur more quickly and dramatically than in adults.
- Maturity of body systems has a great influence on pharmacokinetics.
    - Responses to drugs vary with the age and organ maturity of the infant or child.
        - Some drug effects are unique.
    - Tetracycline should not be given to children because of dental staining.
    - Some aminoglycosides (e.g., gentamicin) have nephrotoxic and ototoxic effects in children.
- Small overdoses may be lethal due to absence of reserve organ capacity, especially in the immature liver and kidney of neonates.
- Dosages are most accurately determined by the child's weight or body surface area.
- Smaller muscle size reduces the volume capacity for IM injections and may affect absorption rate.
    - Until a child is walking, gluteal muscle injection sites should not be used.
    - The vastus lateralis is the preferred site.
- Topical medications may be more rapidly absorbed and have a systemic rather

than local effect due to the thinner skin.

- All caregivers should be taught about a child's medications.
- Nurses have a responsibility to teach parents and caregivers about safe medication storage and administration practices to avoid accidental poisoning.

To the elderly:

- Normal physiologic and anatomic changes with aging alter drug pharmacokinetics, affecting both therapeutic and adverse drug effects.
- Decreased reserve organ capacity, especially of the liver and kidney, make elderly clients vulnerable to adverse effects and drug accumulation to toxic levels.
- Decreased cardiac function and circulation may decrease or delay drug distribution and effectiveness, as well as excretion.
  - Many elders have chronic illnesses and are likely to be taking multiple medications. They may also obtain medical care by more than one health care provider or self- medicate with over-the-counter (OTC) drugs and nutritional supplements.
  - Polypharmacy increases the risk of drug interactions and adverse effects.
- The high cost of medications may make it difficult for clients on fixed incomes to comply with drug regimens.
- Medication side effects such as dizziness, constipation, blurred vision, and mental confusion may be interpreted as changes of aging or organ pathology unless all medications being taken are carefully evaluated.
- Client teaching for safe drug use must be individualized according to the client's physical condition, sensory and mobility status, and memory capacity. Adaptive devices may be necessary to maintain independence.

To client with renal disease:

- Any disturbance of renal function will affect the excretion of many drugs since most drugs leave the body by way of urine.
- Renally excreted drugs may accumulate to toxic levels if given in usual doses.
- Decreased renal function is a chronic complication of many diseases such as diabetes mellitus, atherosclerosis, and hypertension.
- Any condition involving a reduction in blood flow to the kidney will reduce or slow excretion of drugs and their metabolites.
- In states of shock, depleted intravascular fluid volume, and heart failure, drug accumulation occurs.
- Some drugs are potentially toxic to the kidney, especially aminoglycoside antibiotics. Their use requires close monitoring of renal function (serum creatinine, measurement of urine output) to detect toxicity so that dosage adjustments can be made.
- Clients with renal dysfunction should receive either reduced dosage or reduced frequency of administration (or both) for those drugs that are renally excreted.
  - Monitoring of renal function (creatinine clearance) and serum drug levels should be done periodically.
  - Drug references provide guidelines for appropriate dosages based on creatinine clearance.

To client with liver disease:

- Metabolism (biotransformation or detoxification) of most drugs takes place in the liver. Impaired liver function, such as that occurring with hepatitis and cirrhosis, affects the production and effectiveness of the drug metabolizing enzyme systems (hepatic microsomal enzymes) and decreases the production of the drug-binding serum protein albumin. Any disease process causing impaired blood flow to the liver will result in reduced drug metabolism.
- Clients with impaired liver function are at risk for accumulation of drugs to toxic levels due to decreased metabolism and subsequent delayed excretion.
- They should be monitored closely for signs of adverse drug effects and increasing liver malfunction (nausea, jaundice, liver enlargement, increasingly abnormal liver function test results).
- Dosages for drugs that are extensively metabolized in the liver should be reduced. Guidelines for drug selection and dosage reduction are not as well established as they are for renal impairment.
- Some drugs (such as acetaminophen, alcohol, and "statin" antilipidemics) are toxic to the liver, especially if given in large doses or for long periods of time. Liver function tests:
    - Alanine aminotransferase (ALT; also called SGPT: serum glutamic pyruvic transaminase)– an enzyme found primarily in liver cells
    - Aspartate aminotransferase (AST; also called SGOT: serum glutamic oxaloacetic transminase)– an enzyme found in the liver and elsewhere in the body
    - Bilirubin
    - Albumin
    - Prothrombin time (PT)

Substance Abuse

Self-administration of a drug in excessive amounts, such that psychological addiction occurs, is substance abuse. Dependence reduces the individual's ability to function to some degree and involves compulsive drug-seeking behavior. Drugs may be ingested, inhaled, or injected. Most abuse involves drugs that affect the CNS and alter the state of consciousness. They may be depressants or stimulants, including both prescription and OTC drugs, legal and illegal drugs, such as alcohol, sedative-hypnotics, opioid analgesics, nicotine, cocaine, marijuana, and amphetamines. The feelings of pleasure, euphoria, well-being or reduced anxiety caused by the drug's effect on the brain increase the desire to continue taking the drug.

- Physical dependence is physiologic adaptation to prolonged use of a drug. Unpleasant symptoms occur if the drug is stopped suddenly or if its effects are antagonized. Withdrawal (abstinence) produces effects specific to the drug (hyperactivity, salivation, nausea, and agitation, among others). Desire to avoid a withdrawal symptom promotes continued drug use and reinforces psychological dependence.
- Psychological dependence is compulsive drug-seeking behavior to produce pleasurable sensations or feelings, which is at first unrelated to physical needs.

An individual may abuse several drugs at the same time. Drug abuse may lead to dramatic behavioral changes and organ damage, as well as inability to function in society. Clients hospitalized for unrelated health problems may manifest withdrawal symptoms, complicating their care and recovery.

Drug Tolerance

Tolerance is a progressive decrease in a drug's effectiveness over time so that larger doses must be given to achieve the same effect as the original dose. Tolerance may be due to activation of drug-metabolizing enzymes in the liver speeding drug breakdown and excretion. It may also be caused by a decrease in the numbers or sensitivity of receptor sites for the particular drug. Both of these processes would reduce the drug's effect on the target organ. Tolerance develops readily to CNS depressants such as alcohol and narcotic analgesics. Tolerance to one drug within a classification tends to produce cross-tolerance to other drugs in the same classification.

Critical Thinking Exercise: Basic Pharmacologic Principles

Note: *It is recommended the following exercises be reviewed with a partner or in a small group to achieve maximum student interaction and enhance critical thinking skills.*

1. The traditional "five rights" of medication administration include the following:

   a. Medication, client, dose, room number, route of dosage

   b. Medication, dose, strength, route of administration, location

   c. Client, medication, dose, route of administration, time

   d. Client, medication, dose, time, location

2. A nurse should provide which appropriate intervention when administering an intramuscular injection?

   a. Inject needle at a 45-degree angle

   b. Inform client not to massage the site

   c. Select a 25 to 27-gauge needle

   d. Aspirate prior to injection

3. The client's willingness to follow drug therapy is called:

   a. Cooperation

   b. Active participation

   c. Dynamic partnership

   d. Compliance

4. A cream or ointment that is applied to the skin for a therapeutic purpose is classified as a _______________ agent.

   a. Cholinergic

   b. Statin

   c. Topical

   d. Cathartic

Situation: S.S. is a 78-year-old who has been admitted to the ED with severe respiratory distress. After determining the cause of her distress to be pulmonary edema resulting from severe heart failure, the primary care provider orders furosemide (Lasix) 40 mg and then another 40 mg after 30 minutes. As the physician gathers the client's history, he learns the client was diagnosed and treated for breast cancer five years ago and now has metastatic disease, involving her thoracic spine. She has been in chronic pain, taking morphine in the form of morphine sulfate (Roxanol) 30 mg several times per day. In addition, the client takes morphine sulfate (MS Contin) 120 mg HS (at bedtime). The physician then adds the following order: morphine 5 mg IV q 3-4 hrs prn pain.

5. By which route would you expect the furosemide (Lasix) to be ordered?

6. What lab work do you anticipate the doctor will be ordering? Why?

7. Are there any other medications you might anticipate the doctor will order? Why?

8. Why would the doctor order morphine for this client?

9. What kinds of nursing implications are involved with a client who is taking morphine?

R.T. is a 76-year-old admitted to the ED with dehydration related to a gastrointestinal infection that resulted in copious diarrhea for the last 2 days. He has had severe abdominal cramping and can only tolerate small amounts of fluid.

10. Which of the following would be the most appropriate pharmacological intervention? Please provide a rationale for your answer.

    a. IV infusion with 0.45% normal saline at 125 cc/hr

    b. Copious amounts of liquid po to replace depleted body fluids

    c. IV infusion with 0.9% normal saline at 300 cc hr x 3 hrs, then reduce to 150 cc/hr continuously

    d. IV infusion of D5NS with 40 meq KCL/liter to run at 100 cc hr

11. You anticipate R.T. will most likely demonstrate the following labs (explain the nursing principle on which you base your answer):

    a. Elevated sodium and potassium

    b. Increased magnesium and decreased sodium

    c. Elevated BUN and elevated potassium

    d. Decreased potassium levels and elevated urine specific gravity

12. The physician examines the lab results and recommends potassium 40 meq be added to each liter of IV solution. What is the rationale for ordering this medication?

Situation: B.J. is 43 years old. He has worked in construction since he was 16. He was recently admitted to the hospital to treat a herniated disk. Prior to admission, he had been undergoing physical therapy and had been taking oral Vicodin for the last three months as well as muscle relaxants and anti-inflammatories. After surgery to correct the ruptured disk, the physician ordered 75 mg of Demerol with 25 mg Vistaril q 4-6 hours for pain. You have been giving the medication as ordered, but Mr. Johnson states he is receiving only minimal pain relief.

13. What is the most likely explanation for this situation? Discuss the reason for your answer.

a. B.J. has developed a tolerance to the effectiveness of the analgesics and a larger dose of analgesics may be needed to provide adequate pain relief.

b. B.J. has developed psychological dependence on the analgesics.

c. B.J. is anxious and his perception of pain is much more acute.

d. B.J.'s dose of Vicodin needs to be decreased.

CHAPTER 2

Drugs Used to Treat Infection

Key Points

- Anti-infective agents are used to treat infections resulting from pathogens.
- An antibiotic is an anti-infective, antimicrobial, and antibacterial agent used to treat infectious diseases.
  - Not effective against viruses
  - Should not be used for viral infections or infections with minor symptoms.
- A **bactericidal** antibiotic agent kills microorganisms.
- A **bacteriostatic** antibiotic agent inhibits the growth of microorganisms.
- Anti-infective agents include:
  - Penicillins
  - Cephalosporins
  - Aminoglycosides
  - Tetracyclines
  - Sulfonamides
  - Urinary tract antiseptics
  - Macrolides
  - Lincosamides
  - Fluoroquinolones
  - Chloramphenicol
  - Vancomycin
  - Antiviral drugs
  - Antifungal drugs
  - Antitubercular drugs
  - Antiparasitics
- **Gram-negative** infections are potentially life threatening.
- **Gram-negative** organisms include:
  - *Escherichia coli* (*E. coli*)
  - *Proteus*
  - *Pseudomonas salmonella*
  - *Enterococcus*
  - *Klebsiella*
  - *Shigella*
  - *Bacteroides*

- **Gram-positive** organisms include:
    - Streptococcal organisms
    - Staphylococcal organisms
- Anti-infective agents interfere with metabolic or growth processes specific to pathogenic microorganisms. These agents:
    - Inhibit cell wall synthesis
    - Alter membrane permeability, and/or
    - Inhibit protein synthesis
- The choice of an anti-infective agent is usually determined by the results of a culture and sensitivity test.
    - Culture identifies the causative organism and sensitivity determines which drugs are likely to be effective against it.
    - Culture specimens should be obtained before anti-infective drugs are started.
    - Culture and sensitivity tests take 48-72 hours.
    - The drug most likely to be effective should be prescribed and administered until the culture results are available.
- Antibiotics may be given by:
    - PO (mouth)
    - Intramuscular (IM) routes
    - Intravenous (IV) infusion
- Antibiotics should be taken at evenly spaced intervals around the clock.
- The following should be monitored to determine drug effectiveness:
    - Blood levels of the antibiotic
    - Complete blood count (CBC)
    - White blood cell count (WBC)
        - The WBC should return to normal if drug is effective.
- Client should complete taking all medication exactly as ordered, even when symptoms subside.
- Some organisms are becoming resistant to antibiotics because of inappropriate or indiscriminate use of antibiotics, and the failure to complete taking all of the antibiotics as prescribed.
- Antibiotics may cause severe allergic responses.
- Antibiotics may be toxic to the kidney, liver, and bone marrow.
- Broad-spectrum antibiotics may cause yeast infections, which result from disruption in the normal body flora.
    - Manifestations of yeast infection include:
        - Stomatitis (sore mouth, white patches on the oral mucosa, black furry tongue)
        - Monilial vaginitis (rash, itching, vaginal discharge)
- Broad-spectrum antibiotics can cause Clostridium difficile – associated diarrhea (antibiotic-associated pseudomembranous colitis).
    - Manifestations of this bacterial infection include:
        - Bloody diarrhea
        - Foul odor

Overview

The era of antibiotic therapy began with the development of penicillin in the 1940s during World War II. Penicillins are both bacteriostatic and bacteriocidal agents. The penicillins act by binding to the bacterial cell wall, which results in cell lysis and cell death. Penicillins do not penetrate the blood-brain barrier, except when the meninges are inflamed or there is fever. It is generally safe to administer penicillins to children and older adults, as well as during pregnancy.

Penicillins

Uses

- Penicillins are active against:
  - Gram-positive cocci and bacilli (rods)
  - Some gram-negative bacilli
- Penicillins treat a large variety of infections, including:
  - Streptococcal pharyngitis
  - Pneumococcal pneumonia
  - Endocarditis
  - Meningitis
  - Otitis media
  - Sinusitis
  - Syphilis
  - Gonorrhea
- Penicillins are given to prevent rheumatic fever.

Adverse Effects

Drug Allergy

- Penicillins are the most common cause of drug allergies.
- The allergic response may be immediate (2-30 minutes), accelerated (1-72 hours), or late (days or weeks).
- Manifestations of an **allergic response** to penicillin include:
  - Urticarial rash
  - Flushing
  - Diaphoresis
  - Palpitations
  - Fever
  - Arthralgia or myalgia
  - Respiratory distress

Anaphylactic shock may develop in previously sensitized clients.

- This is a life-threatening event
- Manifestations include:
  - Severe respiratory distress
  - Hypotension
  - Tachycardia

  - Cyanosis
  - Convulsions
  - Unconsciousness if no treatment received
- Treatment includes the following
  - A mild allergic reaction is usually treated with diphenhydramine (Benadryl).
  - Anaphylactic shock is treated with airway management and the administration of epinephrine, corticosteroids, and saline or plasma expanders.

Serum sickness is another type of allergic response to penicillin.

- It can develop 7-21 days after treatment is initiated.
- Manifestations include:
  - Fever
  - Arthritis
  - Urticaria
  - Lymphadenopathy
  - Generalized edema
- Treatment includes:
  - Serum sickness is treated symptomatically, although adrenal cortical hormones may be administered in some cases.

Neurotoxicity

- Penicillin can cause convulsions or coma secondary to direct CNS irritation.
- Neurotoxicity is more likely to occur in clients who:
  - Receive large doses of penicillins
  - Have renal impairment
  - Have an underlying CNS disease

Nephropathy

- An inflammation of renal tissue (interstitial nephritis) may develop in clients who receive parenteral penicillin therapy.
- Onset occurs 2-4 weeks after initiating therapy.
- Fever and rash may occur.
- Reaction usually subsides upon discontinuation of the drug.
- Corticosteroids may be given to correct the deterioration in renal function.

Hematologic Effects

- Eosinophilia, hemolytic anemia, and leukopenia may be life threatening unless the penicillin is discontinued.
- Onset is approximately three weeks after starting therapy.
- Effects are reversible upon discontinuation of penicillin.

Immunologic Effects

- Yeast infections result from disruption in the normal body flora.
- Oral thrush (candidiasis) is a secondary infection caused by any species of candida, but usually *Candida albicans*.

Hyperkalemia

- High doses of intravenous penicillin G may cause hyperkalemia, possibly resulting in dysrhythmias or cardiac arrest.
- Monitor serum electrolytes if the client is receiving high intravenous doses, particularly if renal dysfunction is evident.

Gastrointestinal

- Gastrointestinal symptoms are the most common adverse effect associated with penicillin therapy.
  - Mild diarrhea
  - Nausea or vomiting

Precautions

- Penicillin is contraindicated in clients with a history of previous hypersensitivity to penicillins.
- If the client has a mild allergy to the penicillins, a cephalosporin may be administered instead.
  - If the client has a severe reaction to penicillin, the cephalosporins should be avoided because of a 5%-10% cross sensitivity.
- Penicillin should be avoided in clients with severe renal insufficiency.

Important Drugs

Penicillin G is the prototype for the penicillins, and is classified as natural penicillin.

- When penicillin G was first developed, it was effective against:
  - Streptococci
  - Staphylococci
  - Gonococci
  - Meningococci
- Some strains of bacteria are now resistant to penicillin G and other penicillins because they synthesize an enzyme that inactivates penicillin. Most penicillin-resistant infections in hospitalized clients are caused by *Staphylococcal aureus*.

Penicillinase-resistant penicillins include methicillin (Staphcillin) and nafcillin (Unipen).

Broad-spectrum penicillins include amoxicillin (Amoxil) and ampicillin (Polycillin).

Extended-spectrum penicillins include piperacillin (Pipracil) and carbenicillin (Geopen).

Combination drugs include amoxicillin plus clavulanic acid (Augmentin), which protects penicillin from destruction by enzymes and extends its spectrum.

Therapeutic Nursing Interventions

- Question the client concerning history of drug allergies.
- Observe for hypersensitivity and signs of respiratory distress, which may occur 5-30 minutes after injection. Also observe for nausea and vomiting.

- Immediately discontinue the drug at the first sign of an allergic reaction, and notify primary care provider.
- Treat mild allergic reaction with diphenhydramine (Benadryl) as ordered.
- Treat severe respiratory allergic reaction with epinephrine SC or IV as ordered.
- Administer oral penicillin on an empty stomach, one hour before or 1-2 hours after meals, with the exception of amoxicillin, which can be given with food.
- Take with a full glass of water, never with acidic fluids like orange juice.
- Give IM injections deep into a large muscle mass.
    - Shake medication well before injection.
    - Massage the site following injection.
- Change IV sites every 48 hours to prevent phlebitis.
- Administer penicillin around the clock, as ordered.
- Monitor:
    - Immature: total ratio (I:T ratio)
    - Absolute neutrophil count (ANC)
    - Sediment rate
    - C-reactive protein (CRP)
    - WBC counts. WBC count should return to normal if medication is effective.

Client Education

- Take the medication around the clock exactly as ordered to maintain optimum blood levels of the drug.
- Finish taking the drug as ordered, even if condition improves.
    - Failure to complete medication regimen can result in development of antibiotic- resistant strains of organisms.
- Never share this medication because other individuals may be allergic to penicillin and develop a serious reaction.
- Report sore mouth, white patches on oral mucosa, diarrhea, or vaginal discharge and itching to health care professional because these are signs of a yeast infection.
- Ingest yogurt or buttermilk if diarrhea develops to help replace intestinal flora and correct symptoms of yeast infection.
- Notify health professional if symptoms do not improve. The organism may not be sensitive to the prescribed antibiotic, and the health care provider may need to change the dosage or prescribe another antibiotic.
- Always carry an identification card if allergic to penicillins. If you are unconscious or unable to communicate, health care providers will be aware of the allergy and not administer penicillin.

Cephalosporins

Overview

Cephalosporins are bacteriostatic and bacteriocidal. They act effectively on organisms that are multiplying rapidly. Mechanism of action, renal excretion, and allergenicity of cephalosporins resemble those of the penicillins. Cephalosporins primarily act to inhibit bacterial cell wall synthesis. Cephalosporins are used as a second-line therapeutic agent because of the wide availability of equally effective and less expensive alternatives. Compared to penicillins, cephalosporins are less active against gram- positive organisms and more active against gram-negative organisms.

Uses

- Treat urinary tract infections (UTI) caused by E. coli
- Reduce the incidence of surgical wound infections (surgical prophylaxis)
- Treat gram-negative bacterial meningitis
- Treat multiple resistant gram-negative infections
- Treat abdominal and pelvic infections

Adverse Effects

- Cephalosporins are relatively safe.
- Neutropenia, thrombocytopenia, and anaphylaxis may occasionally occur.
- Cephalosporins can cause nephrotoxicity, especially in the elderly and when used with other nephrotoxic drugs.
- Risk of allergy is lower with an oral cephalosporin than with a parenteral one.
- Hypersensitivity (which resembles that of penicillin) is the most frequent adverse effect. Common physical manifestations include:
    - Rash
    - Fever and chills
    - Edema
    - Anal/genital pruritus
- Thrombophlebitis and pain in veins used for injections may occur.
- Superinfection is often manifested by fungal infections of the mouth or vagina.
- Pseudomembranous colitis (PMC) can develop, which can be life threatening. PMC is treated with metronidazole (Flagyl) or oral vancomycin (Vancocin).

Precautions

- Cephalosporins have a cross-sensitivity with penicillin drugs.
- Cephalosporins are contraindicated for clients with a history of severe penicillin allergy.
- Dosage should be adjusted for clients with a history of renal insufficiency.
- Use with caution in clients who are pregnant or lactating.

Important Drugs

First-generation cephalosporins:

- Cefazolin sodium (Ancef, Kefzol) is the prototype: IM or IV
- Cephalexin (Keflex): oral preparation

Second-generation cephalosporins:

- Cefoxitin (Mefoxin): IM or IV
- Cefprozil (Cefzil): PO
- Cefotetan (Cefotan): IM or IV
- Cefaclor (Ceclor): PO
- Cefuroxime (Zinacef): PO, IM or IV

Third-generation cephalosporins—only drugs that are able to penetrate the blood-brain barrier sufficiently to treat CNS infections.

- Cefoperazone (Cefobid): IV or IM
- Ceftriaxone sodium (Rocephin): IM or IV
- Cefotaxime (Claforan): IM or IV
- Ceftazidime (Fortaz): IM or IV
- Cefixime (Suprax): oral suspension or tablets

Fourth-generation cephalosporins—drugs that are active against both gram-positive and gram-negative organisms, and they are more stable than earlier generations.

- Cefepime (Maxipime): IM or IV

Therapeutic Nursing Interventions

- Administer cephalosporins around the clock.
- Give client buttermilk or yogurt with meals to prevent diarrhea.
- Check WBC count regularly to assess effectiveness of drug.
  - WBC should return to normal.
- Calculate the IT ratio (immature to total ratio):

$$I{:}T = \frac{\text{neutrophil bands} + \text{lymphocytes} + \text{monocytes} + \text{eosinophils}}{\text{neutrophil bands} + \text{lymphocytes} + \text{monocytes} + \text{eosinophils} + \text{neutrophil segments} + \text{nucleated red blood cells}}$$

- Monitor laboratory values for CRP, as ordered.
  - Report abnormalities.
  - Follow the trend (improving or worsening)
- Observe the client for hypersensitivity and/or superinfection.
- Monitor I&O and serum creatinine levels in clients with a history of renal insufficiency.
- Monitor IV site for thrombophlebitis (pain, redness, and swelling).
- Change sites every 48-72 hours to prevent phlebitis.
- Simultaneously administer antifungals as ordered if client has a history of vaginitis.
  - Client may be more prone to this infection due to disruption of the normal vaginal flora.

Client Education

- Take the drug around the clock at evenly spaced intervals to maintain optimum blood levels of the drug.
- Finish the prescription completely, even if condition improves.
  - Failure to complete medication regimen can result in development of antibiotic resistant strains of organisms.
- Never double dose because this may cause an adverse reaction.
  - Take a missed dose as soon as possible.
- Take cephalosporins with or without food.
  - Food delays absorption, but it does not affect the amount of the drug absorbed.
  - Food does reduce gastrointestinal irritation.
- Report diarrhea to health care provider.
- Drink buttermilk or eat yogurt with meals to prevent symptoms due to yeast infection.
- Avoid alcohol because it increases sensitivity to the drug.
- Never share medication because other individuals may be allergic to the drug and develop a serious reaction.
- Contact health care provider if symptoms do not improve.
  - The organism may not be sensitive to the prescribed antibiotic, and the health care provider may need to change the dosage or prescribe another antibiotic.

Aminoglycosides

Overview

Aminoglycosides are narrow spectrum, bactericidal antibiotics that are used primarily against aerobic gram-negative bacteria. Aminoglycosides inhibit protein synthesis at the level of the 30S ribosome. Aminoglycosides are often combined with penicillin (usually ampicillin). The combination either expands the therapeutic coverage, or it provides additive or synergistic effects against specific bacteria. When penicillin is added to aminoglycoside therapy, aminoglycosides can more easily penetrate the cell.

Uses

- Treat gram-negative bacterial infections
- Treat staphylococcal infections when penicillin is contraindicated
- Prepare the gastrointestinal tract prior to surgery
  - Kanamycin and neomycin are not well absorbed from the gastrointestinal tract, and are thus used to suppress intestinal bacteria before bowel surgery.
- Treat serious infections such as septicemia
- Treat active tuberculosis in combination with other drugs

Adverse Effects

- Renal impairment is most likely in elderly clients, and in those who receive prolonged aminoglycoside therapy.
- Hearing impairment can develop due to damage to the eighth cranial (acoustic) nerve.

Precautions

- Aminoglycosides are administered cautiously to clients who:
  - Are allergic to aminoglycosides
  - Have a hearing impairment
  - Have kidney disease
  - Are receiving renal toxic agents such as vancomycin
  - Are receiving an anesthetic or muscle relaxant

Important Drugs

Streptomycin was the first systemic antimicrobial drug effective against gram-negative pathogens.

- The drug has limited use today, except for the treatment of tuberculosis. Streptomycin is toxic to the 8th cranial (acoustic) nerve, and can cause hearing loss.

Amikacin (Amikin) is a semi-synthetic derivative of the older drug, kanamycin.

- It is the drug of choice against serious, nosocomial gram-negative infections that are resistant to gentamicin.

Gentamicin (Garamycin) is effective against several gram-positive organisms.

- Penicillins and cephalosporins are more effective and less toxic.

Neomycin (Mycifradin) is administered orally and topically for skin, ear, and eye infections.

Therapeutic Nursing Interventions

- Obtain specimens for culture and sensitivity prior to initiating therapy.
- Separate administration of an aminoglycoside and an extended-spectrum antibiotic by at least two hours to prevent inactivation of the aminoglycoside.
- Provide client with 2000-3000 mL of fluid a day during therapy.
- Monitor intake/output and weight daily throughout therapy.
- Monitor hearing acuity before and throughout therapy.
- Monitor I&O and creatinine levels to assess for nephrotoxicity.
- When ordered IM, give injection deep into a well-developed muscle.
  - Absorption is rapid with IM administration, peaking in 30-90 minutes when tissue perfusion is adequate.
- For preoperative bowel preparation, administer neomycin with erythromycin as ordered, provide a low-residue diet, and administer a cathartic agent or enema.
- Peak serum drug levels should be drawn 30-60 minutes after IV administration and trough serum levels shortly before the next IV dose to avoid over- or under-dosing.

Client Education

- Report ringing in the ears or any change in hearing acuity to health care provider. It is essential to identify hearing loss early to prevent permanent damage to the eighth cranial nerve.
- Report nausea, vomiting, or diarrhea.
- Drink 2000-3000 mL fluid/day, if not contraindicated, to maintain kidney function.
- Finish prescription completely, even if condition improves.
    - Failure to complete medication regimen can result in development of antibiotic resistant strains of organisms.
- Never share medication with other people because other individuals may be allergic to the drug and develop a serious reaction.
- Contact health care provider if symptoms do not improve.
    - The organism may not be sensitive to the prescribed antibiotic, and the health care provider may need to change the dosage or prescribe another antibiotic.

Tetracyclines

Overview

The tetracyclines are broad-spectrum, bacteriostatic antibiotics. Tetracycline stops bacterial protein synthesis at the site of action of the 30S bacterial ribosome. Once inside the bacterial cell wall, tetracyclines inhibit bacterial action. The tetracyclines do cross the blood-brain barrier, but fail to reach therapeutic concentrations in the central nervous system (CNS).

Uses

- Tetracyclines are rarely the drugs of first choice for treating common bacterial diseases.
- They are the drugs of choice for treatment of these more uncommon infections:
    - Rocky Mountain spotted fever
    - Cholera and typhus
    - Endocervical infections caused by chlamydial organisms
    - Nongonococcal pelvic inflammatory disease
    - Acne
    - Traveler's diarrhea—doxycycline (Vibramycin)
    - Lyme disease
    - Anthrax
- Tetracycline is sometimes used as a substitute drug for clients who have gonorrhea or syphilis.
- This classification of antibiotics cannot be substituted for the treatment of strep throat.
- Tetracyclines do not prevent rheumatic fever
- Doxycycline (Vibramycin) is administered to clients with:

- Gonorrhea
- Lyme disease
- Anthrax
- Malaria prophylaxis

Adverse Effects

- Tetracyclines are very irritating to the gastric mucosa.
- Symptoms are:
  - Nausea and vomiting
  - Epigastric burning
  - Stomatitis
  - Glossitis
- Tetracyclines are toxic to the kidneys, especially the earliest forms/derivatives of tetracycline.
- Tetracyclines are highly irritating to the veins, and frequently cause phlebitis and thrombosis.
- Doxycycline (Vibramycin) is often associated with a "sunburn" reaction that appears upon exposure to direct sunlight.

Precautions

- Causes permanent yellow-brown discoloration of the teeth and softening of the bones in children if given in the last trimester of pregnancy, or to children under the age of eight years. The drug binds to newly formed bones and teeth.
- Decreases the effectiveness of penicillin and cephalosporin
- Can cause severe hepatotoxicity during pregnancy
- Contraindicated in clients with renal failure
- May decrease the efficacy of oral contraceptives, and thus increase the risk of pregnancy

Important Drugs

Achromycin is the prototype for the tetracyclines.

Doxycycline (Vibramycin) is a newer tetracycline.

- It is administered to clients with:
  - Gonorrhea
  - Lyme disease
  - Malaria prophylaxis.
- The tetracycline of choice for clients with impaired kidney function.

Therapeutic Nursing Interventions

- Obtain specimens for culture and sensitivity before initiating therapy.
- Do not give tetracycline to children under 8 years, or to women in the last trimester of pregnancy because teeth may be permanently discolored.
- Usually administer tetracyclines orally.
  - Approximately 75% of the drug is absorbed if it is given on an empty stomach.

- Do not give tetracycline with dairy products or antacids.
  - Calcium, magnesium, aluminum, and iron prevent tetracycline absorption.
  - Doxycycline may be given with milk.

Client Education

- Avoid taking tetracycline with antacids, milk products, or iron products because tetracycline combines with metallic ions to form insoluble compounds that cannot be absorbed.
- Avoid strong sunlight and use a sunscreen and protective clothing to prevent photosensitivity reactions.
- Throw away old tetracycline because decomposed tetracycline may cause adverse effects.
  - It is important to check the expiration date on all bottles of medication.
- Report gastrointestinal symptoms to health care provider.
  - Medication may need to be changed or adjusted if gastrointestinal irritation is severe.
- Finish drug completely, even if condition improves.
  - Failure to complete medication regimen can result in development of antibiotic resistant strains of organisms.
- Contact health care provider if symptoms do not improve.
  - The organism may not be sensitive to the prescribed antibiotic, and the health care provider may need to change the dosage or prescribe another antibiotic.

Sulfonamides and Urinary Tract Antiseptic Agents

Overview

Sulfonamides are bacteriostatic agents that inhibit the formation of folic acid in bacterial cells, which results in the suppression of purine synthesis. Bacterial cells cannot survive without purines, which are the building blocks of DNA (deoxyribonucleic acid). Urinary tract antiseptic agents also act by interfering with bacterial enzymes. Urinary tract antiseptic agents have a local effect only. They do not act systemically.

Uses

- The value of the sulfonamides has been greatly reduced by the development of resistance to the drug.
- Sulfonamides are effective in treating:
  - A variety of systemic infections, such as toxoplasmosis
  - Acute uncomplicated urinary tract infections
  - Bronchitis
  - Acute otitis media in children
  - Traveler's diarrhea, ulcerative colitis
  - Gastrointestinal infections caused by shigellae (Shigella enteritis)

    - Pneumocystis carinii pneumonia (PCP)
    - Burn wound infections when administered topically
- Urinary tract antiseptic agents such as nitrofurantoin (Furadantin) are used to treat initial and chronic urinary tract infections (UTIs).

Adverse Effects

- Sulfonamides can cause the following adverse effects:
    - Nausea, vomiting, diarrhea
    - Blood dyscrasias: hemolytic anemia, aplastic anemia, agranulocytosis (a significant decrease in the number of neutrophils)
    - Pneumonitis
    - Peripheral neuropathy
    - Hypersensitivity reactions:
        - Stevens-Johnson syndrome may develop, which is characterized by erythema and ulceration of mucous membranes.
        - Rashes may develop in clients with acquired immunodeficiency syndrome (AIDS). Renal damage that is usually a result of crystalluria caused by precipitation of the sulfonamide or its metabolite in the urinary tract. Maintaining adequate urinary output may reduce this risk.
    - In addition to the adverse reactions listed for the sulfonamides, urinary tract antiseptic agents (e.g., nitrofurantoin) can cause these adverse effects:
        - Dizziness and drowsiness
        - Chest pain
        - Rust/brown discoloration of urine (expected effect)

Precautions

- Sulfonamides are contraindicated for clients who have experienced hypersensitivity reactions to sulfonamides, salicylates, or sulfasalazine.
    - Salicylates increase the toxicity of sulfonamides by displacing them from plasma protein-binding sites, thereby increasing plasma levels of free drug.
- Do not administer sulfonamides or urinary tract antiseptic agents to newborns or pregnant women.
- Do not administer urinary tract anti-infective agents to clients with anuria or oliguria.

Important Drugs

Short-acting drugs that are rapidly absorbed and rapidly excreted:

- Sulfisoxazole (Gantrisin)
- Sulfadiazine (Microsulfon)

Medium-acting drugs that are rapidly absorbed and slowly excreted:

- Trimethoprim/sulfamethoxazole (TMP/SMZ, Bactrim, Septra)

Ultra-long acting drugs, which are combined with pyrimethamine (Daraprim) to treat malaria:

- Sulfadoxine (Fansidar)
- Sulfamylon cream is used to treat burn clients.

    - May cause metabolic acidosis because of systemic absorption

Commonly used urinary anti-infective drugs include:

- Nitrofurantoin (Furadantin), which is used to treat urinary tract infections.
    - Agent of choice in chronic suppression therapy of urinary tract infections
- Nitrofurantoin macrocrystals (Macrodantin) is administered for the same conditions as nitrofurantoin.

Therapeutic Nursing Interventions

- Obtain specimens for culture and sensitivity before starting therapy.
    - The first dose of sulfonamides may be given before receiving test results.
- Ask if client has experienced hypersensitivity reactions to sulfonamides, salicylates, or sulfasalazine. If so, report findings to primary care provider.
- Monitor intake and output (I & O).
- Encourage fluid intake that is sufficient to maintain a urine output of at least 1200-1500 mL daily.
- Administer medication with food if nausea occurs.
- Monitor CBC and urinalysis laboratory results during drug therapy.
    - Observe for low red or white blood cell count, which may indicate anemia or agranulocytosis (a significant decrease in the number of neutrophils).

Client Education

- Drink an adequate amount of fluids in order to maintain a urine output of at least 1200-1500 mL daily to prevent crystalluria and stone formation.
- Avoid driving and other activities that require alertness until reaction to sulfonamide therapy is known.
    - Sulfonamides may cause dizziness.
- Avoid direct sunlight and ultraviolet light, and use a sunscreen and protective clothing when going outdoors to prevent photosensitivity reactions.
- Use aspirin cautiously when undergoing sulfonamide therapy, because salicylates increase the toxicity of sulfonamides.
- Notify health care professional if skin rash, fever, sore throat, mouth sores, or unusual bleeding or bruising develops.
    - A sore throat, fever, or bleeding may indicate agranulocytosis (a significant decrease in the number of neutrophils).
    - A rash may indicate Steven-Johnson syndrome.
- Warn the client who is taking nitrofurantoin that the medication may cause a rust-brown discoloration of the urine.
- Do not administer within one hour of magnesium due to impaired absorption.

Macrolides and Lincosamides

Overview

Macrolides and lincosamides are bacteriostatic; in large doses they are bactericidal. These drugs have similar pharmacologic and therapeutic characteristics, and they act by inhibiting protein synthesis. The most commonly used macrolides are erythromycin ethylsuccinate (EES) and azithromycin (Zithromax). The most commonly used lincosamide is clindamycin (Cleocin).

Uses

- Erythromycin is the drug of choice for acute diphtheria and eliminating the carrier state.
  - Treats mycoplasma pneumonia
  - Substitutes for penicillin to treat respiratory infections caused by Streptococcus *pneumoniae*
  - Substitutes for penicillin to prevent recurrences of rheumatic fever and bacterial endocarditis
  - Treats Legionnaires' disease
  - Prepares the bowel before bowel surgery
  - Prevents whooping cough; erythromycin does not alter the course of the disease but it eliminates the organism responsible, and thus lowers infectivity.
  - Substitutes for penicillin for clients with history of allergy to penicillin
  - Prevents gonorrheal eye infection in newborns (topical)
- Azithromycin (Zithromax) is used to treat:
  - Upper and lower tract respiratory infections
  - Skin infections
  - Cervicitis
  - Gonorrhea
  - Chancroid
- Clindamycin (Cleocin) is used to treat:
  - Respiratory tract infections
  - Skin infections
  - Septicemia
  - Gynecologic infections
  - Osteomyelitis

Adverse Effects

- Erythromycin has a low incidence of adverse effects. These adverse effects have been reported:
  - Nausea, vomiting, diarrhea, cramping
  - Tinnitus
  - Transient hearing loss
  - Superinfections
  - Allergic reactions
  - Hepatotoxicity (jaundice, clay-colored stools, dark urine, enlarged liver)

- Clindamycin is a more toxic drug than erythromycin.
    - The most dangerous adverse effect is the development of pseudomembranous colitis, which can be fatal. Symptoms of pseudomembranous colitis are:
        - Severe diarrhea
        - Fever
        - Stools containing neutrophils and shreds of mucous membrane and blood

Precautions

- Erythromycin is contraindicated in clients with a history of allergy, and should be used cautiously in clients with a history of liver disease.
- Erythromycin and fluoroquinolones should not be given concurrently. Serious ventricular dysrhythmias have occurred.
- Clindamycin is contraindicated in clients with a history of allergy and severe liver disease.

Important Drugs

Macrolides

- **Erythromycin** is considered one of the safest antibiotics.
- Erythromycin is often used as replacement for penicillin G or V for clients with a history of allergy.
- Erythromycin is not stable in the stomach.
- Must be protected from gastric juices so it can be absorbed from the intestine.
    - Tablets are enteric-coated so they can reach the intestines without first dissolving in the stomach.
- **Azithromycin** (Zithromax) and clarithromycin (Biaxin) are more recent macrolides, and they may be used instead of erythromycin.
    - Both azithromycin and clarithromycin require less frequent administration.
    - Single dose or single daily dose therapy is effective.

Lincosamides

- **Clindamycin** (Cleocin):
    - Should be used only in the treatment of conditions for which other antibiotics are inappropriate or ineffective
    - Is the drug of choice for infections caused by Bacteroides fragilis
    - Is well absorbed from the gastrointestinal tract
        - Food does not affect absorption.

Therapeutic Nursing Interventions

- Administer drugs around the clock.
- Give each dose with a full glass of water.
- Observe for any signs of allergic reaction.
- Monitor for:
    - Signs of hepatotoxicity in clients who are taking erythromycin and who have a history of liver disease.

  - Increased:
    - Aalanine aminotransferase (ALT); also called serum glutamic pyruvic transaminase (SGPT)– an enzyme found primarily in liver cells
    - Aspartate aminotransferase (AST); also called serum glutamic oxaloacetic transminase (SGOT)– an enzyme found in the liver, and elsewhere in the body
- Assess client taking erythromycin for gastrointestinal tract symptoms.
- If gastrointestinal symptoms are present, administer erythromycin with food. Otherwise, administer medication on an empty stomach.
- Assess client taking clindamycin for signs of pseudomembranous colitis.

Client Education

- If taking erythromycin, notify health care provider if serious gastrointestinal symptoms develop. Medication may need to be changed or adjusted if gastrointestinal irritation is severe.
- Notify health care provider if diarrhea, abdominal cramping, fever, or bloody stools develop while taking clindamycin. These are signs of pseudomembranous colitis.
- Clients taking macrolides or lincosamides should:
  - Take medication around the clock exactly as ordered to maintain optimum blood levels of the drug.
  - Take each dose with a full glass of water to increase absorption.
  - Take medication with small amounts of food if gastrointestinal symptoms are present.
  - Report signs and symptoms of superinfection to the health care provider.
  - Drink buttermilk or eat yogurt with meals to prevent symptoms due to superinfection.
  - Notify health professional if symptoms do not improve. The organism may not be sensitive to the prescribed antibiotic, and the health care provider may need to change the dosage or prescribe another antibiotic.

Fluoroquinolones

Overview

Fluoroquinolones are broad-spectrum bactericidal antibiotics that are readily absorbed from the gastrointestinal tract. Fluoroquinolones act by interrupting DNA (deoxyribonucleic acid) synthesis.

Uses

- Infections caused by *Escherichia coli* (also called: *E. coli*)
- Urinary tract infections
- Enteritis
- Sexually transmitted diseases
- Bronchitis
- Anthrax

Adverse Effects

- Nausea, vomiting, and abdominal pain
- Allergic reactions with itching, hives, and rashes
- Photosensitivity
- Superinfections
- Renal failure
- Visual disturbances
- Headache, dizziness, and drowsiness

Precautions

- Avoid fluoroquinolones in children and pregnant women.
- Fluoroquinolones should not be administered to clients who have experienced prior hypersensitivity reactions to these drugs.
- Fluoroquinolones should be administered cautiously to clients with renal disorders.

Important Drugs

- The first **quinolone** was nalidixic acid (NegGram), which was developed in 1962.
- Because of serious drug resistance, **fluoroquinolones** have been primarily replaced by the newer fluoroquinolones (fluorinated quinolones).
- Fluoroquinolones allow oral ambulatory treatment of serious infections that primarily required hospitalization for parenteral therapy.
- Commonly used fluoroquinolones include:
  - Norfloxacin (Noroxin), which is highly effective against urinary tract pathogens
  - Ciprofloxacin (Cipro), which is effective against urinary tract pathogens and most gram-positive and gram-negative bacteria
    - Ciprofloxacin should be added cautiously to the regimen of any client receiving theophylline derivatives.
    - Ciprofloxacin is the drug of choice for the treatment of anthrax.
  - Enoxacin (Penetrex), which has the same uses as Cipro
  - Lomefloxacin (Maxaquin), which has the same uses as Cipro
  - Ofloxacin (Floxin), which has the same uses as Cipro
  - Levofloxacin (Levaquin) is used for similar purposes as Cipro and Penetrex and also for many types of pneumonia.

Therapeutic Nursing Interventions

- Obtain specimen for culture and sensitivity before starting drug therapy to ensure selection of the most effective antibiotic.
- Monitor client for allergic reaction to the drug and report reaction immediately.
- Do not administer fluoroquinolones concomitantly with antacids, iron, calcium, zinc, or magnesium supplements.
- Hydrate clients sufficiently; provide 1-2 liters of fluid daily unless contraindicated.

- Monitor I & O.
- Monitor serum creatinine levels. Increased values may indicate renal dysfunction.
- Check the trend of laboratory values indicating liver function.
    - Alanine aminotransferase (ALT); also called serum glutamic pyruvic transaminase (SGPT)–an enzyme found primarily in liver cells
    - Aspartate aminotransferase (AST); also called serum glutamic oxaloacetic transminase (SGOT)–an enzyme found in the liver and elsewhere in the body
- Administer drug on an empty stomach because food may decrease absorption.
- Administer drug with food if client has gastrointestinal symptoms.

Client Education

- Drink at least 1-2 liters of fluid a day to maintain a satisfactory urinary output.
- Take medication on an empty stomach (unless gastrointestinal symptoms are present) to enhance absorption of the drug.
- Avoid taking medication concurrently with antacids, iron, calcium, zinc or magnesium supplements, as these products will significantly decrease absorption.
- Avoid ingesting milk or yogurt concurrently with a quinolone because these products will significantly decrease absorption.
- Avoid drinking products that contain caffeine (coffee, tea, cola) when taking Cipro.
- Cipro inhibits metabolism of caffeine, and can cause symptoms of excessive caffeine stimulation such as nervousness.
- Use protective clothing against sunlight and sunscreen to prevent photosensitivity reactions during drug therapy and for the 5 days following drug therapy.
- Contact primary care provider if inflammation or tendon pain develops.

Antitubercular Drugs

Overview

Tuberculosis is an infectious disease that usually affects the respiratory system, but may also involve the kidneys, meninges, bones, adrenal glands, and gastrointestinal tract. Droplets containing microorganisms spread *Mycobacterium tuberculosis* from person to person. Atypical tuberculosis may be acquired from soil. The only effective treatment for tuberculosis is long-term (6-24 months) drug therapy. Antitubercular drugs act as either tuberculostatic or tuberculocidal agents by interfering with the formation of mycolic acid, an essential metabolite for the *M. tuberculosis*. Combination therapy minimizes the development of bacterial resistance.

Uses

- Prevent or treat tuberculosis
- Treat Hansen's disease (also called leprosy)
- Treat clients exposed to turberculosis

- Treat clients with positive tuberculin tests
- Prevent meningitis (rifampin)

Adverse Effects

- Peripheral neuropathy (tingling in the fingers, hands, and feet)
- Liver damage and jaundice
- Blurred vision
- Nausea, vomiting, and diarrhea
- Rashes
- Irritability and restlessness
- Headache, vertigo, and seizures
- Discoloration of bodily fluids

Precautions

- Antitubercular drugs are contraindicated in clients who have experienced prior hypersensitivity reactions.
- Isonicotinic acid hydrazide, also called isoniazid (INH) is contraindicated for clients with acute liver disease.
- Antitubercular drugs should be used cautiously for clients with a history of liver disease or chronic alcohol ingestion.

Important Drugs

First-line antitubercular agents are the most effective drugs with the least toxicity.

Isoniazid (INH) is used for both prevention and treatment of tuberculosis.

Rifampin (Rifadin) is always used in combination with other drugs to prevent resistance. This is also the drug of choice for prophylaxis of meningitis.

Ethambutol (Myambutol) is usually combined with INH and rifampin.

Pyrazinamide is usually combined with rifampin and isoniazid (INH).

Second-line antitubercular agents are effective but very toxic.

Ethionamide (Trecator-SC)

Para-aminosalicylic acid (PAS)

Cycloserine (Seromycin)

Streptomycin, an aminoglycoside, is used to increase the activities of ethambutol and isoniazid.

Therapeutic Nursing Interventions

- Encourage the client to comply with the drug program, even when condition improves.
- Administer vitamin B6 (pyridoxine) with INH to prevent peripheral neuropathy.
- Assess client for signs of hepatotoxicity (jaundice, clay-colored stools, dark urine, enlarged liver).
- Monitor lab reports which can indicate liver damage:
    - Elevated serum alaine aminotransferase (ALT); also called serum glutamic pyruvid transaminase (SGPT)

    - Elevated serum AST (aspartate aminotransferase); also called serum glutamic oxaloacetic transminase (SGOT)
- Weigh client and assess for weight loss.

Client Education

- Take medications exactly as ordered until the therapy regimen is completed.
- Treatment often requires at least 6 months.
    - This ensures the drug has killed the tuberculosis bacterium and that the organism is not lying dormant developing drug resistance.
- Take drugs on an empty stomach to enhance absorption.
- Avoid co-administration with antacids, as absorption of antitubercular agents may be reduced.
- Weigh self at least weekly, and report changes in weight to health care provider.
    - Weight loss is an important manifestation of tuberculosis.
- Avoid alcohol because antitubercular drugs can damage the liver.
- Plan to eat foods high in vitamin B6 (pyridoxine) to prevent peripheral neuropathy.
    - Sources of vitamin B6 are pork, organ meats, whole wheat bread, potatoes, oatmeal, legumes, and bananas.
- Be aware that rifampin causes a reddish discoloration to urine, tears, saliva, and other body secretions.
    - Client should remove contact lenses to avoid permanent staining.

Chloramphenicol (Chloromycetin)

Overview

Chloramphenicol (Chloromycetin) is a broad-spectrum antibiotic that is bactericidal in high concentrations. Chloramphenicol inhibits protein synthesis and irreversibly binds to a subunit of bacterial ribosomes. This drug is active against gram-negative and gram-positive bacteria, methicillin-resistant *Staphylococcus aureus* (M-RSA), and ampicillin-resistant strains of *Haemophilus influenzae*. Therapeutic concentrations of the drug are readily achieved in the cerebral spinal fluid. Drug levels in the brain may be as much as nine times those in plasma, because chloramphenicol penetrates the cerebrospinal fluid and crosses the blood-brain barrier easily. Chloramphenicol was widely prescribed in the early 1950s, but then lost popularity because it is very toxic to the bone marrow. As a result, safer antibiotics have replaced chloramphenicol.

Uses

- Chloramphenicol is the last drug of choice for the treatment of life-threatening infections that are resistant to other antibiotics.
- It is also used to treat:
    - Typhoid fever
    - Meningitis and other central nervous system (CNS) infections
    - Superficial ocular infections
    - Minor skin abrasions

Adverse Effects

- Bone marrow suppression, resulting in aplastic anemia or in pancytopenia, which is a reduction in all the cellular elements of the blood.
- Gray-baby syndrome, which is characterized by cyanosis and circulatory collapse. Newborns are especially vulnerable.

Precautions

- Chloramphenicol is toxic to the bone marrow, and should be avoided except to treat life-threatening infections that are resistant to other antibiotics.
- Clients receiving chloramphenicol should be hospitalized during therapy for close observation and laboratory study monitoring.

Therapeutic Nursing Interventions

- Monitor for signs of bone marrow toxicity:
  - Low hemoglobin (Hgb)
  - Low hematocrit (HCT)
  - Low platelet count
  - Low lymphocyte count
  - Extreme fatigue and malaise
  - Sore throat
  - Abnormal bleeding or bruising
- Administer oral chloramphenicol on an empty stomach one hour before meals or two hours after meals.
- Convert from IV to oral chloramphenicol as soon as possible to lower risk of bone marrow toxicity.

Client Education

- Take medication on an empty stomach to enhance absorption.
- Immediately report extreme fatigue, malaise, signs of infection (such as sore throat), and abnormal bleeding or bruising to health care provider because these are signs of bone marrow toxicity.
- Never share this medication with other people because they may be allergic to the drug and may develop bone marrow toxicity.

Vancomycin (Vancocin)

Overview

Vancomycin is a narrow-spectrum antibiotic that is active against gram-positive organisms. Vancomycin exerts a action similar to the penicillins. It acts by inhibiting cell wall synthesis, but at a place different from that of the penicillins and cephalosporins. Vancomycin is usually given intravenously (IV). Although oral medication is excreted in the feces, IV Vancomycin is eliminated entirely by the kidneys.

Uses

Vancomycin is used primarily for severe infections caused by penicillin-resistant *Staphylococci*. This drug is also used to treat:

- Infections caused by methicillin-resistant *Staphylococcus aureus* (M-RSA)
- *Clostridium difficile* colitis (oral only)
- Pneumonia
- Septicemia
- Staphylococcal infections

Adverse Effects

- Red-neck or red-man syndrome, a reaction that develops in response to rapid IV infusion of the drug.
  - Characterized by vascular dilatation and skin flushing of the head, neck, and upper body
  - Other symptoms include hypotension, chills, fever, and tachycardia
- Nausea, vomiting, and stomatitis
- Nephrotoxicity (blood urea nitrogen (BUN) greater than 8-18 mg/dL or creatinine greater than 0.6-1.2 mg/dL)
- Ototoxicity
- Irritation to the IV site with possible tissue necrosis

Precautions

- Vancomycin is contraindicated for clients who are allergic to the drug.
- Vancomycin should be administered cautiously to clients with renal disease, hearing impairment, or intestinal obstruction or inflammation.

Therapeutic Nursing Interventions

- Assess client for signs of infection during and throughout drug therapy (e.g., fever, drainage, elevated WBC).
- Administer vancomycin IV over at least 60 minutes to prevent red-man syndrome.
- Monitor blood pressure throughout IV infusion for hypotension, and observe for signs of red-man syndrome.
- Evaluate IV site closely for signs of tissue irritation or damage. Rotate sites on a scheduled basis.
- Measure intake and output, daily weights, BUN, and creatinine levels.
  - Elevated BUN and creatinine levels indicate renal impairment.
- Assess for cloudy or pink urine, which may be a sign of nephrotoxicity.
- Monitor results of audiometry tests, which are ordered to evaluate eighth cranial nerve function.
- Monitor for diarrhea.
  - Assess frequency and consistency of stools.
  - Observe for blood in stools and report this finding to the primary care provider.

- Monitor client for signs of superinfection: sore mouth, black furry tongue, diarrhea.

Client Education

- Immediately report tinnitus or any change in hearing acuity to health care provider. Early intervention is necessary to prevent permanent hearing loss due to drug toxicity.
- Report nausea, vomiting, or diarrhea because dosage may need to be adjusted or another antibiotic may need to be prescribed.
- Report signs of hypersensitivity or superinfection to the health care provider.
- Report cloudy or pink urine to health care provider because this may be a sign of nephrotoxicity.

Antivirals

Overview

Viruses are parasites that only reproduce inside a living cell. Antiviral drugs penetrate human host cells, interfere with production of deoxyribonucleic acid (DNA), and prevent reproduction of the virus. Most antiviral agents are excreted unchanged by the kidneys. A great majority of viral infections occur without any accompanying illness. When a viral infection does produce sickness, the illness is usually self-limited, of short duration, and it results in long-term immunity to the virus involved. Antiviral drugs are generally used when the infection causes CNS, hepatic, or pulmonary symptoms.

Uses

Antiviral drugs are used to treat:

- Mucosal and cutaneous infections caused by the herpes simplex virus (HSV), including shingles
  - HSV-1 causes oral herpes, herpes labialis, and infections around the face.
  - HSV-2 causes genital herpes.
  - Antiviral agents may ease symptoms, but do not eliminate the disease.
- Influenza A and B pneumonia
- Parkinsonism and drug-induced extrapyramidal reactions (e.g., amantadine)
- Hepatitis C

Adverse Effects

Antiviral drugs are generally well tolerated, but when given in higher doses, they can cause the following adverse effects:

- Nausea
- Vomiting
- Diarrhea
- Inflammation and phlebitis at injection site
- Urinary retention
- Depression
- Psychosis

Precautions

- Give high doses of antiviral drugs cautiously because of possible adverse effects.
- Avoid use of antiviral drugs in clients with a history of hypersensitivity to these agents.
- Give antiviral drugs cautiously to pregnant women, children, and clients with a history of renal disease.

Important Drugs

Acyclovir (Zovirax) is effective against herpes simplex type 1 and 2, and varicella-zoster virus (VZV).

- Acyclovir is relatively safe unless administered in high doses.
- Acyclovir IV should be infused slowly over at least one hour to prevent renal damage.
- IV sites should be rotated to prevent injection site reactions.

Amantadine (Symmetrel) is effective against respiratory syncytial virus.

- Amantadine is well tolerated in low dosages.

Foscarnet (Foscavir) is used to treat cytomegalovirus (CMV) retinitis in clients with immunodeficiency.

- Drug is relatively toxic.
  - Can cause renal impairment, electrolyte imbalance, and hypocalcemia.

Ganciclovir (Cytovene) is used to treat CMV retinitis in persons with immunodeficiency and herpes viruses.

- Side effects of ganciclovir include neutropenia and thrombocytopenia.
- Potentially carcinogenic.

Interferons (alpha, beta, gamma) are used most often in the treatment of some of the leukemias, renal cell carcinoma, hepatitis, and Kaposi's sarcoma.

- A flu-like syndrome is the most common adverse reaction to interferons.
  - Other adverse effects include hematologic toxicity, gastrointestinal disturbances, and hypotension.

Antiviral agents used to treat AIDS:

- Nucleoside reverse transcriptase inhibitors (NRTI)
  - Azidothymidine (AZT; also called: zidovudine or Retrovir) is the most important drug currently available to treat HIV infection and AIDS.
  - Most adverse effects involve hematologic toxicities.
- Non-nucleoside reverse transcriptase inhibitors (NNRTI)
  - Nevirapine (Viramune) slows the progression of HIV infection and decreases complications.
- Protease inhibitors
  - Saquinavir (Invirase) slows progression of HIV infection and decreases complications.

Therapeutic Nursing Interventions

- Assess client for signs of an allergic reaction.

- Administer antiviral drugs with food to decrease gastrointestinal side effects.
- Use gloves when administering antiviral drugs IV because lesions may be contagious.
- Monitor IV site for signs of inflammation and phlebitis.
- Rotate IV sites on a scheduled basis.
- Monitor client for signs of renal dysfunction.
- Measure I & O, and monitor laboratory reports for increased BUN and creatinine levels, which may indicate renal dysfunction.

Client Education

- Take oral medication with food to decrease gastrointestinal side effects.
- Immediately report discomfort or pain at site of IV infusion.
- Report nausea, vomiting, or diarrhea to health care provider.
- Dosage may need to be adjusted or another antiviral drug prescribed.
- Report decreased urine output to health care provider because this may be a sign of renal dysfunction.
- Never share medication with other people because they may be allergic to it.

Antifungals

Overview

Antifungal agents act by disrupting the bacterial cell membrane. They adhere to the wall of the membrane, causing it to become semi-permeable. Antifungal agents are poorly absorbed from the intestinal tract. These agents are excreted very slowly by the kidneys, and can be detected in the urine for up to eight weeks following therapy.

Uses

Antifungal agents are used to treat:

- Candidiasis (thrush)
- Coccidioidomycosis
- Blastomycosis
- Histoplasmosis
- Fungal pneumonia
- Tinea capitis (on scalp)
- Tinea corporis (ringworm)
- Tinea cruris (jock itch)
- Tinea pedis (athlete's foot)

Adverse Effects

- Fever and chills
- Nausea and vomiting
- Renal dysfunction
- Thrombophlebitis

Precautions

- Avoid use of antifungal drugs in clients with a history of hypersensitivity.
- Antifungal drugs may not be safe to use during pregnancy.

Important Drugs

Amphotericin B (Fungizone) is one of the most toxic anti-infectives currently in use.

- Given only for life-threatening infections.
  - Nurses know the agent anecdotally as "Amphoterrible."
- Side effects have been referred to as "shake and bake."
- Amphotericin B produces chills and fever with each dose in about 50% of clients.
- Prior to infusion of amphotericin, the client should be premedicated with acetaminophen (Tylenol), diphenhydramine hydrochloride (Benadryl), and glucocorticoids.
- Rapid infusion of amphotericin B beyond the recommended range may precipitate severe cardiovascular symptoms, anaphylaxis, and seizures.
- Amphotericin B may cause severe thrombophlebitis at the injection site.
- Renal dysfunction is common. It is important to monitor urinary output and renal function test abnormalities.
- Many clients receiving amphotericin B therapy develop hypokalemia and hypomagnesemia.
- Amphotericin B may cause a mild anemia due to bone marrow suppression.

Flucytosine (Ancobon) is administered alone or in combination with amphotericin B for serious systemic fungal infections.

- May cause agranulocytosis (a significant decrease in the number of neutrophils).

Nystatin (Mycostatin) may be used orally, topically, or vaginally.

- This drug is administered as a liquid swish and swallow for oral candida infections.
- It is administered vaginally for vulvovaginal candidiasis.
- When applied topically, occlusive dressings should be avoided because they provide a moist environment for fungal growth.

Fluconazole (Diflucan) is used to treat oropharyngeal and esophageal candidiasis, urinary tract infections, peritonitis, pneumonia, and cryptococcal meningitis.

- Fluconazole is generally well tolerated.
- Uncommon reactions are:
  - Nausea and vomiting
  - Rash
  - Elevated liver enzymes:
    - Alaine aminotransferase (ALT); also called serum glutamic pyruvic transaminase (SGPT)
    - AST (aspartate aminotransferase); also called serum glutamic oxaloacetic transminase (SGOT)

Ketoconazole (Nizoral) is a topical antifungal drug used to treat a variety of cutaneous fungal infections, including tinea cruris (jock itch), tinea corporis (ringworm), and tinea pedis (athlete's foot).

- This agent is also effective for coccidioidomycosis and histoplasmosis.
- Ketoconazole can produce life-threatening cardiac dysrhythmias.

Miconazole (Monistat) is used primarily to treat vaginal candidiasis.

- Also prescribed for cutaneous fungus infections.

Therapeutic Nursing Interventions

- Evaluate affected areas prior to and throughout course of antifungal therapy.
- Monitor client for signs of renal dysfunction, measure I & O; and check for BUN and creatinine levels.
- Monitor for:
  - Hypokalemia—Serum potassium level < 3.5 mEq/L
  - Hypomagnesemia—Serum magnesium level < 1.5 mEq/L
  - Muscle weakness
  - Shallow respirations
  - Cardiac dysrhythmias
  - Positive **Chvostek's sign** (twitching of the ipsilateral facial muscles)
  - Positive **Trousseau's sign** (muscular contraction including flexion of the wrist and metacarpophalangeal joints, hyperextension of the fingers, and flexion of the thumb on the palm)
- Assess IV site for signs of phlebitis (e.g., redness, pain, swelling, warmth).
- During IV infusion with amphotericin B, instruct client to report chills, shaking, or dizziness.
- Take vital signs and evaluate heart rhythm throughout therapy because some antifungal drugs cause serious cardiac dysrhythmias.
- Monitor client for fever and chills, and give acetaminophen as ordered for an elevated temperature.

Client Education

- Report immediately to health care provider side effects of drugs, such as:
  - Nausea
  - Vomiting
  - Fever
  - Chills
- Drug dosage may need to be adjusted or another antifungal drug prescribed.
- Symptoms such as muscle weakness or spasms as these may indicate an electrolyte imbalance.
- Health care provider may need to prescribe potassium or magnesium replacement therapy.
- Apply topical creams or lotions in small amounts and cover the affected area completely with the medication.
- Avoid using occlusive dressings or wrappings to cover topical creams because they create a moist environment that encourages fungal growth.

- Notify health care provider if fungal infection does not improve. Another antifungal agent may need to be prescribed.
- Delay eating or drinking after nystatin (Mycostatin) "swish and swallow" to avoid rinsing drug from mucous membranes.

Antiparasitics

Overview

Antiparasitics block the ability of parasites to synthesize chemicals vital to their survival. Antiparasitics are well-absorbed following oral administration and are metabolized in the liver. Major types of antiparasitic drugs are:

Amebicides: Destroy amebae

Anthelmintics: Destroy parasitic worms by disrupting their nervous systems. Worms are found most often in the gastrointestinal tract, but they can migrate to blood, lymph, liver, and other body tissues.

Antimalarials: Active against the parasites that cause malaria

Antiprotozoals: Agents that kill protozoa

Pediculicides: Kill lice

Scabicides: Kill itch mites, the causative agent of scabies

Uses

- Amebicides are used to treat:
  - Amebiasis or amebic dysentery
  - Giardiasis, an intestinal disorder, which is spread by water and food contaminated by feces. This protozoan is also found in untreated well water.
  - *Trichomoniasis vaginalis*, which may be spread by sexual intercourse
- Anthelmintics are used to treat infestations with these parasites:
  - Flatworms
  - Flukes
  - Pinworms
  - Roundworms
  - Tapeworms
- Antimalarials are used to prevent or treat malaria.
- Antiprotozoal agents are primarily used to treat *Pneumocystis carinii* (pneumocystosis).
- Pediculicides (shampoos and creams) are used to treat pediculosis infections of the scalp.
- Scabicides are used to treat scabies, a parasitic skin disorder.

Adverse Effects

Amebicides cause few adverse effects except for nausea and vomiting. Hypersensitivity reactions do occasionally occur.

Anthelmintics cause these adverse effects:

- Nausea, vomiting, dehydration, and anorexia
- Rash
- Anemia

Antimalarials cause these adverse effects:

- Nausea and vomiting
- Agranulocytosis
- Blurred vision, headache, fatigue, agitation

Pentamidine (Pentam-300), a major antiprotozoal agent, causes these adverse effects when administered IV:

- Hypotension, followed by tachycardia and cardiac dysrhythmias
- Renal dysfunction
- Hypoglycemia
- Diabetes
- Nausea and vomiting
- Pruritus
- Hallucinations
- Syncope

Pediculicides

- Can damage the:
    - Heart
    - Kidneys
    - Central nervous system
- Cause drying of the hair

Scabicides and pediculicides

- Can damage the:
    - Heart
    - Kidneys
    - Central nervous system
- Cause skin irritation

Precautions

- Avoid use of amebicides and anthelmintic agents in clients with a history of hypersensitivity.
- The antimalarial drug chloroquine is not recommended during pregnancy.
- The dosage of pentamidine should be reduced in clients with renal insufficiency.
- Metronidazole (Flagyl) is contraindicated during the first trimester of pregnancy.
- Elderly clients should use scabicides and pediculicides cautiously because of increased risk of toxic effects.

Important Drugs

Paromomycin (Humatin) is an amebicide that is active against amebic dysentery.

Metronidazole (Flagyl) is active against anaerobic organisms that survive in the absence of oxygen. Specifically, it is effective against:

- Organisms that cause amebiasis, giardiasis, and trichomoniasis
- *Helicobacter pylori* (also called: *H. pylori*) associated with peptic ulcer disease
- *Clostridium difficile* associated with pseudomembranous colitis
- Gram-negative bacillus (when used in combination with aminoglycoside)

Antimalarial drugs:

- Chloroquine (Aralen)
- Quinine sulfate (Quinamm)
- Hydroxychloroquine (Plaquenil)

Mebendazole (Vermox) is an anthelmintic drug used to treat roundworm, hookworm, and pinworm infestations.

- Pyrantel pamoate (Pin-X) is used to treat pinworm infestations.

Pentamidine is an antiprotozoal diamidine drug used to treat:

- *Pneumocystis carinii* (pneumocystosis), an acute pneumonia-like lung infection, which is caused by the parasite protozoa.
    - This opportunistic infection is a complication of AIDS.
- Leishmaniasis, which is a rare infection in the United States
- Toxoplasmosis, which is an infection found in many mammals and birds, and can be spread by contact with cat feces.

Gamma benzin hexachloride (Kwell) is the most frequently prescribed cream, lotion, and shampoo for scabies.

Lindane shampoo or cream rinse (Nix) is used to treat pediculosis.

Therapeutic Nursing Interventions

Metronidazole (Flagyl)

- Assess clients who are taking anticoagulants concurrently with metronidazole for signs of bleeding. Metronidazole inhibits the metabolism of anticoagulants by the liver.
- Evaluate for rashes, which may indicate an allergic response.
- Assess for thrombophlebitis when metronidazole is given IV.

Anthelmintic drugs

- Treat everyone who is in close contact with the client.
- Monitor complete blood count (CBC) for low red blood cell (RBC) count, which indicates anemia.

Antimalarials

- Clients should start taking antimalarials one to two weeks before traveling to an area where malaria is endemic.
- Monitor for low white blood cell count (WBC) that indicates agranulocytosis (a significant decrease in the number of neutrophils).
- Administer antimalarials with food to decrease gastrointestinal symptoms.

Antiprotozoal drugs (pentamidine)

- Assess site following IM injection for sterile abscess or dermal necrosis.

- Monitor blood pressure, pulse, and ECG (electrocardiogram) during and following IM or IV administration to detect hypotension or cardiac dysrhythmias. Shock and/or cardiac dysfunction have produced fatalities.
- Monitor blood glucose levels during and for several months following therapy. Clients may develop diabetes mellitus.
- Assess BUN and serum creatinine for increased concentrations in clients with a history of renal dysfunction.

Pediculoides

- Treat everyone who is in close contact with clients.
- Use gloves to apply medications to skin and scalp.
- Educate clients about good hygiene.
- Treat all clothing and bedding (including mattresses and furniture).

Scabicides

- Treat everyone who is in close contact with clients.
- Use gloves to apply medications to skin and scalp.
- Educate clients about good hygiene.
- Treat all clothing and bedding (including mattresses and furniture).

Client Education

- Instruct clients taking **antiparasitic** drugs to complete all of the medication exactly as ordered to ensure that the parasite has been killed.
- Inform clients about the side effects that may occur when taking antiparasitic drugs. Emphasize clients should report side effects to their health care provider immediately.
- Instruct clients taking **metronidazole** (Flagyl) to avoid alcohol during drug therapy and for at least 48 hours after treatment is complete.
  - Those who drink alcohol will experience intense flushing, tachycardia, nausea and vomiting, headache, and/or circulatory collapse.
  - Warn clients that metronidazole (Flagyl) can produce a metallic taste and discolor their urine.
- Instruct clients taking **antimalarials** to:
  - Take drug one to two weeks before traveling to an area where malaria is endemic.
  - Take drug with food to decrease gastrointestinal symptoms.
  - Have an eye exam every six months as irreversible blindness is a complication of antimalarial drugs.
- Instruct clients taking **anthelmintic** drugs to:
  - Wash the bedding with hot water and bleach and then put bedding into a hot dryer to kill parasites.
  - Practice good hand washing to prevent reinfection.
- Instruct clients taking **scabicides** or **pediculicides** to:
  - Read instructions and labels on shampoos and creams and follow directions carefully.

- Wash bedding, clothing, hats, and hair accessories with hot water and bleach. Put clothing and bedding into a hot dryer (Items that may shrink may be placed dry into a hot dryer for 20 minutes).

Critical Thinking Exercise: Drugs Used to Treat Infection

Note: *It is recommended that the following exercises be reviewed with a partner or in a small group to achieve maximum student interaction and to enhance critical thinking skills*

Situation: A 26-year-old female comes to the community clinic complaining of a fever, sore throat, and cough. Her posterior pharynx is reddened with patches of purulent exudate and she experiences pain with swallowing. Her cervical lymph nodes are enlarged and tender to touch. The client's vital signs are: temperature, 101.4 orally; pulse, 96; respirations, 22; BP, 122/84. Based on the symptoms and physical examination, the primary care provider suspects a streptococcal infection which is confirmed by a quick strep test performed in the clinic. The client is started on amoxicillin-clavulanate (Augmentin) 500 mg PO q 8h for 10 days.

1. Before administering the first dose of amoxicillin-clavulanate (Augmentin), what additional assessment data should the nurse collect?

2. What teaching do you consider most important for the client taking amoxicillin-clavulanate (Augmentin)?

3. After the first two doses, the client calls and states he is experiencing an itchy rash. What would be your best response and what is your rationale?

Situation: The client returns to the clinic and the physician discontinues the Augmentin and starts the client on cephalexin (Keflex), 250 mg PO q 6h for 10 days. The physician provides samples so the client can begin taking the medication immediately.

4. What would be your best nursing intervention? Explain your rationale.

5. As a nurse, you have particular knowledge about cephalexin (Keflex). List as much information as you can about the drug below.

Situation: Mrs. J, a 46-year-old woman comes to your clinic, stating she has been taking trimethopin-sulfamethoxazole (Bactrim) for a bladder infection, but is concerned because she has developed intense perineal client and a whitish, cheesy appearing vaginal discharge. She is visiting an out-of-state relative and would prefer to see her own doctor, but can't wait because the itching is unbearable.

6. How should the nurse respond to the client's concern?

7. What action do you anticipate from the physician?

Situation: Mr. R comes to the clinic complaining of frequency and burning for the past two days. A preliminary urinalysis reveals the urine is cloudy with moderate sediment and increased white blood cells. The specimen is sent to the lab for a culture and sensitivity. The primary care provider orders nitrofurantoin (Furadantin).

8. Why did the doctor choose this particular medication?

9. What are some of the nursing considerations when giving nitrofurantoin?

CHAPTER 3

Drugs Affecting the Immune System

Key Points

- The immune response is the body's recognition of and reaction to foreign antigens.
  - This response results in the neutralization or destruction of pathogenic antigens, thereby preventing damage to the body.
  - The following types of white blood cells (WBCs) play important roles in the immune response:
    - Neutrophils
    - Monocytes
    - B-lymphocytes
    - T-lymphocytes

Acquired immunity is the second line of defense against infectious agents.

- It is either active or passive.

Active acquired immunity is produced by the person's own immune system in response to a disease caused by a specific antigen from a source outside the body.

Immune serums (immune globulins) and antitoxins are given to provide passive acquired immunity.

Immunity is the state of being protected against infectious diseases.

Immunization is the process of promoting immunity in an individual as a preventive measure against certain infectious diseases.

Immunostimulants, also called immunomodulators, activate or enhance a person's own immune system.

Immunosuppressants act to suppress the immune response.

Natural or innate immunity is present at birth. It is the first line of defense against most infectious agents.

Nucleoside reverse transcriptase inhibitors, nonnucleoside reverse transcriptase inhibitors, and protease inhibitors are used to treat HIV infection and acquired immunodeficiency syndrome (AIDS).

- They may relieve symptoms or delay development of AIDS in HIV-positive persons, but they do not cure, nor do they prevent transmission of viruses.

Passive acquired immunity occurs when antibodies are formed by the immune system of another person or animal, and transferred to the host by means of immunization.

Vaccines and **toxoids** are given to provide active acquired immunity.

Active Immunizing Agents

Overview

Active immunization, also called vaccination or inoculation, involves the injection of killed or weakened (attenuated) microorganisms into the body via vaccines and toxoids. Vaccines contain specific antigens that induce the endogenous production of antibodies, thereby establishing active immunity to a specific infectious disease. Vaccines may contain live microorganisms, or microorganisms that have been killed or inactivated to reduce their virulence. Vaccines provide immunity for a prolonged period of time.

Live vaccines are given for:

- Measles
- Mumps
- Varicella
- Rubella

Killed or attenuated vaccines are given for:

- Cholera
- Typhoid fever
- Pertussis
- Rabies
- Hepatitis B
- Influenza
- Polio

Toxoids are toxins that have been altered to inactivate their toxicity, but are still able to induce the formation of antibodies when injected (e.g., diphtheria toxoid). Active immunity requires 5-14 days to develop following the first immunization. It lasts for at least a year, and can be restored with booster shots. The Centers for Disease Control and Prevention (CDC) website (http://www.cdc.gov) has a current schedule of recommended immunizations for children and adults.

Uses

- Immunizations protect populations who are at high risk of infectious diseases (e.g., elderly clients, chronically ill clients, and health care providers).
  - Vaccines provide active immunization against specific bacterial and viral disorders.
  - Toxoids provide active immunization against tetanus, diphtheria, and pertussis (whooping cough).
  - Immunizations are given to prevent the development and spread of specific communicable diseases and infections that could result in epidemics.

Adverse Effects

Mild:

- Rash
- Raised red area at the injection site
- Pain and swelling at the injection site
- Slight fever
- Irritability
- Malaise

Severe:

- Anaphylactic reactions (MMR)
- Convulsions
- Encephalitis (DTP)
- Serum sickness
- Guillain-Barré syndrome
- Paralysis (oral polio vaccine (OPV))
- Manifestations of the disease
- Death

Precautions

- Vaccinations are contraindicated for clients who:
  - Have had a previous anaphylactic reaction
  - Have a moderate or severe acute illness with or without a fever
  - Are pregnant (with some vaccines)
  - Are breast-feeding (with some vaccines)
  - Are immunocompromised due to cancer, leukemia, lymphoma, or the use of immunosuppressive drugs
- Contrary to popular belief, vaccines can be given:
  - During mild illness
  - While on antimicrobial therapy
  - With diarrhea
  - Following mild local reactions to previous vaccines
  - During convalescence
  - To premature infants
  - After recent exposure to an infectious illness
  - With a personal or family history of allergies

Important Drugs

Bacterial Vaccines

- Bacillus Calmette-Guerin (BCG) vaccine
- Pneumococcal polysaccharide vaccine
- Haemophilus B conjugate vaccine
- Cholera vaccine

- Typhoid vaccine
- Anthrax vaccine

Viral Vaccines

- Hepatitis A vaccine (HAV)
- Hepatitis B vaccine (HBV)
- Poliovirus vaccine
- Influenza virus vaccine
- Measles, mumps, rubella (MMR)
- Varicella (chicken pox)
- Mixed respiratory vaccine
- Smallpox vaccine

Toxoids

- Tetanus toxoid
- Diphtheria toxoid
- Diphtheria, tetanus toxoid, and pertussis (DTP) vaccine
    - DTaP, introduced in 1997, is about 10 times less likely to cause certain adverse reactions (such as fever, vomiting, and mild seizures) than DTP. The DTP vaccine contains the whole, inactivated pertussis bacteria, while the DTaP uses only the parts of the bacteria that help develop immunity to it and leaves behind all the other parts that may have been responsible for many of DTP's adverse effects. (The "a" in DTaP stands for "acellular," which means there are no whole pertussis bacteria in the vaccine.)

Therapeutic Nursing Interventions

- Schedule clients to maintain vaccinations as recommended by the Advisory Committee on Immunization Practices (ACIP).
- Check the expiration date on all vials of vaccine before administering vaccine.
- Store vaccines according to instructions from the manufacturer.
    - Most vaccines and toxoids are refrigerated.
    - Do not store vaccines in the refrigerator door because the temperature is higher than usually recommended.
- Prior to immunizing a client, obtain a history of previous allergic reactions to specific vaccines.
    - Check with the client for allergies to eggs.
        - If the client is allergic to eggs, do not administer the live form of the vaccine. When administering the killed form, provide an antihistamine prior to the injection to prevent or lessen an allergic reaction.
- Administer most vaccines per injection into the upper arm.
- Have the client remain in the office/clinic for 30 minutes after receiving a vaccine.
    - If an allergic reaction occurs, it is usually within 30 minutes.
    - Signs and symptoms include difficulty breathing, collapse, shock, and urticaria.

  - Treatment: subcutaneous epinephrine 0.5 mL for adults, 0.01 mL/kg for children.
- Report unusual reactions to vaccines or toxoids to the U.S. Food and Drug Administration (FDA).
- Always aspirate before giving a parenteral vaccine to prevent accidental intravenous injection.
- Be sure epinephrine 1:1000 is available for immediate treatment of allergic reactions.
- OPV can be given to infants with a dropper, on a sugar cube, in milk or in distilled water.
- MMR
  - Reconstitute exactly as directed by manufacturer.
  - Use within 8 hours of reconstitution.
  - Give subcutaneously.
- Give infant DPT vaccine in lateral thigh muscle.
- Administer HBV intramuscularly.
  - Infants and young children: anterolateral thigh
  - Adults and older children: deltoid
- Maintain accurate records.

Client Education

- Encourage clients to receive recommended vaccinations prior to foreign travel.
- Instruct clients to immediately report any serious reaction to an immunization.
- Instruct clients who develop a slight fever to rest, drink fluids, and take acetaminophen to reduce mild discomfort.
- Encourage older clients to get an influenza vaccine every three years and the pneumococcal vaccine if at risk of developing pneumonia.
- Encourage all adolescents and adults to have a tetanus-diphtheria booster shot every 10 years if they received the primary series earlier.
- A mild local reaction and low fever are common.
- Instruct clients to keep their vaccination records, as they may have to present it to their school or employer.

Passive Immunizing Agents

Overview

Artificially acquired passive immunity involves immunization with antibodies against an organism that have been obtained from another human or animal (e.g., injections of immune globulins or serums).

Antitoxins are agents manufactured from prepared animal serum. They contain antibodies that neutralize the effects of specific toxins released by pathogens into the bloodstream (e.g., diphtheria, tetanus, and gas-gangrene are caused by toxins).

Antivenins are suspensions also manufactured from prepared animal serum. They also contain antibodies that neutralize venom from snake and spider bites and prevent secondary infection.

Live virus vaccines are usually administered 14-30 days before or 6-12 weeks after the injection of immune globulins to help foster the development of immunity.

Passive immunization with immune globulins provides immediate but temporary protection against an infectious disease. The half-life of injected antibodies is approximately 7 days.

Uses

Immune globulins are used to treat:

- Immunodeficiency syndromes
- Idiopathic thrombocytopenia purpura
- Tetanus
- Rabies
- IgG (immunoglobulin, Class G) deficiency
- Wounds contaminated with Clostridium tetani
- Clients following renal transplant
- Clients following exposure to hepatitis A or hepatitis B
- Varicella zoster
- Non-sensitized Rh-negative women who are pregnant or who have delivered an Rh- positive baby (Rho [D] immune globulin)
  - The mother's body detects the Rh factor in the fetus' blood as a foreign substance and begins to develop antibodies to the fetus' blood. The antibodies pass from the mother's blood and begin to attack the red blood cells of the fetus.
  - Not required for Rh-positive women who have delivered a Rh-negative baby, or where the mother and baby are both Rh-positive, or both Rh-negative
- Respiratory syncytial virus (RSV) immune globulin for high-risk premature infants and children

Antitoxins and antivenins are used to treat:

- Tetanus
- Rabies
- Diphtheria
- Gas gangrene
- Black widow bites
- Snake bites

Adverse Effects

- Mild local discomfort
- Anaphylaxis (rare)
- Chills and fever
- Headache
- Serum sickness

Precautions

- Immune globulins are not used during pregnancy unless clearly indicated.
- Immune globulins may be contraindicated for clients with coagulation disorders and thrombocytopenia, because these products are administered IM.

Important Drugs

Immune globulins

- Tetanus immune globulin
- Hepatitis B immune globulin
- Cytomegalovirus immune globulin
- Varicella-zoster immune globulin (VZIG)
- RhoD immune globulin (RhoGAM)
- Rabies immune globulin
- Vaccinia immune globulin (VIG) given to treat adverse effects from smallpox vaccine
- RSV immune globulin (RSV-IVIG)

Antitoxins

- Tetanus antitoxin
- Diphtheria antitoxin

Therapeutic Nursing Interventions

- Prior to giving serum globulin or an antitoxin, obtain a history of previous allergic reactions to these agents.
- Prior to administration of immune globulins, assess body temperature and vital signs because client may develop a fever following administration.
- Administer most serum globulins or antitoxins per injection into the upper arm.
- Most immune globulins or serum may be given IV.
- Monitor clients following injection for any untoward reactions.
- If agent is given IV and client develops chest pain or chills, stop infusion and notify primary care provider.

Client Education

- Provide a full history of any previous allergic reactions to immune globulins or antitoxins.
- Notify health care professional if chills, generalized rash, dyspnea, or chest pain develop while receiving immune globulin IV.

Immunostimulants

Overview

Immunostimulants (also called immunomodulating agents) activate or enhance a person's own immune system. The goal of immunostimulants is to restore normal function to the immune system, and to increase the ability of the immune system to eliminate potentially harmful invaders. The three most important immunostimulants are:

Colony-stimulating factors (CSF): Stimulate growth and function of hematopoietic cells

Interferons: Antiviral, antiproliferative, and immunoregulatory agents. They interfere with the ability of viruses in infected cells to replicate and spread.

Interleukins: Stimulate growth of early lymphoid stem cells into lymphocytes

Uses

- Interferons are used to treat cancer and viral infections.
- Interleukins are used to treat renal cell carcinoma, malignant melanoma, and lymphoma.
- Colony-stimulating factors are used to treat renal disease, leukemias, and lymphomas.

Adverse Effects

Colony-stimulating factors

- Anorexia, nausea, vomiting, diarrhea, headache, fever
- Cough, dyspnea, sore throat
- Blood dyscrasias
- Bone pain
- Hypertension
- Edema

Interferons

- Flu-like syndrome is most common. Symptoms are fever, chills, nausea, vomiting, fatigue, and malaise.
- Dizziness and confusion
- Renal dysfunction with increased BUN and creatinine levels
- Liver dysfunction
- Nausea, vomiting, diarrhea, anorexia
- Neutropenia and thrombocytopenia

- Cardiac dysrhythmias
- Alopecia

Interleukins

- Flu-like syndrome is most common. Symptoms are fever, chills, nausea, vomiting, fatigue, and malaise.
- Capillary leak syndrome: Capillaries leak vital proteins into the surrounding tissues, resulting in fluid retention with excessive weight gain, edema, pulmonary congestion, congestive heart failure, cardiac dysrhythmias, and acute myocardial infarction.
- Disorientation
- Renal failure with oliguria and anuria
- Anemia

Precautions

Colony-stimulating factors should be administered cautiously to clients receiving antineoplastics because adverse interactions may develop.

Interferons:

- Should be administered cautiously to clients with hepatic disease or neurologic disorders because these agents are potentially hepatotoxic and neurotoxic.
- Should be administered cautiously to clients receiving aminophylline therapy because adverse interactions may develop.
- Are contraindicated for clients who are allergic to eggs or neomycin. However, if a client has had a mild allergic reaction, and the client requires interferon therapy, then interferons should be administered with antihistamines to prevent severe allergic reactions.

Interleukins:

- Should be administered in an intensive care unit because of the risk of a severe adverse reaction.
- Should be administered cautiously to clients receiving antihypertensives, corticosteroids, some antibiotics, and some chemotherapeutic agents.
- Are contraindicated during pregnancy and lactation.

Important Drugs

Colony-stimulating factors

- **Epoetin alfa** (Epogen) is usually classified as a blood modifier rather than an immunostimulant. It is used to treat anemia caused by chronic renal failure and cancer chemotherapy.
- **Granulocyte colony-stimulating factor**, filgrastim (Neupogen), stimulates neutrophil production.
    - Prescribed for clients with cancer to fight infection.
    - Granulocyte-macrophage colony-stimulating factor, sargramostim (Leukine), stimulates production of granulocytes and macrophages.
    - Prescribed for clients undergoing bone marrow transplantation.

Interferons

Interferon-alpha (Roferon-A) is the agent most commonly used for treatment of cancer and viral infections. A clinical response to this agent occurs in 1-3 months.

Interferon-beta (Betaseron)

Interferon-gamma (Actimmune)

Interleukins

Interleukin-2 (aldesleukin) (IL-2) is the only interleukin available for clinical use.

- Causes leukocytosis (an increase in the number of leukocytes)
- Produces cytokines
- Inhibits tumor growth

Therapeutic Nursing Interventions

Colony-stimulating factors

- Monitor for elevated blood pressure.
- Monitor for signs of edema.
- Assess for cough and sore throat.
- Monitor CBC for signs of bone marrow failure.
- Administer a non-opioid analgesic for minor symptoms.

Interferons

- Administer interferons by injection because they are proteins. Proteins will be destroyed if given orally.
- Monitor for increased BUN and creatinine levels, which could indicate renal dysfunction.
- Monitor CBC count for indications of bone marrow suppression. Assess for anemia, neutropenia, and thrombocytopenia.

Interleukin-2

- Monitor for capillary leak syndrome; assess for cardiac dysfunction, edema, weight gain, and pulmonary congestion.
- Monitor for increased BUN and creatinine levels, which could indicate renal dysfunction.
- Monitor for changes in mental status.
- Administer non-opioid analgesics PRN for symptoms of flu-like syndrome.
- Inform client that temporary visual symptoms may develop after starting this drug.

Client Education

Colony-stimulating factors

- Clients should report cough or sore throat to their health care provider.

Interferons

- Notify health care provider if bleeding or infection occurs. This agent may cause a low platelet and white blood cell count.

- Minimize flu-like symptoms by taking medication at bedtime.
- Avoid being immunized without a primary care provider's order because interferons lower the body's resistance to infection.
- Avoid contact with people who have recently been immunized with live virus vaccine because interferons lower the body's resistance to infection.

Interleukin-2

- Report flu-like symptoms to the health care provider.
- Avoid drinking alcohol or taking medication containing aspirin (acetylsalicylic acid) or nonsteroidal anti-inflammatory drugs (NSAIDs) as these products may cause gastric bleeding.
- Use a non-hormonal birth control method while taking this drug.

Immunosuppressants

Overview

The role of the immune system is to protect the body against internal and external threats. Autoimmune disorders occur when the immune system reacts to normal body tissue as if it were foreign. These inappropriate immune responses can have devastating effects on affected tissues. Examples of autoimmune disorders are rheumatoid arthritis, systemic lupus erythematosus, and inflammatory bowel disease. It is necessary to suppress the immune system when clients receive transplanted organs; without immune suppressants, they will probably reject the organ. Immunosuppressants include corticosteroids, cytotoxic antineoplastic drugs, antirejection drugs, antibody preparations, and others. Corticosteroids are discussed in a later chapter. The prototypes are the cytotoxic antineoplastic agents methotrexate and azathioprine.

Immunosuppressive drugs act to suppress the immune response by suppressing the production and activity of lymphocytes. Lymphocytes are white blood cells that fight infection and eliminate abnormal cells that may become malignant. Immunosuppressive drugs are grouped according to their primary mode of action:

- Anti-inflammatory agents
- Antimetabolites
- Cytotoxic agents
- Antibodies
- Polypeptide antibiotics

Uses

- Treat autoimmune disorders (e.g., systemic lupus erythematosus [SLE] and rheumatoid arthritis).
- Prevent organ rejection following organ transplantation.
    - The goal is to provide adequate but not excessive immunosuppression.
    - T-lymphocytes of the recipient react against the antigens of the donor organ.
    - The organ graft can be destroyed unless the immune system is adequately suppressed.

- Acute rejections may occur in 2 weeks.
- Chronic rejection may occur after months or years, and is characterized by slow progressive organ failure.

Adverse Effects

- All **immunosuppressants** place the client at risk for:
  - Infection
  - Malignancy, most often lymphoma with long-term therapy
- Adverse effects of **methotrexate** include:
  - Bone marrow suppression
  - Oral and gastrointestinal ulcers
  - Pulmonary infiltrates and fibrosis
  - Nausea and vomiting
  - Nephrotoxicity (with high dosage)
  - Fetal malformation
- Adverse effects of **azathioprine** include:
  - Gastrointestinal distress
  - Hepatotoxicity
  - Bone marrow suppression
  - Serum sickness, fever, and chills

Precautions

- Immunotherapy should not be given at the same time as live vaccines. Serum sickness may develop 2-3 weeks after therapy. Symptoms of serum sickness are:
  - Fever
  - Skin rash
  - Joint pain
  - Swollen lymph nodes
- These drugs should be avoided during pregnancy and lactation.

Important Drugs

Cytotoxic agents

- Azathioprine is used primarily to prevent organ or tissue rejection reactions. It may be used for rheumatoid arthritis.
- Methotrexate is used to treat some autoimmune disorders, such as rheumatoid arthritis and psoriasis, as well as some types of cancer.

Conventional antirejection agents

- Cyclosporine is used to prevent rejection reactions for inhibiting T-lymphocytes and B-lymphocytes.
- Mycophenolate is used to prevent rejection of cardiac and renal transplants.
- Tacrolimus is used to prevent rejection reactions and to treat autoimmune disease.

Corticosteroids suppress growth of all lymphoid tissue and, thereby, decrease formation and function of antibodies and T-cells.

Antibody preparations

- Polyclonal antibodies
- Monoclonal antibodies
  - Muromonab-CD3 (Orthoclone OKT3) is a monoclonal antibody that acts as an immunosuppressant agent by interfering with T-lymphocyte function. It is used to reverse organ transplant rejection.

Other

- Etanercept (Enbrel)
- Leflunomide (Arava)

Therapeutic Nursing Interventions

- Auscultate the client's lungs for adventitious sounds.
- Monitor complete blood count (CBC) for signs of bone marrow suppression.
  - These signs include a reduction in the counts of:
    - Hemoglobin (Hgb)
    - Hematocrit (Hct)
    - Leukocytes
    - Platelets
- Monitor liver enzyme tests for an elevation that could indicate liver dysfunction.
- Assess:
  - For signs of hepatic failure at least weekly
    - These signs include jaundice, ascites, and upper right quadrant abdominal tenderness.
  - For signs of transplant rejection, which vary with the involved organ or tissue
  - For the development of infections
  - Oral cavity for pallor and bleeding gums
  - Ability to swallow
- Report an elevated temperature to the primary care provider.
- Observe IV site at least hourly for signs of infiltration of IV fluid or infection.
- Explain to clients undergoing organ transplantation that they will likely need lifelong immunosuppressant therapy to prevent transplant rejection.
- Review the signs and symptoms of organ rejection with clients.
  - Signs are specific for each tissue or organ.
  - General manifestations include:
    - Fever
    - Fatigue
    - Altered vital signs (VS)
    - Tenderness over the graft site
- Assess for the development of infections. Signs may be subtle due to the effects of immunosuppressants.
- Be alert for allergic reaction or sign of anaphylaxis.

- Azathioprine: Monitor renal, hepatic, and hematologic function.
- Methotrexate: Monitor respiratory, hepatic, and hematologic function.

Client Education

- Take oral medications with food or milk to avoid gastrointestinal upset.
- Contact health care provider if a fever of 99° F or higher develops because this may indicate organ rejection or an infection.
- Avoid contact with persons with infectious diseases.
- Avoid crowds because of increased exposure to infectious diseases.
- Wear sunscreen and protective clothing to decrease risk of skin cancer.
- Schedule routine follow-up laboratory tests to identify the development of liver disease or bone marrow failure.
- Avoid vaccinations with live vaccines because of the risk of developing serum sickness.
- Avoid other drugs (prescription or OTC) without immunosuppressant drug prescriber's permission, due to numerous effects these drugs can have and interactions.
- Avoid pregnancy during therapy and for a prescribed period of time thereafter.
- Notify the primary care provider of:
  - Any signs of infection (e.g., fever, cough, sore throat)
  - Unusual bleeding or bruising
- Methotrexate (Folex)
  - Do not double up if you miss a dose.
  - Do not drink alcohol or take NSAIDs while on this drug.
  - You may have hair loss while taking this drug.
- Azathioprine (Imuran)
  - If you take the drug only once a day and miss a dose, do not double up.
  - If you take this drug several times a day, you can take the missed dose with the next dose.
  - Take drug with or after meals to reduce gastrointestinal symptoms.
  - Lifelong therapy will be needed to prevent rejection.
  - After kidney transplant: Immediately report fever or chills, back or side pain, urinary symptoms, severe diarrhea, black stools, and bloody urine to primary care provider.

Agents Used to Treat HIV Infection and AIDS

Overview

HIV is the retrovirus that causes AIDS (acquired immunodeficiency disease syndrome). HIV is able to incorporate itself into the normal cell's ribonucleic acid (RNA), resulting in the replication of HIV cells rather than normal cells. HIV tends to bind to the human CD4 molecule found on T4 lymphocytes and monocytes, with resulting cellular destruction and compromised cellular immune function. HIV cells are covered with a protective coating that makes them difficult to destroy. Major categories of drugs used to destroy HIV cells and treat HIV infection and AIDS are:

- **Non-nucleoside reverse transcriptase inhibitors (NNRTI)**: These agents bind with reverse transcriptase and inhibit the enzyme.
- **Nucleoside reverse transcriptase inhibitors (NRTI)**: These agents inhibit reverse transcriptase, an enzyme required in HIV infection to convert ribonucleic acid (RNA) into deoxyribonucleic acid (DNA).
- **Protease inhibitors**: These agents inhibit the action of HIV protease and block the formation of viral protein, which is needed for the viruses to replicate.

Uses

Non-nucleoside reverse transcriptase inhibitors (NNRTI) are used in combination therapy with other anti-HIV agents to treat HIV infection and AIDS.

Nucleoside reverse transcriptase inhibitors (NRTI) are used to treat HIV infections and to decrease maternal transmission of HIV to the fetus.

Protease inhibitors are used in combination therapy with other anti-HIV agents to treat HIV infection and AIDS.

Adverse Effects

NNRTI may cause these adverse effects:

- Nausea, vomiting, diarrhea
- Skin rash

NRTI may cause these adverse effects:

- Neurologic problems such as insomnia, confusion, peripheral neuropathies, and seizures
- Bone marrow suppression resulting in granulocytopenia and anemia
- Pancreatitis

Protease inhibitors may cause these adverse effects:

- Nausea, vomiting, diarrhea, and abdominal cramping
- Kidney stones
- Insomnia and headache

Precautions

- NNRTI are contraindicated for clients with impaired hepatic function. These agents should always be administered in combination with other drugs to slow the development of drug resistance.

- NRTI must be given cautiously to:
  - Clients with renal insufficiency, because these agents are excreted by the kidneys.
  - Clients who are concomitantly taking medications causing peripheral neuropathy (e.g., chloramphenicol, isoniazid, and nitrofurantoin).

Protease inhibitors are contraindicated for children and for pregnant or lactating women.

  - These agents should be used cautiously for clients with liver disease.
  - These agents should not be given in combination with didanosine (Videx), which is a nucleoside reverse transcriptase inhibitor.

Important Drugs

Non-nucleoside reverse transcriptase inhibitors (NNRTI):

Nevirapine (Viramune) slows the progression of HIV infection and decreases complications.

Delavirdine mesylate (Rescriptor) slows the progression of HIV infection and decreases complications.

Nucleoside reverse transcriptase inhibitors (NRTI):

Zidovudine (AZT, Retrovir) is the most important drug currently available to treat HIV infection and AIDS. Most adverse effects involve hematologic toxicities.

Zalcitabine (Hivid) is prescribed for clients with advanced HIV disease, and is given only in combination with zidovudine.

Stavudine (Zerit/d4T) is prescribed for advanced HIV disease when clients have become resistant or very toxic due to the prolonged administration of zidovudine.

Didanosine (Videx) is prescribed for adults and children six months or older who are intolerant to zidovudine.

Protease inhibitors

Saquinavir (Invirase) slows progression of HIV infection and decreases complications.

Ritonavir (Norvir) slows progression of HIV infection and decreases complications.

Indinavir (Crixivan) helps to prevent HIV infection after known exposure. This drug should be used in combination with other antiretrovirals.

Therapeutic Nursing Interventions

- Monitor CD4 counts to determine if client is responding properly to the drug.
- A reduced CD4 count indicates that HIV is still destroying cells.
- Another agent may need to be added to the drug regime, or a new drug may need to be prescribed.
- Monitor complete blood counts, renal function tests, and liver function tests for signs of bone marrow failure, renal failure, or liver dysfunction.
- Measure intake and output (I & O). Assess color and general appearance of urine.
- Assess client for dysuria that may indicate renal dysfunction.

- Administer antiemetic or antidiarrheal PRN for nausea, vomiting, and diarrhea.
- Perform a neurologic examination before starting client on drug therapy, and on a scheduled basis throughout therapy. Assess for insomnia, confusion, peripheral neuropathies, and seizures.
- Ask family members to report any subtle changes in the client's personality that could indicate the development of these neurologic complications.
- Give non-opioid analgesics PRN for discomfort.
- Provide emotional support to clients on antiretroviral drug therapy. Responses to therapy and an improvement in symptoms may take weeks.

Client Education

- Take medications as close to scheduled time as possible to enhance positive effects of drugs.
- Take medications at least 2 hours before or after eating.
- Immediately report bleeding to health care provider. Bleeding may indicate bone marrow suppression.
- Report infections immediately to health care provider. Clients are at risk of infection because they are in an immunocompromised state.
- Report stomach pain, nausea, diarrhea, or loss of appetite to health care provider. The medication dosage may need to be changed or a new medication prescribed.
- Report tingling or loss of feeling in fingers or toes, and pain in the hands or feet. These symptoms may indicate peripheral neuropathy.
- Eat a nutritious diet and get sufficient rest. These measures will augment the medication regime.

Critical Thinking Exercise: Drugs Affecting the Immune System

Note: *It is recommended that the following exercises be reviewed with a partner or in a small group to achieve maximum student interaction and to enhance critical thinking skills.*

Situation: R.G. is a 22-year-old pregnant female who has been diagnosed with advanced acquired immunodeficiency syndrome (AIDS). Her CD4 cell count is 145. Her primary care provider has prescribed zidovudine 200 mg tid to be administered with zalcitabine (Hivid) 0.75 mg PO tid. Before starting R.G. on combination therapy, the nurse performed a neurologic assessment. Throughout her course of therapy, the nurse continued to closely monitor R.G.'s neurologic status, and CBC and CD4 count.

1. Why is it important to monitor the CD4 cell count in clients who are being treated for HIV infection?

2. Why do you want to closely monitor the CBC of clients taking zidovudine (AZT)?

3. The client informs you she is experiencing burning and tingling in her fingers and toes. What might this indicate?

4. What are some of the important nursing considerations related to this client?

Drugs that Affect the Immune System - Key Concepts

Locate the appropriate terms in the word scramble below.

R M H T B O J M X B M J C B J K J J N T P Z A G D

K M C I Y T B Q I T E I I K Z L A Q R V W O S Y U

W Q D N X E A V V M H H K V A C C I N A T I O N G

I X I F S V P I M M U N O S U P P R E S S A N T S

A A G E I M M U N O S T I M U L A N T S P K D R V

X Q P C W B Y M B I V N S Q D L O I X S J C D N D

L Q L T A J L S A X O G L A I N N A T E Q R N Y G

W A K I Q C G D F P V F G S W U L I C Q G C E K L

G Q A O J G Q P P R E F R I G E R A T E R R Z L N

J O C N E F Q U Z I N O E Q H R H A P G V V K M T

Y X T H P Q N C I D L Y S B C N L P Q C R L O U L

Q X I V K C R K L R C O K D K R X O T K Z F I O J

E X V M C B B Z T W E E P B Q M P O V J C K N V X

L G E D I C E P P Y U D U G L P E F Y D P M L W E

U Q V F L D T R V D O U E E Y R J A X Y N V L Q N

U I M L U N O S S P P R E S S A N T S D N H I W K

M Y L W V O U P X I B B E Z W P G L P E Q R S A M

1. ____________________act to suppress the immune response.
2. Drugs that activate or enhance a person's own immune system.
3. Most vaccines and toxoids are kept in the ______________.
4. Involves the injection of killed or weakened (attenuated) microorganisms into the body via vaccines and toxoids.
5. All immunosuppressants place a client at risk of _______________.
6. What kind of immunity is the second line of defense against infectious agents?
7. The first line of defense present at birth.
8. What kind of immunity is produced by the person's own immune system?
9. The nurse should ask a client who is receiving a vaccine if they have an allergy to ___________.
10. MMR is an example of a _______________ vaccine.
11. Bone marrow suppression would be most easily measured by this test.

CHAPTER 4

Drugs for Pain and Inflammation

Key Points

- **Analgesics** are drugs that relieve pain.
- Analgesics include narcotic (opiate) analgesics, non-narcotic (non-opiate) analgesics, and antimigraine drugs.
    - Anti-inflammatory drugs also provide analgesia.
- Narcotic or **opiate analgesics** are drugs that suppress the central nervous system (CNS), thereby relieving pain and promoting sleep.
- Opiates are drugs derived from the juice of the opium poppy.
- Opioids are synthetic substitutes that have opium-like properties.
- Morphine, the major narcotic contained in the opium plant, still serves as the ultimate standard of analgesic effectiveness.
- Most narcotics are Schedule II drugs, and cannot be sold without a medical prescription.
- Major side effects of **narcotic (opiate) analgesics** include:
    - Respiratory depression
    - Constipation
    - Inhibition of cough reflex
    - Pinpoint pupils
    - Postural hypotension
- Use of narcotic (opiate) analgesics may result in:
    - Drug tolerance (decreased sensitivity to subsequent doses of the same substance)
    - Drug dependence
    - Drug addiction
- Signs of withdrawal from narcotics include:
    - Nausea
    - Intestinal cramps
    - Vomiting
    - Fever
    - Anorexia
    - Syncope or light-headedness
- **Narcotic (opiate) antagonists** reverse the effects of narcotic (opiate) analgesics.
- **Anti-inflammatory drugs** include:
    - Salicylates
    - Anti-gout drugs
    - Corticosteroids
    - Disease-modifying antirheumatic drugs (DMARDs)
    - Nonsteroid anti-inflammatory drugs (NSAIDs)
- Some anti-inflammatory drugs also act as antipyretics and reduce body temperature.
- Acetaminophen (Tylenol) is a non-narcotic analgesic/antipyretic agent.

Analgesics

Narcotic (Opiate) Analgesics

Overview

Narcotic (opiate) analgesics are natural, semisynthetic, or synthetic alkaloid derivatives of opium. Narcotic (opiate) analgesics are classified as opiate agonists or opiate agonist-antagonists. Narcotic analgesics are administered for medical purposes by oral, rectal, subcutaneous, intramuscular, and intravenous routes. When abused, narcotics should be smoked, injected or applied to the nasal mucosa as snuff, which can be inhaled. The effects of oral administration vary, because many narcotics undergo significant metabolism in the liver immediately after intestinal absorption:

- When analgesics are taken orally, liver enzymes largely deactivate morphine and related compounds. This reduces their effectiveness.
- Meperidine, codeine, and methadone are more effective than morphine when administered orally.
- The kidneys excrete narcotics and their metabolites.

Narcotic (Opiate) Agonists

Overview

Narcotic opiate agonists are drugs that stimulate opiate receptors. The opiate agonists include natural opium alkaloids, such as morphine and codeine; semisynthetic analogs, such as hydromorphone (Dilaudid) and synthetic compounds or opioids, such as meperidine (Demerol).

Opiates and opioids act by binding to opiate receptors in the CNS, causing inhibition of ascending pain pathways and altering the perception of pain at the spinal cord and higher levels in the CNS. Opiates and opioids are readily absorbed from the gastrointestinal tract and nasal mucosa, the surface of the lung, and the peripheral tissues following injection.

Uses

- Morphine and meperidine (Demerol) are used for severe pain.
- Codeine and related compounds are used for moderate pain.
- Codeine is also used for its antitussive effect.
- Methadone (Dolophine) is used primarily to treat withdrawal syndrome in heroin- or morphine-dependent individuals.

Adverse Effects

Respiratory Effects

- Decreased rate and depth of respirations, resulting in respiratory depression and carbon dioxide retention
- Irregular or periodic breathing due to depression of medullary and pontine centers in the brain

- Decreased cough due to inhibition of the cough reflex
- Bronchoconstriction due to the release of histamine

Cardiovascular Effects

- Postural hypotension due to histamine release and peripheral vasodilatation

Skin Effects

- Flushing due to peripheral vasodilatation
- Increased perspiration due to histamine release
- Pruritus due to histamine release

Gastrointestinal Effects

- Nausea and vomiting due to increased vestibular sensitivity and stimulation of the vomiting center
- Delayed passage of stools due to decreased secretion of bile and pancreatic juice, increased spasticity of valves and sphincters, and decreased peristaltic patterns

Urinary System Effects

- Urgency due to increased tone of detrusor muscle
- Urinary retention due to increased sphincter tone
- Reduced attentiveness for need to void
- Increased water absorbed in kidney due to release of vasopressin

Reproductive System Effects

- Interrupted or prolonged labor
- Decrease in oxytocin-induced hyperactivity of the uterus
- Respiratory depression in the newborn because the drug crosses the placenta to depress the fetal respiratory center
- Decreased motility of sperm, volume of ejaculate, and testosterone levels
- Inhibition of the pituitary hormone luteotropin

Endocrine Effects

- Fluid retention due to enhanced antidiuretic hormone release by the pituitary

Musculoskeletal Effects

- Increased muscle rigidity due to stimulation of the spinal cord (rare)

Ocular Effects

- Pupillary constriction due to excitation of autonomic fibers of the oculomotor nerve
- Pinpoint pupils are a characteristic of narcotics dependency.
- Pupil remains pinpoint even in dim light, and will only dilate when a life-threatening respiratory depression develops.

CNS Effects

- Inability to concentrate due to depression of the cortex
- Lethargy and sleep due to depression of reticular formation
- Mood elevation and euphoria due to depression of limbic system and brain stem

- Lowered body temperature due to resetting of the hypothalamic temperature-regulating mechanism
- EEG activity decreases due to increased voltage and decreased frequency of electrical activity in the brain.

Precautions and Contraindications

- Narcotic analgesics are contraindicated for clients with a history of drug allergies or sensitivities.
- Narcotic analgesics are contraindicated for clients with a head injury and increased intracranial pressure (IICP).
    - Administration of narcotic analgesics in clients with head injury causes increased intracranial pressure (IICP), cerebral vasodilatation, and hypotension, which can aggravate brain injury.
    - Clients with IICP should be closely monitored for decreased consciousness, decreased respiratory rate, and altered reaction to light, all masked by effects of narcotics.
- Narcotic analgesics are contraindicated for clients with acute asthma, chronic airway problems, or respiratory depression (less than 10 breaths per minute) due to chronic obstructive pulmonary disease (COPD), cystic fibrosis, or neuromuscular disorders that affect the respiratory system.
- Narcotic analgesics should be administered with caution to elderly clients and clients with severe renal disease, pulmonary disease, congestive heart failure (CHF), liver disease, hypothyroidism, alcoholism, undiagnosed pain, or prostatic hypertrophy.
- In large doses, morphine decreases venous return and afterload in pulmonary edema and CHF.
- Opiate analgesics may lead to drug tolerance, dependence, and addiction.

Important Drugs

Natural opium alkaloids

Morphine sulfate

- Morphine still serves as the ultimate standard of analgesic effectiveness.
- Morphine not only alleviates pain, but it also alters the perception of pain.
- Relatively little morphine passes the blood-brain barrier in adults, but this fraction is responsible for its central actions.
- Morphine is used to treat pain and relieve anxiety caused by myocardial infarction.
- Morphine is the drug of choice for pulmonary edema because it relieves anxiety and causes vasodilatation, which reduces the workload on the heart.
- When morphine is given orally, higher doses are necessary because a portion of the oral drug is metabolized in the liver before it reaches systemic circulation.
    - Concentrated solutions (Roxanol) and controlled release tablets (MS Contin) have been developed for oral administration of high doses.
- Morphine may also be given by continuous IV infusion.

- Peak effects are:
  - Intravenous route: 10-20 minutes
  - Intramuscular route: 30 minutes
  - Oral route: 30-60 minutes
  - Subcutaneous route: 60-90 minutes
- Severe sedation is dangerous and should be reported to the primary care provider.

Codeine sulfate

- Codeine is used to manage mild to moderate pain.
- It can be added to cough medicine to suppress cough reflex.

Semisynthetic Analogs

Hydromorphone (Dilaudid)

- Hydromorphone is a semisynthetic derivative of morphine.
- It is more potent, but shorter-acting than morphine.

Oxycodone is a semisynthetic drug.

- It is more potent than codeine (Percocet - oxycodone with acetaminophen; and Percodan - oxycodone with aspirin).

Synthetic Compounds

Meperidine (Demerol)

- The first of the synthetic narcotic analgesics.
- 80-100 mg of meperidine is approximately equivalent to 10 mg of morphine.
- Oral meperidine is only half as effective as a parenteral dose, because about 50% is metabolized in the liver and never reaches the systemic circulation.
- Differs from morphine in these ways:
  - Shorter duration of action
  - Less respiratory depression in the newborn when used for obstetric analgesia
  - Less smooth muscle spasm
- Toxic to the CNS; may cause tremors, hallucinations, and seizures
- May produce serious interactions with monoamine oxidase (MAO) inhibitors and antipsychotic drugs, such as phenothiazine.

Fentanyl (Sublimaze)

- Fentanyl is an analgesic adjunct to general anesthesia, which may be administered IM or IV.
- Fentanyl is administered during open heart surgery to protect myocardium from excessive demands for oxygen.

Methadone hydrochloride (Dolophine)

- Methadone is used for severe pain.
- It suppresses withdrawal symptoms during narcotic drug detoxification and maintenance.
- It is administered only in approved drug rehabilitation programs.

Mixtures

- Brompton's cocktail
  - Brompton's cocktail is a mixture of morphine, cocaine, dextroamphetamine, and alcohol.
  - Mixture is given to terminally ill clients for relief of severe cancer pain.

Therapeutic Nursing Interventions

- Monitor respiratory rate, and withhold drug if respiratory rate is less than 10 breaths per minute or if breaths are shallow or labored.
- Monitor blood pressure and withhold drug if systolic blood pressure is less than 90 mmHg.
- Take measures to ensure client's safety.
  - Place bed in a low position and put up side rails.
  - Narcotics may cause dizziness and orthostatic hypotension.
- Measure client's response to medication by using a pain intensity scale, with 0 indicating no pain, and 10 indicating the most severe pain. Speak with the primary care provider if the client is still experiencing severe pain after taking a narcotic analgesic.
- Monitor bowel elimination patterns and assess for constipation.
- Increase fluids and bulk in diet to prevent constipation.
- Administer stool softeners and laxatives as needed.
- Administer antiemetics if client develops nausea and vomiting.
- Observe for the development of tolerance, which is signaled by the client's report that the analgesic effect of the drug is not lasting as long.
- To slow the development of tolerance, change client to a different analgesic as ordered.
- Fentanyl is measured in mcg; therefore, to prevent inadvertent overdose, precaution is warranted.

Client Education

- Request pain medication from health care provider before pain becomes severe.
- Encourage client to push button on patient-controlled analgesia (PCA) pump before pain becomes severe.
- Report to health care provider if medication fails to lessen or alleviate pain.
- Drink at least 8 cups of water a day and eat high-fiber foods to prevent constipation.
- Make position changes slowly to prevent orthostatic hypotension.
- Avoid driving and activities that require alertness until the effects of the drug are known.
- Report side effects of narcotic analgesics to health care provider.
- Avoid concurrent use of alcohol and other CNS depressants.
- Use sugarless gum, mouthwash, and good oral hygiene to reduce dry mouth.
- Use nonpharmacologic methods for controlling pain, such as guided imagery, relaxation therapy, deep breathing, meditation, massage, and heat/cold applications.

- Discourage "PCA by proxy" (family members administering PCA doses for the client).

All caregivers (clients and family members) need education regarding the proper use of PCA. The danger of having others press the PCA button (PCA by proxy) need to be understood by all involved in the client's care. Written instructions should be given to family members emphasizing PCA doses by proxy are not to be given.

Narcotic (Opiate) Agonists-Antagonists

Overview

An opiate agonist-antagonist is a drug that stimulates some opiate receptors, but antagonizes other opiate receptors. Opiate agonist-antagonist drugs depress the CNS and alter the client's perception of and response to pain. Because of their antagonistic characteristics, these drugs have a reduced potential for narcotic abuse. Opiate agonist-antagonists are not antitussives, and they produce fewer gastrointestinal side effects than opiate agonists.

Uses

Opiate agonist-antagonists are used to relieve moderate to severe pain.

Adverse Effects

- Similar to the effects of opiate agonists
- Opiate agonist-antagonists produce withdrawal symptoms in clients addicted to narcotics:
  - Anorexia
  - Nausea
  - Vomiting
  - Intestinal cramps
  - Fever
  - Syncope or light headedness

Precautions

- Do not give to clients with liver failure because drug metabolism occurs in the liver. Acetaminophen causes liver toxicity in overdoses and liver damage in alcoholics, and can be problematic in the elderly even when administered within the usual dosage range.
- Opiate agonist-antagonists should not be administered to clients who frequently use opiates or are dependent on narcotics.
- Pentazocine (Talwin, Talwin-Nx) can produce life-threatening side effects when given by injection to clients addicted to narcotics.
- Opiate agonist-antagonists should not be abruptly discontinued.

Important Drugs

Pentazocine (Talwin, Talwin-Nx) is used to treat moderate to severe pain, and may be administered to control pain during labor.

Nalbuphine hydrochloride (Nubain) is a potent drug that provides analgesia equivalent to morphine.

Dezocine (Dalgan) provides analgesia that is equivalent to morphine. It is not classified as a controlled substance.

Butorphanol (Stadol) provides analgesia that is 3-5 times more potent than morphine and is used for moderate to severe pain, and as an adjunct to anesthesia.

Buprenorphine (Buprenex) provides analgesia that is 30 times more potent than morphine, but has a low potential for abuse.

Therapeutic Nursing Interventions

- Assess the client's mental status and responsiveness to drug therapy.
- Measure the client's perception of pain using pain rating scales.
    - Adjustment in dosage may be necessary depending on the drug's effectiveness.
- Assess for signs of respiratory depression.
    - Have resuscitative equipment and narcotic antagonist available.
- Assess for signs of central nervous system (CNS) side effects, including confusion and dizziness.
- Administer stool softeners and laxatives as needed.
    - Provide a diet high in fiber with liberal fluids as tolerated during hospitalization.
- Take measures to protect client while sedated.
    - Make sure the bed is in a low position and side rails are up.
- Opiate agonist-antagonists should not be abruptly discontinued.
    - Weaning dose is less likely to produce abstinence symptoms.

Client Education

- Avoid use of alcohol during treatment.
    - An increased respiratory depressant effect may occur.
    - These drugs are metabolized in the liver.
    - Alcohol can cause liver dysfunction, which further potentiates the drug effects.
- Do not take butorphanol (Stadol) with MAO inhibitors or buprenorphine (Buprenex) because of drug interaction effects.
- Avoid activities that require concentration or mental alertness due to the sedative effects.
- Prevent constipation with a liberal fluid intake, high-fiber diet, and active lifestyle.
- Use non-pharmacologic methods for controlling pain, such as:
    - Guided-imagery
    - Progressive relaxation therapy
    - Deep breathing
    - Meditation
    - Massage
    - Heat/cold applications

Narcotic (Opiate) Antagonists

Overview

Narcotic antagonists compete with narcotics for receptor sites, which then block the effects of opiates. Narcotic antagonists cause withdrawal in people who are physically dependent on narcotics.

Uses

- Diagnose opioid toxicity
- Reverse CNS and respiratory depression caused by narcotics
- Treat babies born to addicted mothers

Adverse Effects

- Severe withdrawal symptoms in people who are physically dependent on narcotics
- Withdrawal symptoms in infants of mothers who are dependent on narcotics
- Nausea and vomiting
- Abdominal cramps
- Tachycardia
- Hypertension
- Headache
- Reversal of analgesia and return of pain

Precautions

- Narcotic (opiate) antagonists are contraindicated for clients who are addicted to narcotics because they precipitate withdrawal.

Important Drugs

Naloxone (Narcan)

- Naloxone is the drug of choice for respiratory depression caused by a suspected overdose of a narcotic.
- Therapeutic effects occur within minutes after parenteral injection and last 1-2 hours.
- Naloxone does not exert any pharmacologic action of its own; it is a pure narcotic antagonist.

Nalmefene hydrochloride (Revex) may not completely reverse narcotic-induced respiratory depression.

Therapeutic Nursing Interventions

- Assess level of pain and implement interventions to relieve pain. Narcotic antagonists reverse respiratory depression, but also reverse analgesia.
- Make certain that resuscitation equipment, oxygen, vasopressors, and mechanical ventilation are available to supplement narcotic antagonist therapy.
- Assess every 5 minutes:
  - Blood pressure

    - Respiratory rate, rhythm, and depth
    - Pulse
    - Level of consciousness
- Notify primary care provider if heart rate remains higher than 120 bpm, and BP is over 140/90 mmHg.
- Assess for relapse of respiratory depression, which may occur 15-20 minutes following administration of narcotic antagonists.
- Repeat dose PRN within 30-60 minutes if respiratory depression recurs; usually administer narcotic antagonists IV push.
- Monitor clients closely for signs of narcotic withdrawal, which may develop within a few minutes to two hours following administration.
- Administer a different pain medication with less respiratory depression effects if severe pain returns.
- Explain purpose of narcotic antagonist therapy to client.

Client Education

- Do not share narcotic antagonist with others, even those dependent on opioids.
- Do not take opioids to overcome the effects of the antagonists. Severe CNS toxicity, including coma or death, may occur.
- Follow-up visits with health care provider are necessary to determine hepatic function. Liver function tests may need to be followed if long-term use is needed.
- Opioid medication used for pain relief, cough suppression, or diarrhea will not be therapeutic because the antagonist counteracts its effects.
- Report increasing intensity of pain or signs of narcotic withdrawal.

Non-Narcotic (Non-opiate) Analgesics

Overview

Non-narcotic (non-opiate) analgesics inhibit the formation of prostaglandins in inflamed tissues, thereby preventing stimulation of pain receptors. Non-narcotic analgesics lower body temperature by resetting the hypothalamus. Non-narcotic analgesics include aspirin (acetylsalicylic acid), nonsteroidal anti-inflammatory drugs (NSAIDs), and acetaminophen (Tylenol, Datril, Panadol).

Acetaminophen

Overview

Acetaminophen is discussed under analgesics because it has no significant anti- inflammatory effects. Acetaminophen may be combined with opioids for an additive effect to provide greater pain relief. Acetaminophen inhibits the formation of prostaglandins that act as mediators of pain and fever, mainly in the central nervous system. Acetaminophen (Tylenol, Datril, Panadol) may be purchased OTC. Acetaminophen is equal to acetylsalicylic acid (aspirin) in analgesic and antipyretic effects, but lacks the anti-inflammatory and anti-platelet actions of aspirin. Also, acetaminophen does not upset the gastrointestinal system.

Uses

- Acetaminophen is used to reduce pain and fever.
- For children with high fever, acetaminophen and ibuprofen are altered q 3-4 hours.

Adverse Effects

- Hepatic failure in high doses
- Nephrotoxicity with chronic overdose

Precautions

- Acetaminophen causes liver toxicity in overdoses, and liver damage in alcoholics and the elderly even when administered within the usual dosage range.
- Acetaminophen is contraindicated in clients who are malnourished and who chronically abuse alcohol.
- Death occurs as a result of acute hepatic failure in about 10% of individuals who overdose.
- Antidote must be administered within 24 hours of overdose.

Important Drugs

- Tylenol, Datril, and Panadol are trade names for **acetaminophen**.
- **Propoxyphene** is a synthetic drug combined with acetaminophen (Darvocet-N) and is chemically related to the narcotic methadone.
- **Tylox** is a combination of acetaminophen and the narcotic oxycodone hydrochloride.
- **Vicodin** is a combination of acetaminophen and the narcotic hydrocodone bitartrate.

Therapeutic Nursing Interventions

- Assess hepatic and renal function tests at the beginning and throughout the course of prolonged high-dose therapy.
- Assess type, intensity, and location of pain prior to and throughout administration.
- Assess body temperature prior to and throughout administration.
- Administer acetaminophen with a full glass of water.
- In the emergency management of hepatotoxic overdose of acetaminophen, administer acetylcysteine (Mucomyst) within 24 hours (either orally or IV) as an antidote.

Client Education

- Carefully read labels of over-the-counter drugs because many of these drugs contain acetaminophen.
- Avoid drinking alcohol because of the risk of toxic effects on the liver.
- Avoid taking salicylates or NSAIDs concurrently with acetaminophen because of toxic effects.
- Carefully check dosage of liquid preparations because errors have resulted in severe liver damage.

- Use acetaminophen under a doctor's supervision if taking the drug for more than 10 days (adult) and 5 days (child).
- Report to health care provider if body temperature does not decrease or return to normal after taking two doses of acetaminophen.
- Instruct the parent to administer the proper dose at the appropriate interval based on age and weight of the child.

Anti-inflammatory Drugs

Anti-inflammatory/Antipyretic Drugs

Overview

Anti-inflammatory/antipyretic drugs include the **salicylates** and **nonsteroidal anti-inflammatory drugs (NSAIDs)**. Ibuprofen is the prototype for NSAIDs. Anti-inflammatory drugs act by inhibiting prostaglandin formation. In the inflammatory process, prostaglandins potentiate the pain and edema caused by the release of bradykinin, histamine, and other substances into areas of tissue damage. Prostaglandins also regulate many cell functions.

- Regulate smooth muscle in blood vessels and the gastrointestinal, respiratory, and reproductive systems
- Protect gastrointestinal mucosa from the erosive effects of gastric acid
- Regulate renal blood flow
- Inhibit platelet function (platelet aggregation)
- Increase cardiac output
- Stimulate uterine contractions
- Stimulate erythropoietin production
- Suppress the immune response

Salicylates and NSAIDs do not produce tolerance, or physical or psychologic dependence. Also, these agents do not alter the course of the disease for which they are prescribed. Antipyretics act by inhibiting the formation of pyrogens, which reset the hypothalamic thermostat, thereby lowering body temperature and reducing fever.

- Antipyretic agents do not cure, but induce comfort.
- The most common route of administration of antipyretics is by mouth. However, the rectal route is indicated for clients unable to take the medication orally (e.g., infants, toddlers, debilitated clients, and clients following oral surgery).
- Aspirin is the prototype for antipyretic drugs.

Uses

Anti-inflammatory/antipyretic drugs are used to treat:

- Mild to moderate pain
- Discomfort following minor surgical procedures
- Inflammatory processes
- Arthritis

  - Dysmenorrhea
  - Fever
  - Cardiovascular disorders (stroke, deep vein thrombosis)
  - During catheterization procedures
  - Also given with anticoagulants (heparin) or anti-platelets for an additive effect

Antipyretics not only help to restore temperatures to normal, but they reduce the discomfort and physiologic depletion characterized by prolonged fever.

Adverse Effects

- Nausea
- Vomiting
- Heartburn (gastritis)
- Gastrointestinal bleeding
- Gastric ulcer formation (especially aspirin and other salicylates)
- Salicylism (adverse effects caused by toxic doses of aspirin and other salicylates):
  - Tinnitus (ringing in the ears)
  - Confusion
  - Adverse changes in liver, kidney, and respiratory function
  - Increased uric acid production
- Reye's syndrome
  - Syndrome occurs in children under 15 years old who received aspirin while they had varicella (chicken pox) or influenza-like viral illnesses.
  - Syndrome is characterized by encephalopathy and fatty infiltration of the liver.
- Bone marrow depression, anemia, and thrombocytopenia
- Hypersensitivity reactions to NSAIDs are:
  - Skin rashes
  - Angioedema
  - Urticaria
  - Dyspnea

Precautions

- Because of the risk of Reye's syndrome, aspirin is contraindicated for children under 15 years old who have high fevers or viral infections.
- Salicylates and NSAIDs are contraindicated for clients with gastrointestinal disorders or who are hypersensitive to these drugs.
- Salicylates and NSAIDs should be avoided or given cautiously to clients with bleeding disorders because they prolong bleeding time.
- Pregnant women should not take aspirin or other NSAIDs because they can cause intrauterine growth impairment and fetal loss.
- Large doses of aspirin can be very toxic.
  - Early signs of toxicity are tinnitus and decreased hearing ability, along with nausea, vomiting, confusion, and lethargy.

- Severe intoxication is characterized by abnormal breathing patterns progressing to respiratory failure, convulsions, and coma.
- Hypoprothrombinemia can also result from large doses of aspirin.

- Administration of salicylates and NSAIDs should be stopped 24-48 hours prior to surgery to decrease the risk of hemorrhage during or after surgery.
  - Clients who take daily aspirin should stop the medication 1-2 weeks prior to surgery to prevent bleeding following surgery.
  - Immediately after a post-cardiac procedure, the client is restarted on aspirin, anti- platelets, or anticoagulants (heparin or warfarin).
- Antipyretic drugs, if administered before diagnosis, can make a definitive diagnosis difficult because they eliminate the cardinal symptom of fever.

Important Drugs

Acetylsalicylic acid (aspirin)

- Other forms of aspirin include Halfprin, Bufferin, Alka-Seltzer, Ecotrin, and BC Powder.
- A newer "super-aspirin" tirofiban hydrochloride (Aggrastat) is used primarily for coronary artery disease, angina, post-MI, and cardiac procedures.
- Therapeutic uses of aspirin are:
  - Analgesic
  - Anti-inflammatory
  - Antiplatelet (one tablet can double bleeding time for about one week)
- Aspirin is administered every 3-4 hours for adults.
- Aspirin can be absorbed from both the stomach and duodenum, but is absorbed faster from the duodenum.
- Action is slower when aspirin is taken with food because the pyloric sphincter closes and traps aspirin in the stomach.
- Salicylate is metabolized in the liver shortly after its absorption. The liver furnishes glycine that inactivates the salicylate. Glycine is limited, so if the dosage is too great, toxicity may result.
- Aspirin is not indicated for hangovers because it contributes to the gastric irritation already caused by alcohol.
- Low doses of aspirin decrease uric acid excretion; high doses (5 gm/day) increase uric acid excretion.
- Gastric irritation is the major adverse effect of aspirin. Taking enteric-coated tablets can reduce irritation.
- aspirin can produce serious allergic reactions.
- aspirin is associated with Reye's syndrome in children.

Other nonsteroidal anti-inflammatory drugs (NSAIDs)

- NSAIDs tend to have similar therapeutic effects.
- Selection of an NSAID depends on how well the client responds, and the price of the drug.
- Costs vary widely.
- Side effects of the following NSAIDs differ in intensity from aspirin, but are generally the same as for aspirin.

- All of the following drugs are ulcerogenic (ulcer-causing).
  - Ibuprofen (Advil, Motrin) can be purchased over-the-counter. It is more expensive than aspirin. While ibuprofen is better tolerated than aspirin, it may cause all of the same adverse effects.
  - Naproxen (Naprosyn) is used for moderate to severe arthritis. It is also administered for mild to moderate pain.
  - Ketorolac (Toradol) is indicated for managing pain, but not for inflammation. This is the only injectable NSAID, and it is available for short-term IM or IV use. The drug may also be given orally.
  - Piroxicam (Feldene) is used to treat arthritis.
  - Phenylbutazone (Butazolidin) is used to treat arthritis. It can produce severe adverse side effects such as bone marrow depression.

Selective COX-2 (cyclo-oxygenase-2) Inhibitor Drugs

- These newer prescription NSAIDs block production of the prostaglandins, which cause pain, but they do not block the prostaglandins that help to protect the gastric mucosa.
  - The newest COX-2 is valdecoxib (Bextra). It is primarily used for rheumatoid arthritis, osteoarthritis, and dysmenorrhea. The pain control effects are similar to NSAIDs.

Therapeutic Nursing Inteventions

- Assess type, intensity, and location of pain prior to and throughout administration of aspirin (acetylsalicylic acid) and other NSAIDs.
- Assess body temperature prior to and throughout administration of drugs.
- Administer with a full glass of water, food, or antacids if client is prone to gastrointestinal irritation.
- Monitor CBC, hemoglobin, hematocrit, and platelet count because NSAIDs can cause bone marrow suppression.
- Do not give these drugs 24-48 hours prior to surgery unless otherwise ordered by the primary care provider because of the risk of bleeding and hemorrhage.
- To treat aspirin overdose:
  - Transport client to ED as quickly as possible.
  - Prevent further systemic absorption of any drug left in the stomach by inducing emesis or lavaging client.
  - Hasten elimination of absorbed salicylate with a diuretic.
  - Provide supportive therapy.

Client Education

- Take medication with food or antacids to prevent gastrointestinal irritation.
- Never crush or chew enteric-coated tablets.
- Throw away tablets that have an acetic (vinegar) odor.
- Avoid concurrent consumption of alcohol because alcohol can increase gastric irritation.
- Report gastric irritation, tendency to bleed, and/or symptoms of "salicylism" to health care provider.

- Never administer aspirin to children or adolescents with varicella (chicken pox) or influenza-like viral illnesses because of the risk of Reye's syndrome.
- Report to health care provider if body temperature does not decrease or return to normal after taking two doses of aspirin or other NSAIDs.
- Educate the parent that alternating acetaminophen with an NSAID may reduce fever more quickly.

Anti-inflammatory Corticosteroids

Overview

Anti-inflammatory corticosteroids are produced by the adrenal cortex. Anti-inflammatory corticosteroids help to reduce acute inflammation of the joints associated with rheumatoid arthritis. They also reduce the inflammatory process in other diseases.

Uses

- Rheumatoid arthritis
- Bursitis
- Polymyalgia
- Tendinitis
- Nephrotic syndrome
- Pericarditis
- Myocarditis
- Ulcerative colitis
- Dermatitis
- Systemic lupus erythematosus
- Ocular inflammatory processes
- Hypersensitivity reactions to bee stings, hay fever
- Organ rejection
- Respiratory infections
- Respiratory conditions, such as:
  - Allergies
  - Asthma
  - Chronic obstructive pulmonary disease (COPD)
  - Croup
- Meningitis

Adverse Effects

- Corticosteroids are relatively safe for short-term treatment of self-limiting conditions.
- Sometimes corticosteroids are given every other day to reduce adrenal suppression and other adverse effects.
- Topical corticosteroids can have systemic effects, and even toxicity, with significant absorption through skin or mucus membranes.

- Adverse effects of pharmacologic doses (risk increases with dosage and duration of therapy):
  - Adrenal insufficiency
  - Increased risk of infection
  - Increased blood glucose
  - Muscle weakness
  - Cataracts and open-angle glaucoma
  - Osteoporosis
  - Abnormal fat distribution ("buffalo hump," "moon face," "potbelly")
  - Mood swings, hallucinations
  - Increased gastric acid and pepsin; decreased gastric mucus and blood flow
  - Fluid and electrolyte imbalances
    - Water and sodium retention: edema and increased blood pressure
    - Hypokalemia: muscle weakness, cardiac dysrhythmias
- Adverse effects of topical corticosteroids are most likely to be local and may include:
  - Skin rash
  - Burning and dryness
  - Increased hair growth
  - Loss of pigmentation

Precautions

- Anti-inflammatory corticosteroids are contraindicated for clients with hypersensitivity reactions.
- Long-term topical application of glucocorticoids can result in systemic absorption of the agent, which can cause hypothalamic-pituitary-adrenal suppression of glucocorticoid secretion, and a glucocorticoid deficiency.
- Corticosteroids are contraindicated with active untreated infections.
- If corticosteroid therapy is stopped abruptly, the client may develop acute adrenal insufficiency.
- During times of stress such as surgery or trauma, the client with adrenal insufficiency may die if not given supplemental glucocorticoids.
- Clients taking corticosteroids should not be given vaccinations.
  - The vaccine may be ineffective because the client cannot manufacture adequate antibodies.
  - Live-virus vaccines may introduce the infection they were intended to prevent.
- Corticosteroids must be used cautiously with:
  - Pregnancy
  - Lactation
  - Children
  - Clients at high risk for infection
  - Osteoporosis, peptic ulcer disease, cardiac or renal failure, diabetes mellitus, hypertension, and myasthenia gravis

- Significant drug interactions include:
  - Increased risk of hyperkalemia with potassium-sparing diuretics
  - Increased risk of digitalis toxicity with hypokalemia
  - Increased risk of gastric ulcers with NSAIDs
- Do not use ophthalmic preparations with fungal or viral eye infections.

Important Drugs

Corticosteroids typically have both glucocorticoid and mineralocorticoid activity.

Systemic

- Cortisone (Cortone) is a short-acting corticosteroid.
- Prednisone (Deltasone) is an intermediate-acting corticosteroid.
- Betamethasone (Celestone) is a long-acting corticosteroid.
- Fludrocortisone (Florinef Acetate) is a potent mineralocorticoid.

Topical: Hydrocortisone (Cortaid)

Inhaled: Beclomethasone (Vanceril)

Ophthalmic: Prednisolone (AK-Pred)

Therapeutic Nursing Interventions

For all clients on corticosteroid therapy:

- Corticosteroids come in many preparations for various routes of administration; be careful to select the correct preparation.
- Assess for adverse effects, although serious systemic effects are not expected with physiologic doses.

For clients receiving pharmacologic dosages:

- Monitor the effects of the corticosteroids on the condition being treated.
- Assess for subtle signs of infection.
- Implement safety measures to prevent falls and fractures.
- Monitor clients with diabetes for hyperglycemia.
- Monitor growth in children.
- Assess for psychologic disturbances.
- Assess for fluid and electrolyte imbalances.
- Monitor clients taking digitalis for toxicity.
- Assess stools for melena.

For parenteral corticosteroids:

- Be certain you have the correct preparation.
- Shake suspensions to mix thoroughly.
- Do not give suspensions intravenously.
- Do not dilute with other solutions.

Client Education

All clients on corticosteroid therapy:

- Always wear a medical alert tag noting that you take corticosteroids.

- Always have an emergency supply of your medication with you.
- Never stop taking this medication without medical supervision.
- Corticosteroids require gradual withdrawal by tapering the dose with the exception of 3 to 5 day burst therapy.
- Take oral medications with food or milk to minimize gastrointestinal irritation.
- Resistance to infection is low; avoid people with active infections.
- Notify your primary care provider of the following:
    - Any sign of infection
    - Weight gain, edema
    - Blurred or cloudy vision
    - Pregnancy
    - Dark or tarry stools, abdominal pain

Clients receiving physiologic dosages:

- For Addison's disease:
    - It is important to take two-thirds of the daily dosage in the morning, and the remainder in the afternoon.
    - Lifelong corticosteroid therapy will be required.
    - Increased dosage will be required during times of stress (surgery, trauma, infection).

Clients receiving pharmacologic doses:

- Avoid activities that could cause bone fractures.
- Do not take NSAIDs (aspirin, ibuprofen, etc.) unless directed by the primary care provider.
- Do not have any vaccinations while on corticosteroids without primary care provider approval.
- Increase dietary intake of protein, calcium, and potassium; reduce intake of sodium and carbohydrates; avoid alcohol.

Antimigraine Drugs

Overview

Migraines are associated with dilatation of arteries of the scalp and face. **Antimigraine drugs** are used either to prevent attacks by inhibiting vascular dilatation, or to terminate attacks by constricting the dilated vessels. Antimigraine drugs include **ergot alkaloids**, triptans, serotonin antagonists, narcotics, aspirin, acetaminophen, and NSAIDs. Ergot alkaloids are alpha-adrenergic blockers that reduce extracranial blood flow, which helps to control headache. **Triptans** and **serotonin antagonists** stimulate the receptors that are present on the basilar artery and in the vessels of the dura mater. This results in vasoconstriction of vessels and the relief of migraine headache pain.

Uses

- Antimigraine drugs are used to treat mild to moderate pain caused by migraine headaches.

Adverse Effects

- Antimigraine drugs produce adverse effects specific to the drug or drug group.
  - Adverse effects for narcotics, non-narcotics, aspirin, and acetaminophen have been previously discussed.
- Ergot alkaloids may produce these adverse effects:
  - Early signs:
    - Nausea
    - Vomiting
    - Abdominal cramps
    - Confusion
  - Later signs:
    - Circulatory stasis with itching
    - Coldness and numbness in fingers and hands, leading to gangrene of the nose, digits, and ears
    - Seizures, rapid irregular pulse, and confusion
- Triptans and serotonin antagonists may produce these adverse effects:
  - Nausea
  - Malaise
  - Dizziness
  - Weakness
  - Angina
  - Hypertension
  - Palpitations
  - Dry mouth
  - Nasal congestion

Precautions

Ergot Alkaloids:

- Contraindicated for:
  - Hypersensitivity
  - Sepsis
  - Vascular disease
  - Hepatic or renal disease
  - Marked atherosclerosis
  - Hypertension
  - Anemia
  - Pregnant clients due to uterine stimulation and compromised uteroplacental circulation
- Should be administered cautiously to women who are lactating, elderly clients, and children

Triptans and serotonin antagonists:

- Contraindicated for clients with cardiovascular disease, and should be administered cautiously to clients with liver or kidney disease.
- Should not be given within 24 hours of administration of ergot alkaloids.

Important Drugs

Ergot Alkaloids

- Ergotamine tartrate (Ergostat) is a vasoconstrictor. It is poorly absorbed orally, and is also given sublingually, by rectal suppository, or by inhalation.
- Ergotamine with caffeine (Cafergot) is a common antimigraine that combines caffeine with ergotamine.

Triptans

- Sumatriptan (Imitrex) is a vascular headache suppressant that is used to treat acute migraine headaches and cluster headache episodes.
- Zolmitriptan (Zomig) constricts cranial vessels, thereby relieving migraine headache.
- Rizatriptan (Maxalt) is a newer drug used to provide relief of migraine headache, with or without a preceding aura, by causing vasoconstriction of cranial blood vessels.

Serotonin antagonist

- Methysergide (Sansert) prevents or aborts vascular headaches.

Therapeutic Nursing Interventions

- Assess clients for sensitivity to antimigraine medications.
- Administer antiemetic medication prior to giving antimigraine medication, as ordered.
- Assess for early signs of ergotism in clients taking ergot alkaloids, and notify primary care provider of any manifestations.
- Assess pulse and blood pressure, and report an irregular heartbeat and/or increased blood pressure to the primary care provider.
- Do not administer triptans and serotonin antagonists if client received an ergot alkaloid within 24 hours.
- Assess degree of pain relief obtained from antimigraine drugs.
- Do not increase the dosage of antimigraine drugs, or administer more medication than ordered without consulting with the primary care provider.
- Monitor the amount of medication that is taken within one month.

Client Education

- Lie down in a quiet, dark room for 2-3 hours following administration of drug to augment medication effects.
- Notify health care provider if adverse effects develop.
- Avoid smoking and exposure to cold because these activities further constrict blood vessels and increase pain.
- Avoid driving and other activities that require concentration for 3-5 hours after taking antimigraine drugs. These medications may cause dizziness and confusion.

- Notify health care provider if pregnancy is suspected or planned. Ergot preparations are contraindicated in pregnancy because they stimulate the uterus.
- Advise the client to take the antimigraine medication at the first sign of this type of headache or when the aura is present.
- Encourage the client to keep a record of headache occurrences, foods, and specific triggers (stress, fatigue, dairy products, caffeine, and chocolate).

Anti-gout Drugs

Overview

Gout is a type of acute arthritis that is characterized by joint inflammation. Gout is caused by a metabolic disturbance of purine metabolism that results in hyperuricemia. Gout symptoms develop when the serum uric acid level is > 6 mg/dL. Anti-gout drugs act to prevent and treat attacks of gouty arthritis.

Uses

- Reduce inflammation in the joints
- Decrease the production of uric acid
- Increase the excretion of uric acid by the kidneys

Adverse Effects

- Gastrointestinal symptoms such as:
  - Diarrhea
  - Abdominal pain
  - Nausea
  - Vomiting
- Kidney stones
- Renal failure
- Hypotension
- Arrhythmias
- Bone marrow suppression
- Anemia

Precautions

- Contraindicated for clients with hypersensitivity, gastrointestinal disorders, hepatic disorders, blood dyscrasias, or kidney disease
- Should be administered with caution to elderly or debilitated clients

Important Drugs

Colchicine

- Colchicine is effective for acute attacks of gouty arthritis pain.
- Colchicine is not an analgesic. The major action is to reduce inflammation in the joint.
- It can be given by mouth or intravenously.

- The client should not take aspirin (acetylsalicylic acid) at the same time as colchicine without consulting the primary care provider.

Ibuprofen (Advil, Motrin, Nuprin) and **Naproxen** (Naprosyn)

- These medications have largely replaced colchicine in the treatment of acute gout.
- Ibuprofen and naproxen are highly effective with minimal toxicities.

Allopurinol (Zyloprim)

- Allopurinol is used for gout and hyperuricemia that develop secondary to chemotherapy. It is used to treat chronic acute gouty arthritis.
- Allopurinol reduces uric acid synthesis.
- Clients should be well hydrated when taking allopurinol.

Probenecid (Benemid) and **sulfinpyrazone** (Anturane)

- These anti-gout agents inhibit the tubular reabsorption of uric acid in the kidney and increase the renal excretion of uric acid.
- When probenecid is used to treat gout, it should not be given with aspirin because this combination of drugs decreases elimination of uric acid.
- Sulfinpyrazone is not effective in treating acute gout, but is used as a preventative agent.

Therapeutic Nursing Interventions

- Obtain baseline uric acid levels and CBC.
    - Monitor laboratory reports throughout drug therapy.
        - A decrease in serum uric acid is a positive therapeutic result.
        - A decrease in blood cells and platelets signal bone marrow suppression due to the toxic effects of anti-gout drugs.
- Administer anti-gout drugs with food to prevent gastrointestinal side effects.
- Encourage fluid intake of at least 3000 mL per day.
- Encourage rest and immobilize the inflamed joints during acute attacks.
- Arrange for physical therapy, as ordered, once pain and swelling have subsided.

Client Education

- Take medications with food to prevent gastrointestinal irritation.
- Drink at least 3000 mL of water a day (if there are no contraindications) to prevent formation of uric acid stones by the kidneys.
- Avoid excessive alcohol intake.
- Avoid taking aspirin at the same time as probenecid without consulting the primary care provider. Taking these drugs concurrently decreases the excretion of uric acid.
- Notify health care provider if rash, sore throat, fever, or bleeding develops.
- Eat a low purine diet to prevent recurrent gouty arthritis attacks. The client should avoid red and organ meats, lunch meats, shellfish, sardines, anchovies, and meat gravies.
- Test urinary pH with nitrazine paper between attacks, and report to primary care provider if urinary output of uric acid decreases. Client may need to start anti-gout medication immediately to prevent a new attack of gout.

Disease-Modifying Antirheumatic Drugs (DMARDs)

Overview

Disease-modifying antirheumatic drugs (DMARDs) are used to slow the progression of rheumatoid arthritis. Rheumatoid arthritis is a chronic immunologic disease that causes inflammatory changes in the joints, resulting in pain, reduced mobility, and even shortened longevity. Currently, there is no cure for rheumatoid arthritis. Thus, attention has focused on medications.

Major classifications of drugs used to treat rheumatoid arthritis are:

- DMARDs
- Gold compounds
- Chelating agents
- Antimalarial drugs
- Cytotoxic immunosuppressant drugs

Uses

- DMARDs are used to relieve the inflammation, pain, stiffness, and swelling of joints associated with rheumatoid arthritis.
- These drugs help to slow or arrest the progression of rheumatoid arthritis, thus producing a partial or complete remission.
- DMARDs take 6 weeks to 6 months longer to produce an improvement than do NSAIDs.

Adverse Effects

- Gold preparations produce adverse effects in about 40% of clients who have received a cumulative dose of 400-800 mg of parenteral gold. Adverse effects include:
  - A metallic taste, stomatitis, mouth ulcers, thrombocytopenia, and nephrotic syndrome
  - Pruritus and other skin changes due to deposits of gold in the tissues
  - Gold deposits in the eyes (less common)
- Chelating agents such as penicillamine (Cuprimine) produce many dangerous toxic effects including gastrointestinal disturbances, bone marrow depression, alopecia, and skin friability.
- The antimalarials may produce macular degeneration in clients who take these drugs for extended periods.
- Cytotoxic immunosuppressant drugs may produce gastrointestinal disturbances, bone marrow depression, increased risk of infection, liver failure, and skin rash.

Precautions

- Gold preparations are contraindicated in clients who are allergic to heavy metals.
- Gold preparations should not be given to clients with renal or liver disease, congestive heart failure, uncontrolled diabetes, and acute hepatitis because gold deposits in the tissues worsen these conditions.

- Chelating agents such as penicillamine are contraindicated in pregnancy, blood dyscrasias, and renal disease. Drugs should be discontinued if client develops a fever.
- Antimalarials are not recommended during pregnancy.

Important Drugs

Examples of **gold compounds** are:

- Gold sodium thiomalate (Myochrysine).
- Aurothioglucose (Solganal).
- Auranofin (Ridaura).

Organic gold compounds are given parenterally for rheumatoid arthritis.

- A significant number of clients experience some form of toxicity, and must stop therapy.
- Dermatitis is the most common side effect.

D-penicillamine (Cuprimine) is a chelating agent that helps to reduce the titer of the rheumatoid factor.

Chloroquine hydrochloride (Aralen) is an antimalarial drug that is used to treat rheumatoid arthritis.

Methotrexate (Rheumatrex) is a cytotoxic drug used for rheumatoid arthritis.

- Also a potent immunosuppressive drug at anticancer doses

Azathioprine (Imuran) is a cytotoxic drug used to treat severe rheumatoid arthritis that has not responded to more conservative therapy.

- Liver function tests should be done every three months.

Cyclophosphamide (Cytoxan) is a cytotoxic and immunosuppressant agent that is used to treat severe, active rheumatoid arthritis.

- A major toxic effect is hemorrhagic cystitis.

Cyclosporine (Neoral) is an immunosuppressant agent used to treat severe, active rheumatoid arthritis.

- Causes major nephrotoxicity

Therapeutic Nursing Interventions

- Assess client with rheumatoid arthritis for pain and range of motion at the beginning of and throughout drug therapy.
- Monitor CBC for signs of bone marrow suppression before starting and throughout drug therapy. These signs include a reduction in the hemoglobin, hematocrit, leukocyte count, and platelet count.
- Monitor liver enzymes tests for an elevation that could indicate liver dysfunction.
- Monitor for increased BUN and creatinine levels, which could indicate renal dysfunction.
- Shake bottle of gold medication before withdrawing it into a syringe to ensure adequate suspension. Use a 20- or 21-gauge needle.
- Inject gold preparations deep into the gluteal muscle. Have the client lie down for at least 30 minutes following the injection.

- Keep gold medications in a tightly closed, light-resistant container.
- Do not administer gold preparations that are darker than pale yellow.
- Immediately refer clients who are receiving gold preparations and who develop mouth ulcers to their primary care provider.
- Assess client taking chelating agents for fever, which is the first sign of an allergic reaction.
- Schedule clients who are taking antimalarials for periodic eye examinations because these agents may cause macular degeneration.

Client Education

- Take medications exactly as ordered and immediately report any adverse effects to the health care provider.
- Protect skin from overexposure to the sun to prevent photophobic reactions.
- Schedule periodic lab tests, physical examinations, and eye appointments to assess for adverse effects.
- Inspect mouth for signs of redness and ulceration, and report these signs immediately to the primary care provider.
- Use a soft toothbrush to prevent mouth irritation.

Critical Thinking Exercise: Drugs for Pain and Inflammation

Note: *It is recommended that the following exercises be reviewed with a partner or in a small group to achieve maximum student interaction and to enhance critical thinking skills.*

Situation: D.S. is a 76-year-old woman who had a total hip replacement yesterday. Her pain is managed by patient-controlled analgesia (PCA). She has an epidural catheter in place and is receiving fentanyl (Duragesic) and bupivacaine (Marcaine) via the PCA.

1. D.S. is very worried she will give herself too much medication and become addicted. What do think would be an appropriate nursing intervention? Provide a rationale for your answer.

2. What are the most important assessment parameters for any client who is receiving narcotic analgesics?

3. The plan is to discontinue the epidural catheter in 48 hours and order oxycodone/acetaminophen (Percocet 7.5/500), 1 tab PO q 6h PRN pain management. Your nursing knowledge provides you with important information regarding the side effects of this medication. Discuss some of the implications this has in relation to your nursing assessments and interventions.

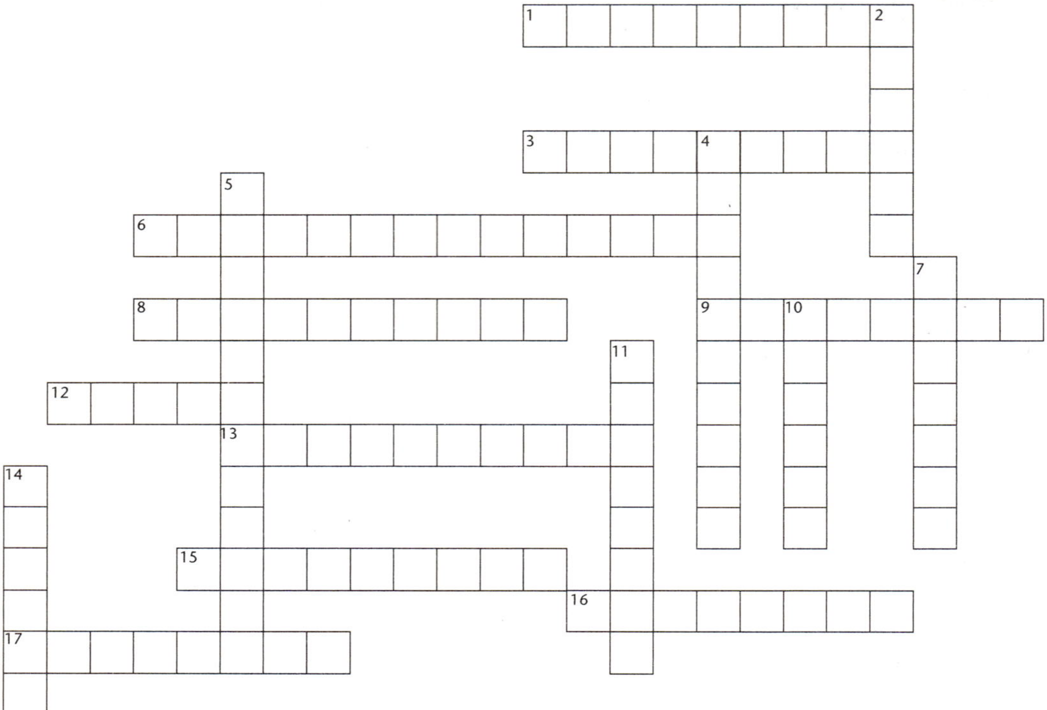

Across

1. Gout is a type of acute __________.
3. Decreased sensitivity to subseqent doses of the same substance is called___________.
6. This drug in high doses is extremely toxic to liver (generic name).
8. An commonly used sythetic narcotic analgesic is (generic name) ___________.
9. This drug may be given by continuous IV infusion.
12. Opiate agonists-antagonists such as Talwin, or Nubain are metabolized in the___________.
13. Drugs that relieve pain are classified as:
15. Salicylates ane NSAIDS are safer medications because they do not produce__________ .
16. Opiates may excite the autonomic fibers of the oculomotor nerve resulting in ___________pupils.
17. Drugs that stimulate opiate receptors are called ________.

Down

2. Morphine and meperidine are used for ___________ pain.
4. Anti-inflammatory corticosteroids help reduce acute inflammation of the joints associated with _____________ arthritis.
5. The nurse must monitor clients on opiate analgesics closely because these drugts may supress ______________.
7. Narcotics and their metabolites are excreted by the __________.
10. Some anti-inflammatory drugs are used in fever because they may _________the body temperature.
11. Topical corticosteroids may have larger or ___________ effects.
14. The drug of choice that reverses respiratory depression during a narcotic overdose is (trade name) ________.

CHAPTER 5

Drugs Affecting the Nervous System

Key Points

- Drugs that affect the nervous system act upon the:
  - Autonomic nervous system (ANS)
  - Central nervous system (CNS)
  - Neuromuscular system
- The ANS is a regulatory, self-governing system that functions (without conscious thought) to maintain the internal environment of the body at an optimal level (homeostasis).
- The ANS is divided into:
  - **Sympathetic** system
    - Helps us to "fight or flight" when faced with stress
  - **Parasympathetic** system
    - Which is restorative and vegetative
- Most organs are innervated by both the sympathetic and parasympathetic branches, and the opposing actions of each balance one another.
- **Adrenergic (sympathomimetic)** drugs mimic the action of the sympathetic nervous system. Epinephrine (Adrenalin), an emergency drug, is the prototype for adrenergic drugs.
- **Anti-adrenergic (sympatholytic)** drugs block the action of the sympathetic nervous system.
- Anti-adrenergic drugs are divided into:
  - Alpha-adrenergic blockers
  - Beta-blockers
  - Ganglionic blockers
- **Cholinergic (cholinomimetic)** drugs stimulate the parasympathetic nervous system, while anticholinergic drugs inhibit parasympathetic nervous system function.
- **Skeletal muscle relaxants** are prescribed to relax skeletal muscles and sedate the client.
  - Used to relieve musculoskeletal pain and muscle spasms.
- **Neuromuscular blocking agents** prevent the transmission of nerve impulses, causing total relaxation of muscles and flaccid paralysis.
- These agents are used to facilitate surgical anesthesia, endotracheal intubation, mechanical ventilation, and electroconvulsive therapy.
- CNS stimulants act to stimulate the respiratory system, the heart, and the general metabolism.

  - Major classifications of CNS stimulants are:
    - Analeptic stimulants
    - Psychomotor stimulants such as the amphetamines
    - Non-amphetamine anorexiants
- CNS depressants depress the central nervous system. They include:
  - Sedatives
  - Hypnotics
  - Anxiolytics
- **Sedatives and hypnotics** are usually classified as:
  - Barbiturates
  - Non-barbiturates
  - Benzodiazepines
- **Anxiolytic (anti-anxiety)** drugs counteract or relieve anxiety. They are also used to treat anxiety disorders, which include phobias, obsessive-compulsive behaviors, and generalized anxiety disorder.
- **Antidepressants** are prescribed to treat major depressive illness as well as panic disorder and enuresis in children. Major groups of antidepressants are:
  - Tricyclic antidepressants
  - Selective serotonin reuptake inhibitors (SSRIs)
  - Monoamine oxidase (MAO) inhibitors
  - Atypical antidepressants
- Lithium is the mood-stabilizing drug of choice for the long-term management of bipolar disorder (also called manic-depressive disorder).
- **Antipsychotic drugs** are used to treat psychosis, most commonly schizophrenia. These agents are also used to treat delusions; visual, auditory, or olfactory hallucinations; and extreme agitation.
- **Anti-seizure drugs (anticonvulsants)** are prescribed to treat epilepsy and other seizure disorders. These agents depress abnormal electrical activity in the brain, control seizure activity, and allow the client to live a normal life.
- Parkinson's disease is a progressive, idiopathic, neurologic disorder caused by depletion, degeneration, or destruction of dopamine in neurons located in the basal ganglia of the brain.
  - The two major categories of drugs used to treat Parkinson's disease:
    - Dopaminergic drugs
    - Anticholinergic drugs (antimuscarinics)
- **Antimyasthenic agents** treat myasthenia gravis (an autoimmune neuromuscular disorder), but they do not cure this disease. The goal of antimyasthenic therapy is to help the client maintain as normal a lifestyle as possible. Cholinesterase inhibitors comprise the major group of antimyasthenics.
- Anesthetic agents cause partial or complete loss of sensation, with or without loss of consciousness.
- **General anesthetics** are usually administered by injection or inhalation.
- The major types of anesthetic agents are general anesthetics and local anesthetics.
- Balanced anesthesia is the use of a combination of drugs to produce anesthesia.

Drugs Affecting the Sympathetic Nervous System

Adrenergic (Sympathomimetic) Drugs

Overview

Adrenergic (sympathomimetic) drugs mimic the actions of the sympathetic nervous system. The sympathetic nervous system prepares the body to meet stress with either a fight or flight reaction. Major therapeutic uses and adverse effects of adrenergic drugs stem from drug effects on the heart, lungs, and blood vessels. Some adrenergic drugs act on both heart and lung receptors. Stimulation of the sympathetic nervous system increases the heart rate, dilates the bronchioles, and takes blood from the gastrointestinal tract, sending it to the skeletal muscles. Norepinephrine, which is synthesized from the amino acid tyrosine, is the primary neurotransmitter for the sympathetic system. Adrenergic agents mimic functions of the sympathetic nervous system by stimulating alpha-adrenergic, beta-adrenergic, and dopaminergic receptors.

Adrenergic receptors and their functions are further subdivided:

- Alpha-receptors are primarily found in blood vessels.
    - Activation results in vasoconstriction, which then raises blood pressure and decreases nasal congestion. Activation also causes contraction of gastrointestinal and bladder sphincters.
- $Beta_1$-receptors are found primarily in the heart.
    - Activation results in increased heart rate, increased force of heart contraction, and increased automaticity and conduction velocity.
- $Beta_2$-receptors are found primarily in the lungs and peripheral blood vessels.
    - Activation in the lungs results in bronchodilation.
    - Activation in the blood vessels results in vasodilation, with increased blood flow to skeletal muscles, the heart, and the brain.
        - The body needs this increased blood flow for fight or flight reactions.

Adrenergic drugs are either:

- Catecholamines
    - A group of chemically similar compounds
    - Cannot cross the blood-brain barrier or be taken orally
    - Catecholamines are:
        - Endogenous: Norepinephrine, dopamine, and epinephrine (adrenalin)
        - Exogenous (synthetic): Dobutamine and isoproterenol
- Noncatecholamines
    - Can cross blood-brain barrier
    - Ephedrine, albuterol, and phenylephrine are noncatecholamines

Uses

- Adrenergic drugs are primarily emergency drugs.
- Are given to treat the following acute cardiovascular, respiratory, and allergic disorders:
    - Cardiac arrest—given to stimulate the heart
    - Hypotension—given to increase blood pressure
    - Congestive heart failure (CHF)—given to increase force and contraction of the heart
    - Bronchial asthma—given to open the bronchioles
    - Upper respiratory congestion—given as a decongestant
    - Allergic reactions—given for vasoconstriction and decongestant effects that relieve edema
    - Hypoglycemia—given to stimulate glycogen release from the liver and skeletal muscles
    - Local bleeding—given to constrict blood vessels and stop bleeding
    - Obstetrics—given to relax the uterus
    - Eye disorders—given for vasoconstriction and mydriasis
- Adrenergic drugs may also be administered as local anesthetics to prolong anesthesia; for example, with the use of novocaine by dentists.

Adverse Effects

Catecholamines

- Nervousness and restlessness
- Angina
- Hypertension
- Tachycardia
- Hyperglycemia
- Nausea and vomiting

Noncatecholamines

- Severe anxiety and insomnia
- Tachycardia and palpitations
- Dysrhythmias
- Muscular weakness and cramps

Precautions

Contraindications

- Cardiac dysrhythmias
- Angina
- Hypertension
- Narrow-angle glaucoma
- Pregnant women
- Use cautiously with children.

Important Drugs

Catecholamine drugs

Epinephrine hydrochloride (Adrenalin Chloride) is:

- The prototype of the adrenergics
- The drug of choice for anaphylaxis
- The active ingredient in OTC asthma preparations
- Effects:
  - Stimulates both alpha- and beta-receptors
  - Increases blood pressure
  - Increases heart rate
  - Increases blood flow to brain, heart, and skeletal muscles
  - Constricts peripheral vessels
  - Relaxes gastrointestinal smooth muscle
- Administered by:
  - Intramuscular injection
  - Subcutaneous injection
  - Inhalation
  - Injection directly into the heart (intracardially)
  - Cannot be given orally because gastrointestinal enzymes destroy it

Norepinephrine (Levophed)

- Potent vasoconstrictor
- Used to treat:
  - Hypotension
  - Cardiac arrest

Dopamine hydrochloride (Intropin)

- The immediate precursor of norepinephrine
- Dosage effects:
  - Low doses cause renal perfusion
  - Low to moderate doses cause increased cardiac output
  - Higher doses increase peripheral resistance and blood pressure

Dobutamine hydrochloride (Dobutrex)

- A synthetic catecholamine
- Acts directly on the heart muscle to increase the force of contraction

Isoproterenol hydrochloride (Isuprel)

- A synthetic catecholamine
- A bronchodilator
- Stimulates both $beta_1$- and $beta_2$-receptors
- Used to control shock and some dysrhythmias
- Absorption effect
  - Good by injection or aerosol
  - Poor by oral or sublingual

Noncatecholamine drugs

Ephedrine

- Less potent, but longer acting drug than epinephrine
- Used as a bronchodilator and nasal decongestant during allergic reactions

Pseudoephedrine (Sudafed)

- Related to ephedrine, and has similar actions

Phenylephrine hydrochloride (Neo-Synephrine)

- Stimulates the alpha-receptor, which results in vasoconstriction and nasal decongestion
- Acts as a bronchodilator

Albuterol (Proventil)

- Used to produce bronchodilation

Therapeutic Nursing Interventions

- Monitor:
  - Vital signs and electrocardiogram (ECG) for increased heart rate, increased blood pressure, and dysrhythmias
  - Respirations and lung sounds for bronchial congestion and dyspnea
  - Blood glucose levels for elevated blood sugar
  - Input and output (I & O) for signs of mild renal failure
  - For severe anxiety and insomnia in clients receiving noncatecholamines
- Avoid infiltration of intravenous infusion into the tissues, especially when infusing norepinephrine bitartrate (Levophed), which can cause tissue necrosis, resulting in possible amputation of the involved extremity.
  - Inspect the intravenous site every 15 minutes for edema and coolness.
  - Compare the injection site with the opposite extremity.
  - Observe for a decreased or stopped drip rate.
  - Discontinue the infusion immediately and notify the primary care provider if infiltration is suspected.
- Report any adverse drug effects to the primary care provider immediately.

Client Education

- Take the medication exactly as ordered and do not exceed the dosage. Overdosage may result in severe adverse effects.
- Report to health care provider shortness of breath that remains unrelieved by the medication.
- Avoid smoking or alcohol while taking these medications as the combination can precipitate adverse effects.
- Consult with health care provider before taking over-the-counter medications concurrently with adrenergics.
- Drink at least 2000-3000 mL of fluid daily to help liquify thick respiratory tract secretions.
- Correctly self-administer inhalants, and properly use aerosolization equipment, intermittent positive pressure breathing (IPPB), and metered-dose inhalers.

- Avoid spraying inhalers near the eyes.
- Notify health care provider if contents of one canister of inhalent are used up in less than two weeks.
- Save inhaler because it may be possible to purchase refill canisters.

Antiadrenergic Drugs

Overview

Antiadrenergic drugs (adrenergic-blocking agents or sympatholytics) are used to block the sympathetic system in whole or in part. Blocking agents can prevent the action of naturally occurring or externally administered catecholamines. The goal of antiadrenergic drug therapy is to suppress pathological responses to activity, stress, or other stimuli—not the normal physiological responses.

The three major types of antiadrenergic drugs are:

- Alpha-adrenergic blocking agents
- Beta-adrenergic blocking agents
- Ganglionic blockers

Alpha-Adrenergic Blocking Agents

Overview

The alpha-adrenergic blocking agents block the effects of alpha-receptors, primarily in blood vessels. Alpha-adrenergic blockers are developed from natural sources such as ergot and its derivatives, or they are manufactured synthetically.

These drugs act to:

- Block sympathomimetic agents
- Dilate vessels in smooth muscles
- Lower peripheral vascular resistance

$Alpha_2$ adrenergic blocking agents inhibit the release of norepinephrine in the brain, decreasing sympathetic stimulation and blood pressure.

Uses

- Mild to moderate hypertension
- Benign prostatic hypertrophy (BPH)
- Migraine headaches
- Pheochromocytoma
- Congestive heart failure (CHF) when used in conjunction with cardiac glycosides and diuretics
- Peripheral vascular disorders (e.g., Raynaud's disease and frostbite)

Adverse Effects

- Ergotism:
  - Early signs include nausea, vomiting, abdominal cramps, and confusion

    - Later signs include:
        - Circulatory stasis with itching
        - Coldness and numbness in fingers and hands leading to acute or chronic gangrene of the extremities, nose, digits, and ears
        - Seizures, rapid irregular pulse, and confusion
- Nasal congestion
- Nausea
- Vomiting
- Sudden tachycardia
- Postural hypotension

Precautions

- Alpha-adrenergic blocking agents should be administered cautiously to clients with coronary or cerebral arteriosclerosis, renal impairment, or peptic ulcer disease.
- Ergot alkaloids
    - Contraindicated for:
        - Hypersensitivity
        - Sepsis
        - Vascular disease
        - Hepatic or renal disease
        - Marked atherosclerosis
        - Hypertension
        - Anemia
        - Pregnant clients, because they stimulate the uterus and can harm the fetus
    - Should be administered cautiously to women who are lactating, elderly clients, and children

Important Drugs

Phentolamine mesylate (Regitine)

- The prototype for alpha-adrenergic blocking agents
- Used to prevent tissue necrosis following extravasation of intravenous norepinephrine
- Prevents and controls hypertension caused by pheochromocytoma, which is a tumor that releases excessive amounts of catecholamines
- When administered by intravenous infusion, the nurse should monitor:
    - Blood pressure
    - Pulse
    - Electrocardiogram (ECG) every two minutes until stable

Ergotamine tartrate (Ergostat) is a vasoconstrictor that is used to treat migraine headaches. It is poorly absorbed orally, and is given sublingually, by rectal suppository, or by inhalation.

Ergotamine tartrate with caffeine (Cafergot) is a common antimigraine medication that combines caffeine with ergotamine.

Doxazosin (Cardura) is a peripherally acting antiadrenergic drug that is used to treat hypertension or BPH. It acts by blocking post synaptic alpha 1-adrenergic receptors.

Prazosin (Minipress) is a peripherally acting, antiadrenergic drug that is used to treat hypertension or BPH. It acts by blocking post-synaptic alpha1 adrenergic receptors.

Terazosin (Hytrin) is a peripherally-acting antiadrenergic drug that is used to treat hypertension or BPH. It acts by blocking post-synaptic alpha 1-adrenergic receptors.

Sumatriptan (Imitrex) is a vascular headache suppressant used to treat migraines.

Therapeutic Nursing Interventions

- Monitor blood pressure with the client in the lying, sitting, and standing positions.
- Have clients remain supine throughout intravenous administration of phentolamine mesylate (Regitine).
- Assess clients for:
  - Sensitivity to medications containing ergot alkaloids
  - Early signs of ergotism in clients taking ergot alkaloids, and notify primary care provider of any manifestations
  - Degree of pain relief obtained from antimigraine drugs
- Do not increase the dosage of medication or administer more medication than ordered without consulting with the primary care provider.

Client Education

- Change positions slowly to prevent orthostatic hypotension.
- Notify health care provider if chest pain occurs during intravenous infusion of phentolamine mesylate.
- Take antimigraine medications immediately upon development of a headache.
- Notify health care provider if early signs of ergotism or other adverse effects develop.

Beta-Adrenergic Blocking Agents

Overview

Beta-adrenergic blocking agents act to block adrenergic stimulation to $beta_1$ or $beta_2$ receptors by competing with norepinephrine for available beta-adrenergic receptor sites. Beta-blockers that block $beta_1$-receptors cause a decrease in blood pressure, contraction of the heart muscle, and cardiac output. These agents are used to control angina pectoris. Beta-blockers that block $beta_2$-receptors cause vasodilatation in skeletal muscle arterioles. They are used to control angina pectoris and lower blood pressure.

Uses

Angina: Given to decrease oxygen demand, myocardial contractility, heart rate, and blood pressure

Dysrhythmias: Given to slow sinus node and prolong conduction through the AV (atrioventricular) node, thereby slowing ventricular response

Hypertension: Given to lower blood pressure

Myocardial infarction: Given to decrease the incidence of catecholamine-induced dysrhythmias following attack

Glaucoma: Given to reduce intraocular pressure by binding to beta-adrenergic receptors in the eye, thereby decreasing the formation of aqueous humor

Migraine headache: Given to prevent migraines; mechanism of action is unclear

Palpitations and tremor: Aassociated with anxiety; however, they have not yet been approved as antianxiety drugs

Adverse Effects

- Bradycardia
- Shortness of breath
- Edema
- Reduced tolerance to exercise
- Hypoglycemia
- CHF
- Orthostatic hypotension
- Fatigue
- Nausea
- Vomiting
- Diarrhea
- Bronchospasm
- Impotence
- Depression
- Sleep disorders

Precautions

- Should be administered cautiously to clients with:
    - Diabetes, who are taking insulin or oral hypoglycemic agents because they may mask the symptoms of hypoglycemia
    - Peripheral vascular insufficiency, because they constrict peripheral blood vessels and thus reduce blood flow to the extremities
    - Kidney or liver disease, because they accumulate in the serum of clients with these diseases, and cause toxic effects
- Should not be stopped abruptly, particularly in clients with ischemic heart disease
    - These agents are titrated down slowly, usually over a period of 1-2 weeks.

    - Clients with angina who abruptly discontinue beta blockers are at four times greater risk of developing an anginal attack or a mild myocardial infarction within 30 days of discontinuation.
- Should not be taken with alcohol, central nervous system depressants, or over-the-counter decongestants
- Beta blockers are not always effective for African-American clients, and thus are usually combined with a diuretic. The reason why this combination is therapeutic is not clearly understood.

Important Drugs

Propranolol hydrochloride (Inderal)

- The prototype for beta-adrenergic blocking agents
- Used to treat hypertrophic subaortic stenosis, hypertension, angina, dysrhythmias, and myocardial infarction
- Available in a wide dosage range
    - Clients vary greatly in the amount of oral drug that survives hepatic metabolism to reach the systemic circulation.

Metoprolol tartrate (Lopressor) is used to treat hypertension and dysrhythmias.

Atenolol (Tenormin) is used to treat hypertension, angina, and myocardial infarction.

Sotalol (Betapace) is used to treat dysrhythmias.

Timolol maleate (Timoptic) is an eye drop medication used to treat glaucoma.

Therapeutic Nursing Interventions

- Obtain a baseline weight before starting the administration of beta blockers.
- Check the client's pulse rate before administration, because beta blockers slow the sinus rate and may produce bradycardia.
- Monitor the client's blood pressure for hypotension.
- Monitor for hypoglycemia, which is indicated by a blood glucose level of less than 60 mg/dL.
- Assess breath sounds and listen for wheezing.
- Carefully evaluate the effect of the medication. Because the first dose of a beta blocker is almost completely metabolized by the liver, the dosage may need to be increased for a therapeutic effect.

Client Education

- Learn to take pulse and blood pressure, and identify lowered blood pressure and pulse rate.
- Learn to monitor blood sugar level for low blood sugar. Beta blockers may mask the symptoms of hypoglycemia in clients who are diabetic and are taking insulin or oral hypoglycemic agents.
- Change positions slowly to prevent orthostatic hypotension.
- Never stop medication abruptly because of the risk of an anginal attack or myocardial infarction.
- Take beta-blockers at the same time each day.

- Avoid taking beta blockers with antacids without the primary care provider's permission because of the risk of a drug interaction.
- Avoid taking beta blockers and over-the-counter drugs at the same time without the primary care provider's permission.
- Avoid prolonged exposure to the sun, taking hot showers, sitting in hot tubs, or visiting locations with very hot climates.
- Use caution when driving a vehicle or operating heavy machinery because beta blockers can cause dizziness.
- Avoid drinking alcoholic beverages because the interaction of alcohol and beta blockers may cause adverse effects.
- Store beta blockers in dry, moisture-proof, childproof bottles.

Ganglionic Blocking Agents

Overview

Ganglionic blocking agents stop the delivery of both sympathetic and parasympathetic nerve impulses through the ganglia. Ganglionic blockers compete with acetylcholine to occupy receptor sites in the autonomic ganglia. These agents act to decrease arterial pressure and lower blood pressure.

Uses

- Ganglionic blockers are used to treat clients who are in the advanced stages of hypertension, or in hypertensive crisis when other medications have failed to control the disease process.
- Ganglionic blockers are also used to treat pulmonary edema—a complication of severe hypertension.
- Ganglionic blockers are seldom used today because other, more effective medications, which have fewer side effects, are available.

Adverse Effects

- Hypotension
- Bradycardia
- Dry mouth
- Dilated pupils
- Decreased gastrointestinal and urinary tract mobility

Precautions

- Contraindicated for clients with glaucoma
- Should be used cautiously for clients with heart disease

Important Drugs

Mecamylamine hydrochloride (Inversine) is the ganglionic blocker of choice in the United States.

Therapeutic Nursing Interventions

- Monitor blood pressure every five minutes and observe for a rapid decrease.
- Immediately report to the primary care provider if the client's systolic blood pressure goes below 60 mmHg.
- Measure input and output (I & O) and report any decrease in urinary output.
- Provide ice chips or saliva substitutes to relieve dry mouth.

Client Education

- Learn to take own pulse and blood pressure and identify low blood pressure and pulse rate.
- Report side effects of drugs to health care provider; dosage may need to be adjusted.
- Use ice chips, hard candies, and saliva substitutes to relieve dry mouth.

Drugs That Affect The Parasympathetic Nervous System

Cholinergic Drugs

Overview

The **parasympathetic nervous system** coordinates with the sympathetic nervous system to maintain homeostatic balance. 75% of all parasympathetic fibers are in the vagus nerves. Parasympathetic nervous system functions are resting, reparative, and vegetative. This system is involved in:

- Digestion
- Excretion
- Cardiac deceleration
- Anabolism

Stimulation of the parasympathetic nervous system causes:

- Constricted pupils
- Contractions of the smooth muscle of the gastrointestinal tract
- Constricted bronchioles
- Bradycardia
- Increased glandular secretion, except for the sweat glands

The neurotransmitter for the parasympathetic nervous system is acetylcholine. The two types of cholinergic receptors are:

- **Nicotinic** action which resembles the effects of nicotine, including tachycardia, elevated blood pressure, and peripheral vasoconstriction
- **Muscarinic** action which is like that of muscarine, an alkaloid obtained from a toadstool. Effects include slowed heart rate, decreased blood pressure, and increased saliva.

There are two types of cholinomimetic (cholinergic) drugs:

- Direct-acting cholinomimetic drugs
- Indirect-acting cholinomimetic drugs

Direct-Acting Cholinomimetic Agents

Overview

Direct-acting cholinomimetic drugs are synthetic derivatives of choline. The effects may be global, but most therapeutic agents are selective in action. Direct-acting agents directly stimulate cholinergic receptors and mimic acetylcholine. Specific effects are:

- Decreased heart rate
- Increased tone of gastrointestinal muscle and relaxation of sphincters
- Increased tone of bladder and relaxation of sphincters
- Increased respiratory secretions
- Constriction of pupils

These agents are absorbed from most sites of administration.

Uses

- Direct-acting cholinomimetic drugs are used to treat:
  - Glaucoma
  - Accommodative esotropia (an eye disease)
  - Postoperative atony
  - Gastrointestinal reflux disease
  - Neurogenic bladder
  - Atrial dysrhythmias
- Direct-acting cholinomimetic drugs prevent nausea and vomiting related to chemotherapy.

Adverse Effects

- Nausea and vomiting
- Diarrhea
- Wheezing and shortness of breath
- Bradycardia
- Hypotension
- Headache
- Increased salivation
- Increase sweating
- Impaired vision
- Poor night vision
- Anxiety and restlessness
- Sleep disturbances
- Convulsions
- Coma

Precautions

- Direct-acting cholinomimetic drugs are contraindicated for clients with these disorders because they aggravate symptoms in persons with:
  - Diabetes mellitus
  - Coronary artery disease
  - Myocardial infarction
  - Heart block
  - Gangrene
- These agents are contraindicated for clients with intestinal obstruction, ulcerative colitis, or peptic ulcer because they increase gastrointestinal contractions and secretions.
- Direct-acting cholinomimetic drugs should be administered cautiously to clients with respiratory disorders or asthma because they cause bronchial constriction and increase bronchial secretions.
- These agents should be administered cautiously when given concomitantly with adrenergic drugs, because there is a risk of an adverse interaction.

Important Drugs

Acetylcholine is the prototype for the direct-acting cholinomimetic drugs.

Bethanechol chloride (Urecholine) is used for urinary retention and atony because it contracts the smooth muscle of the bladder, and stimulates gastric motility in paralytic ileus. It is also used to treat open-angle glaucoma.

Pilocarpine hydrochloride (Pilocar) is used to lower intraocular pressure in glaucoma by constricting the pupil.

Carbachol intraocular (Miostat) is used to treat simple glaucoma and open-angle glaucoma.

Metoclopramide hydrochloride (Reglan) is used to prevent chemotherapy-induced nausea and vomiting, and to treat heartburn and delayed gastric emptying due to reflux esophagitis.

Therapeutic Nursing Interventions

- Monitor heart rate and rhythm.
- Monitor respiratory rate and breath sounds.
- Monitor for abdominal distention, constipation, or diarrhea.
- Assess for abnormal bowel sounds.
- Monitor intake and urinary output, and assess for urinary frequency and retention.
- Report gnawing, aching, burning, or epigastric pain to the primary care provider. Direct-acting cholinomimetic drugs can cause or exacerbate peptic ulcer.
- When administering direct-acting cholinomimetic drugs concomitantly with adrenergic drugs, have atropine sulfate on hand to counteract a potential dangerous drug interaction.

Client Education

- Take the medication before or after eating to lessen gastrointestinal problems.
- Report gnawing, aching, burning, or epigastric pain, which could indicate peptic ulcer.
- Report constipation, diarrhea, urinary retention, or urinary frequency to health care provider, who may prescribe another drug or adjust the dosage.
- Instill eye drops, as ordered, using the correct procedure.
- Drive cautiously at night because direct-acting cholinomimetic eye drops constrict the pupil of the eye, decreasing night vision.

Indirect-Acting Cholinomimetic Drugs

Overview

Indirect-acting cholinomimetic drugs (anticholinesterase agents or cholinesterase inhibitors) are drugs that inhibit the action of acetylcholinesterase. **Acetylcholinesterase** is an enzyme that breaks down acetylcholine. Indirect-acting cholinomimetic drugs prolong the effect of acetylcholine by inhibiting acetylcholinesterase. These drugs are the active ingredients in many insecticides and nerve gases. Exposure to these products causes salivation, tearing, increased peristalsis, weakness, hypotension, nausea and vomiting, slurred speech, convulsions, and paralysis.

Uses

- Myasthenia gravis: improves muscle strength
- Glaucoma: reduces intraocular pressure
- Postoperative bladder distention: promotes bladder emptying
- Postoperative paralytic ileus: increases intestinal muscle tone
- Also used to counteract the neuromuscular blockade caused by muscle relaxants employed for anesthesia

Adverse Effects

- Hypotension
- Miosis
- Vasodilation
- Bradycardia
- Intestinal spasm
- Nausea and vomiting
- Increased salivation
- Diaphoresis
- Bronchial secretions and spasm
- Weakness and muscular paralysis
- Paralysis of the diaphragm
- Respiratory arrest

Precautions

- Indirect-acting cholinomimetic drugs are contraindicated for clients with the following disorders because they can aggravate symptoms:
  - Diabetes mellitus
  - Coronary artery disease
  - Heart block
  - Ulcerative colitis
  - Hypothyroidism
  - Gangrene
- These agents are contraindicated for clients with intestinal or urinary tract obstruction.
- Indirect-acting cholinomimetic drugs should be administered cautiously to clients with respiratory disorders or asthma, because they increase bronchial secretions and constrict the smooth muscles of the bronchioles.
- These agents should be not be given with ganglionic blocking agents because the combination of drugs can cause severe hypotension.

Important Drugs

Neostigmine bromide (Prostigmin)

- Neostigmine is used to treat urinary retention and paralytic ileus.
- It also is the drug of choice in the treatment of myasthenia gravis, which is a neurologic disease characterized by decreased neuromuscular transmission, and accompanied by increased weakness and fatigue of skeletal muscles.

Edrophonium chloride (Tensilon)

- Used to diagnose myasthenia gravis
- This agent is also used to differentiate between myasthenia crisis (not enough medication is being administered) and cholinergic crisis (too much medication is being administered).
- Antidote for pancuronium (Pavulon), which is a neuromuscular blocker

Pyridostigmine bromide (Mestinon) is the maintenance drug of choice for myasthenia gravis.

Atropine sulfate is used as an antidote to counteract the adverse effects of cholinergic agents.

Therapeutic Nursing Interventions

- Assess for signs and symptoms of myasthenia gravis (drooping of the upper eyelid, double vision, and difficulty chewing and swallowing).
- Assess for tremor, restlessness, confusion, convulsions, and other signs of neurologic toxicity; ensure client safety.
- Monitor respiratory rate and quality of respirations; listen for increased bronchial secretions and diminished breath sounds.
- Assess for abdominal cramps, vomiting, and diarrhea. Provide an antiemetic, if ordered.
- Assess vital signs for changes in heart rate and blood pressure.
- Measure I & O and assess for urinary frequency and incontinence.

Client Education

- Plan on taking medication for the rest of life if myasthenia gravis is diagnosed.
- Carry an identification card at all times that details medication regimen for myasthenia gravis.
- Take medication as scheduled to prevent myasthenic crisis or cholinergic crisis.
- Report adverse effects of drugs to health care provider.

Anticholinergic Drugs

Overview

Anticholinergic drugs, sometimes called muscarinic antagonists, block parasympathetic nerve impulses by competing with acetylcholine for sites on muscarinic receptors. These agents depress the central nervous system, and they affect the skin, eyes, gastrointestinal tract, bladder, bronchi, and heart rate.

Uses

- Anticholinergic drugs have widespread effects on the body, and this limits their clinical value.
- These agents are used to treat gastrointestinal disorders that are characterized by increased gastric mobility, excessive secretion of gastric acid, and abdominal pain.
- Anticholinergic drugs are also prescribed for:
  - Genital urinary disorders—given for their antispasmodic action
  - Eye disorders—given to produce cycloplegia (paralysis of the ciliary muscle) and mydriasis
  - Respiratory disorders—given for bronchodilation
  - Cardiac disease—given to treat bradycardia
  - Parkinson's disease—given to decrease salivation, tremors, and spasticity, and also to treat the side effects of some psychoactive medications
- Anticholinergic drugs are also administered preoperatively to prevent vagal stimulation and to decrease secretions during head and neck surgery.

Adverse Effects

- Dry mouth
- Constipation
- Blurred vision
- Difficult urination
- Tachycardia
- Intolerance to heat
- Contact dermatitis of the eyelids and conjunctiva
- Confusion
- Delusions

Precautions

- Anticholinergic drugs are contraindicated in clients with glaucoma because they may precipitate an attack by dilating the pupil.
- These agents are also contraindicated in clients with a history of hypersensitivity to these drugs.
- Anticholinergics should be given cautiously to clients with:
    - Chronic lung, renal, or hepatic disease
    - Myasthenia gravis
    - Heart disease
    - Paralytic ileus
    - Ulcerative colitis
- Anticholinergics should be administered cautiously to older clients who may develop severe adverse effects, and to clients who are taking central nervous system depressants, antidysrhythmics, and antihypertensives.

Important Drugs

Atropine sulfate

- Atropine is the prototype for anticholinergic drugs.
- It is a naturally occurring belladonna alkaloid that can be extracted from the belladonna plant or prepared synthetically.
- Atropine is used:
    - Preoperatively to dry secretions
    - To treat bradycardia
    - As an antidote for cholinergic drugs
    - As an antidote for insecticide poisoning

Belladonna tincture, an ingredient in several drug mixtures, is used to treat gastrointestinal disorders.

Homatropine (Spectro-Homatropine) eye drops are used to produce mydriasis and cycloplegia.

Trihexyphenidyl (Artane) is used to treat Parkinson's disease, and the Parkinson-like symptoms that occur with some psychoactive drugs.

Oxybutynin chloride (Ditropan) is used to increase bladder capacity and to decrease the frequency of voiding in clients with neurogenic bladders.

Scopolamine hydrobromide (Hyoscine) is used to treat motion sickness, manage the nausea and vomiting that accompanies general anesthesia, and produce preoperative amnesia.

Therapeutic Nursing Interventions

- Monitor pulse and blood pressure regularly, and report changes in heart rate or blood pressure to health care provider.
- Assess elderly clients carefully for complications arising from drug side effects.
- Encourage fluids to prevent constipation.
- Provide ice chips and oral hygiene to prevent discomfort from dry mouth.

Client Education

- Use ice chips, good oral hygiene, chewing gum, or hard candy to relieve the discomfort of a dry mouth.
- Drink at least 8 cups of water a day to decrease the risk of constipation.
- Take the drug 30-60 minutes before traveling to prevent motion sickness.

Drugs That Affect The Neuromuscular System

Skeletal Muscle Relaxants

Overview

Skeletal muscle relaxants are prescribed to relax the skeletal muscles, which are striated (striped) muscles attached to the skeletal frame. The function of skeletal muscles is to contract, enabling the skeleton to move. Skeletal muscle relaxants reduce skeletal muscle hyperactivity, while neuromuscular blocking agents cause skeletal muscles to completely relax during surgery, intubation, and mechanical ventilation. Skeletal muscle relaxants are also used to relieve musculoskeletal pain or spasm. Muscle spasm is an involuntary contraction of a muscle that is accompanied by pain. Muscle spasms may develop due to irritation, injury, or an inflammatory process. Prolonged muscle spasticity may result in severe pain, contractures, and disability. The majority of skeletal muscle relaxants act on the CNS, while others act directly (or peripherally) on the skeletal muscles. The primary therapeutic effect provided by skeletal muscle relaxants is sedation without loss of consciousness.

Central Skeletal Muscle Relaxants

Overview

While the exact mechanism of action is unknown, central skeletal muscle relaxants may act to depress polysynaptic reflexes in the CNS, as well as certain areas in the brain that control skeletal muscles. The primary therapeutic value of central skeletal muscle relaxants is to sedate the client, rather than directly relax tense muscles. These drugs are usually administered in conjunction with rest and a program of physical therapy.

Uses

- Relieves musculoskeletal pain
- Relieves severe musculoskeletal spasticity caused by inflammation, trauma, or some surgical procedures
- These agents are also used to treat the acute, painful muscle spasticity associated with:
    - Multiple sclerosis
    - Cerebral palsy
    - Cardiovascular accident (CVA)
    - Spinal cord injuries

Adverse Effects

- Drowsiness
- Dizziness
- Light-headedness
- Nausea and vomiting
- Constipation or diarrhea
- Flaccid muscles
- Dependence (rare, but may occur with large doses)

Precautions

- Central skeletal muscle relaxants should be administered cautiously to elderly or debilitated clients. Initially, dosage should be lower than the usual adult dosage.
- Central skeletal muscle relaxants should be administered cautiously to clients with liver or renal disease, because these agents are biotransformed in the liver and excreted in the urine.
- Discontinuation of central skeletal muscle relaxants should be very gradual if the client has developed a dependence on these agents. Abrupt discontinuation could cause seizures.
- These drugs should not be taken concomitantly with alcohol or other central nervous system depressants because toxic drug interactions may occur.

Important Drugs

Carisoprodol (Soma) is prescribed as an adjunct to rest and physical therapy in the treatment of muscular spasm caused by acute musculoskeletal conditions.

Cyclobenzaprine hydrochloride (Flexeril) manages muscular spasm and severe pain associated with musculoskeletal conditions. It is similar in structure to the tricyclic depressants.

Baclofen (Lioresal) is used to alleviate signs and symptoms of spasticity resulting from multiple sclerosis, spinal cord injuries, and other spinal cord diseases. High doses may produce ataxia (lack of normal muscle movements).

Orphenadrine (Norflex) is less commonly used than other central-acting skeletal muscle relaxants.

Therapeutic Nursing Interventions

- Assess the client's muscle strength, spasticity, gait, and degree of physical impairment prior to starting and throughout drug therapy.
- Assess for allergies prior to starting drug therapy.
- Measure I & O and monitor for urinary retention.
- Use safety precautions after administrating central skeletal muscle relaxants. Place the client's bed in low position and raise the side rails.

Client Education

- Take medication with meals to prevent gastrointestinal symptoms.
- Avoid alcohol and other CNS depressants.

- Perform activities involving alertness (driving or working with machines) with caution, as drug causes drowsiness.
- Ask for assistance when ambulating.
- Get sufficient rest, apply heat, and meet with a physical therapist as prescribed to reduce pain and muscle spasms.
- Notify health care provider if signs of allergy to the drug (rash, hives, dyspnea) develop.

Direct-Acting Skeletal Muscle Relaxants

Overview

Direct-acting or peripheral-acting skeletal muscle relaxants act directly on skeletal muscles. These agents produce skeletal muscle relaxation by interfering with the release of calcium from the sarcoplasmic reticulum, which then weakens the force of skeletal muscle contractility.

Uses

- Spasticity associated with:
  - Spinal cord injuries
  - Cerebral injuries
  - Multiple sclerosis
  - Cerebral palsy
  - Stroke
- Malignant hyperthermia crisis, a condition that may develop when clients are exposed to anesthetic agents such as halothane, succinylcholine, and methoxyflurane.

Adverse Effects

- Drowsiness
- Muscle weakness
- Slurred speech and drooling
- Headache
- Vomiting, diarrhea, anorexia, and hepatotoxicity
- Photophobia
- Yellow discoloration of skin and eyes

Precautions

- Dantrolene sodium (Dantrium) is contraindicated for clients with severe liver disease. The risk of developing hepatitis is greatest for women, for clients older than 35 years, and for clients who are taking 800 mg or more of dantrolene daily.
- This drug is contraindicated for clients with skeletal muscle spasms caused by rheumatic disorders.
- Dantrolene should be administered cautiously to clients who are lactose-intolerant because dantrolene contains lactose.

- Dantrolene should not be taken concomitantly with alcohol, other central nervous system drugs, or over-the-counter drugs that contain alcohol. Adverse drug interactions may occur.

Important Drugs

- Dantrolene acts directly on skeletal muscles to treat conditions associated with spasticity.
  - This is the drug of choice to treat malignant hyperthermia crisis.
  - May be administered with diazepam to augment its effect, but this combination causes drowsiness.

Therapeutic Nursing Interventions

- Place client in recumbent position for intravenous administration of dantrolene.
- Monitor laboratory studies for signs of liver abnormalities.
- Give medication with food if gastric irritation is a problem. Add oral suspensions to fruit juice, mix, and administer immediately.

Client Education

- Use caution when driving or operating machinery, especially if combining dantrolene with diazepam, which produces drowsiness.
- Wear protective clothing and sunscreen when in the sun to guard against photophobia.
- Notify health care provider if adverse effects develop.
- Never double the dose of this medication if a dose is missed because of the increased risk of hepatotoxicity.

Neuromuscular Blocking Agents

Overview

Neuromuscular blocking agents interrupt the transmission of nerve impulses at the neuromuscular junction by competing with acetylcholine for receptor sites. Acetylcholine is a neurotransmitter. These agents also act by either blocking depolarization or causing depolarization. This blockade of nerve impulses results in the relaxation of muscles and total flaccid paralysis. Neuromuscular blocking agents do not affect the central nervous system, and thus do not diminish pain. For this reason, these drugs must be administered concurrently with adequate anesthesia, opioid narcotics, and/or sedatives. Neuromuscular blockers must always be administered parenterally because they do not easily cross membranes. Neuromuscular blockers are used to:

- Relax smooth muscles as an adjunct to surgical anesthesia.
- Lessen convulsive muscle spasms during electroconvulsive therapy.
- Facilitate intubation of clients who require laryngectomy, bronchoscopy, or esophagoscopy, or who are under anesthesia.
- Facilitate the use of mechanical ventilation.

Only highly trained personnel, such as anesthesiologists and nurse anesthetists, should administer neuromuscular blocking agents. Following administration, clients need to be continually monitored. Equipment for endotracheal intubation, oxygen therapy, and reversal drugs must be available in case of emergency. Neuromuscular blocking agents should be administered cautiously to disabled clients, elderly clients, and clients with neuromuscular disorders or respiratory disorders. The two types of neuromuscular blocking agents are nondepolarizing agents and depolarizing agents.

Nondepolarizing Neuromuscular Blocking Agents

Overview

Nondepolarizing neuromuscular blocking agents block the transmission of nerve stimuli to muscles by blocking depolarization or by competing with acetylcholine for receptor sites at the neuromuscular junction. These agents cause muscle paralysis, but they do not relieve pain. Clients require anesthesia, narcotic analgesics, or sedatives for pain relief. Administering anticholinesterase agents (e.g., neostigmine), which allow acetylcholine to build up, reversing the action of nondepolarizing blockers.

Uses

Nondepolarizing agents are administered to cause muscle relaxation for performance of these procedures:

- Endotracheal (ET) intubation
- Surgical anesthesia
- Mechanical ventilation
- Electroconvulsive therapy

Adverse Effects

- Prolonged weakness or paralysis of muscles needed for ventilation
- Hypotension
- Dysrhythmias
- Bronchospasm
- Dyspnea and apnea
- Excessive salivation

Precautions

- These agents are contraindicated for clients who are pregnant or lactating, or who are hypersensitive to the drug.
- Nondepolarizing agents should be administered with caution to clients with asthma, endocrine disorders, lung cancer, underlying cardiac disease, impaired renal function, severe obesity, and neuromuscular diseases such as myasthenia gravis.
- These agents should be administered with caution to clients taking antibiotics because antibiotics can intensify their muscle blocking effects.

Important Drugs

Pancuronium bromide (Pavulon) is used to cause skeletal muscle paralysis during intubation following induction of anesthesia.

Vecuronium bromide (Norcuron) is used to facilitate endotracheal intubation and mechanical ventilation.

Tubocurarine chloride (Tubarine) is given to lessen the intensity of muscle contractions during electroshock therapy and to assist with the diagnosis of myasthenia gravis.

Atracurium (Tracrium) is given prior to endotracheal intubation or surgery.

Rocuronium (Zemuron) is given prior to endotracheal intubation or surgery.

Mivacurium (Mivacron) is given prior to endotracheal intubation or surgery.

Therapeutic Nursing Interventions

- Have suction and intubation equipment on hand when neuromuscular blockers are being administered.
- Monitor clients receiving continuous intravenous neuromuscular blockers with train-of-four (TOF) testing to determine the extent of neuromuscular blockade. TOF testing:
  - The client receives mild electrical shocks to a motor nerve from a peripheral nerve stimulator.
  - The client's response to four consecutive shocks (train of 4) indicates the extent of neuromuscular blockade.
  - One twitch indicates a 90% blockade; 2 or 3 twitches indicate a 75-90% blockade; and no twitches indicates no blockade.
  - The goal is for an 85-90% level of blockade.
  - Too large a dose of neuromuscular blockers can result in too large or deep a blockade and prolonged paralysis.
- To alleviate pain and produce conscious sedation, administer morphine, fentanyl (Sublimaze), or benzodiazepines to the client as ordered.
- Monitor vital signs continuously and assess for respiratory depression if the client is not receiving mechanical ventilation.
- Place a notice at the head of the client's bed that indicates the reversing agent to be administered should an emergency arise.
- During the period of paralysis, patch the client's eyes, and administer artificial tears.
- Once the procedure is over, administer anticholinesterase agents such as neostigmine, as ordered. Anticholinesterase allows acetylcholine to build up, which then reverses the action of the neuromuscular blockers.
- Administer atropine prior to or concurrently with anticholinesterase agents to decrease the side effects of acetylcholine buildup, which include bradycardia, bronchospasm, and excessive salivation.
- When the client is able to raise his/her head and keep it raised for 5 seconds, the effects of the blockade have been reversed.

Client Education

- Understand the purpose of neuromuscular blockers.
- Know that a skilled professional person will be in continuous attendance.
- Reassure the client that movement and communication skills will return once the blockade is reversed.

Depolarizing Agents

Overview

Depolarizing agents imitate the action of acetylcholine by depolarizing the muscle end plate, which then prevents the end plate from repolarizing, and thus stops muscle contraction. Succinylcholine chloride (Anectine) is a short-acting depolarizing agent that rapidly relaxes skeletal muscles. There is no specific antidote for succinylcholine. While anticholinesterase drugs are not used to reverse the effects of depolarizing agents, they do delay the pharmacological effects of succinylcholine.

Uses

Because it is a short-acting drug, succinylcholine is used to relax muscles during:

- Endotracheal intubation
- Electroconvulsive therapy
- Short orthopedic procedures

Adverse Effects

- Bradycardia or tachycardia
- Hypertension or hypotension
- Dysrhythmias
- Increased intraocular pressure
- Respiratory depression and apnea
- Excessive salivation
- Postoperative stiffness

Precautions

- Succinylcholine is contraindicated for clients with acute narrow-angle glaucoma because it raises intraocular pressure.
- This agent is also contraindicated for clients with malignant hyperthermia, which is a rare and sometimes fatal disorder characterized by an elevated body temperature.
- Succinylcholine should be administered cautiously to clients with fractures or muscle spasms because this agent may cause additional trauma.

Important Drugs

Succinylcholine (Anectine) is a short-acting depolarizing agent.

Therapeutic Nursing Interventions

- Assess client for a history of malignant hyperthermia before administering succinylcholine.
- Monitor client for signs of malignant hyperthermia throughout therapy: tachycardia, tachypnea, hypercarbia, jaw muscle spasm, lack of laryngeal relaxation, and hyperthermia.
- If malignant hyperthermia develops, immediately alert the primary care provider, discontinue the succinylcholine and the anesthesia, perform cooling

measures, administer an infusion of iced saline, and administer dantrolene sodium (Dantrium) as ordered. Dantrolene helps to prevent malignant hyperthermia.

- Other therapeutic nursing interventions are the same as for nondepolarizing agents.

Client Education

- Explain the purpose of neuromuscular blockers to the client.
- Reassure the client that a skilled professional person will be in continuous attendance.
- Reassure the client that movement and communication skills will return once the blockade is reversed.

Drugs That Stimulate The Central Nervous System

Overview

Central nervous system (CNS) stimulants act to stimulate the respiratory system, heart, and general metabolism. Small doses of CNS stimulants increase alertness and impart a feeling of well-being. Large doses of CNS stimulants produce insomnia, tremors, and restlessness. Toxic doses of CNS stimulants produce convulsions, cardiac dysrhythmias, and possibly death. Prolonged use of these agents results in exhaustion, hypertension, and drug abuse. There are many drugs that stimulate the central nervous system, but few are used clinically. Major classifications of CNS stimulants are analeptic stimulants, psychomotor stimulants (such as the amphetamines), and non- amphetamine anorexiants.

Analeptic Stimulants

Overview

Analeptic stimulants include caffeine, doxapram (Dopram), and the methylxanthines. These short-acting stimulants act on the cerebral cortex and medullary centers. They are absorbed orally. General effects of analeptic stimulants on the body include:

- Central nervous system stimulation
- Slight increase in basal metabolic rate
- Wakefulness
- Increased alertness
- Diuresis
- Cardiac stimulation
- Euphoria after ingestion

Analeptic stimulants have limited clinical use. Caffeine is incorporated in many headache preparations because it constricts cerebral vessels, thus reducing blood flow to the brain.

Uses

- Increase alertness and wakefulness
- Reverse the effects from an overdose of central nervous system depressants
- Treat migraine headaches
- Treat respiratory depression

Adverse Effects

- Dysrhythmias
- Severe tachycardia
- Severe hypertension
- Clonic-tonic seizures that may be fatal
- Severe muscle spasms (opisthotonos)
- Fetal abnormalities
- Tolerance and abuse

Precautions

- Analeptic stimulants are contraindicated in clients who are hypersensitive to these agents.
- Analeptic stimulants should be discontinued slowly; rapid discontinuation may produce nausea, vomiting, and headaches.

Important Drugs

Caffeine

- In low to moderate amounts, caffeine increases alertness and decreases fatigue.
- Two to three cups of coffee (250 mg or more of caffeine) may cause excessive stimulation of the CNS, resulting in nervousness, restlessness, and insomnia.
- Caffeine is found in coffee, tea, some soft drinks (e.g., Coca-Cola, Dr. Pepper, Pepsi, Diet Pepsi), analgesics (Anacin, Cafergot, Darvon, Excedrin), stimulants (No-Doz, Vivarin), menstrual drugs (Midol), cold tablets (Dristan Decongestant), chocolate, and foods containing chocolate (e.g., chocolate milk, chocolate cake).
- Caffeine acts as a weak diuretic, and can increase the basal metabolic rate.
- Caffeine is also a methylxanthine, which is a xanthine derivative. Xanthine derivatives are used primarily to treat respiratory diseases.

Doxapram hydrochloride (Dopram) is a respiratory stimulant that is used to treat respiratory depression.

Theophylline, a methylxanthine, is primarily used to treat respiratory diseases.

Therapeutic Nursing Interventions

- Assess client for amount of daily intake of caffeine in drinks and over-the-counter (OTC) drugs.
- Assess client for signs and symptoms of adverse responses to analeptic drugs.

Client Education

- Limit amount of caffeine intake per day to avoid symptoms of caffeinism.
- If ingesting excessive amounts of caffeine, reduce caffeine intake gradually in order to avoid withdrawal symptoms (nausea, vomiting, and headaches).
- Check labels of OTC drugs to see if they contain caffeine.

Psychomotor Stimulants

Overview

Psychomotor stimulants include the amphetamines and other drugs that are pharmacologically similar to amphetamine. Amphetamines are primarily stimulants of the cerebral cortex. They also act as anorexiants. **Anorexiants** suppress the appetite, and were once used extensively for weight control. The practice of giving amphetamines for weight control is no longer accepted as good practice. While psychomotor stimulants have limited use today, they are prescribed for severe obesity, narcolepsy, and ADHD (attention deficit hyperactivity disorder). ADHD is characterized by a level of activity that is excessive.

Uses

- ADHD
- Narcolepsy
- Weight reduction when all other methods of weight control have failed
- Depression
- Symptoms of withdrawal from addictive drugs that have been abused

Adverse Effects

- Nervousness, irritability, and extreme talkativeness
- Insomnia
- Headaches
- Tachycardia and other cardiac dysrhythmias
- Anorexia, weight loss, and fatigue
- Vomiting and diarrhea
- Dry mouth
- Increased libido
- Tolerance and dependence

Precautions

- Psychomotor stimulants, such as amphetamines, are contraindicated in clients with hyperthyroidism, hypertension, hyperexcitability, cardiovascular diseases, glaucoma, and hypersensitivity to amphetamines.
- These drugs should be taken with caution when driving a vehicle or operating machinery.
- Amphetamines should be administered with caution to clients taking antidepressants because antidepressants increase the effects of amphetamines.

- Amphetamines can be dangerous because clients may abuse them along with alcohol and other drugs.
- Health care professionals and those who work late or irregular shifts are particularly susceptible to amphetamine abuse.

Important Drugs

Methylphenidate (Ritalin)

- Methylphenidate, a Schedule II drug, is the agent of choice for treating narcolepsy and ADHD.
- Structured treatment interruptions (drug holidays) for children should coincide with school vacations.
- The rationale for giving this drug is that minimal brain dysfunction arises from a disruption of norepinephrine metabolism.
  - By stimulating norepinephrine release, methylphenidate can restore brain chemistry to a normal state.

Pemoline (Cylert), a Schedule IV drug, is used also used to treat ADHD, but it is not as effective as other psychomotor stimulants.

- It is similar in structure to the amphetamines.
- Liver function tests should be monitored during long-term therapy.

Amphetamine sulfate is used to treat narcolepsy and attention deficit disorder.

Methamphetamine hydrochloride (Desoxyn) is used to treat ADHD and obesity.

Dextroamphetamine sulfate (Dexedrine) is used to treat ADHD and narcolepsy.

Therapeutic Nursing Interventions

Weight reduction

- Encourage a planned weight loss and exercise program for clients taking amphetamines to reduce weight.
- Weigh clients prior to and weekly throughout the program; obtain height and bone structure measurements.
- Have client maintain a diet history and record of all food and fluid intake.
- Monitor for cardiac symptoms, hyperexcitability, hypertension, and signs of hyperthyroidism throughout the program.

Narcolepsy

- Obtain a complete history of sleep irregularities and seizures.
- Assess the client's neurologic status and provide a complete baseline neurologic examination.
- To decrease episodes, suggest a varied, stimulating daily routine at work and home.
- Refer the client to a counselor if the person is having problems interacting with family and business associates.

ADHD (attention-deficit hyperactivity disorder)

- Obtain the child's history and conduct a physical examination.
- Assess the child for motor incoordination and clumsiness.
- Obtain school records. Note how the child performs in reading and writing activities. Question how the child interacts with teachers and fellow students.

- Obtain the family history and assess for a familial pattern of ADHD.
- Administer drugs in the morning and again at noon, as required.
- Monitor children closely for weight loss.
- With the parents, plan drug-free holidays for the child.
  - These should be on weekends or holidays.
  - During these periods, evaluate the effectiveness of the drug and the dosage.
- Children may need to take these drugs for several years for maximum therapeutic effect.

Client Education

- If taking psychomotor stimulants for weight loss:
  - Develop a realistic goal and time frame for losing weight.
  - Follow a weight-reduction diet and exercise daily while taking the medication.
  - Realize that psychomotor stimulants are a temporary adjunct to diet and exercise.
  - Take medication to suppress appetite 30-90 minutes before meals because drug action peaks around an hour following administration.
  - Avoid drinking caffeinated drinks and taking other stimulating drugs.
  - Avoid taking amphetamines close to bedtime because they cause insomnia.
- If taking psychomotor stimulants for narcolepsy:
  - Avoid routine, boring tasks if possible.
  - Avoid air travel and shift work because these activities cause a greater number of narcolepsy attacks.
  - Take medication around times of peak sleepiness for maximum effect.
- Advise families of children who are taking psychomotor stimulants for ADHD to:
  - Monitor the effects of different drug dosages in order to find the dosage needed for optimum therapeutic effect.
  - Plan for drug-free holidays with the nurse or primary care provider.
  - Evaluate their child for improvement in relationships, self-image, and learning skills.

Nonamphetamine Anorexiants

Overview

Anorexiants are classified as sympathomimetic drugs. Anorexiants suppress the appetite by depressing the central nervous system appetite center in the brain. The practice of routinely giving anorexiants for weight control is no longer accepted.

Uses

- Exogenous obesity on a short-term basis
- Nasal congestion

Adverse Effects

- Stroke
- Seizure
- Heart attack
- Arrhythmia
- Psychosis
- Death
- Hypersensitivity
- Eating disorder

Precautions

- Epilepsy
- Hyperthyroidism
- Some cardiac disorders
- Hypertension
- Glaucoma
- Depression

Important Drugs

Phentermine hydrochloride (Fastin) is used in the short-term management of obesity.

Phenmetrazine (Preludin) has the same uses as phentermine hydrochloride.

Diethylpropion hydrochloride (Tenuate) has the same uses as phentermine hydrochloride. This drug has precipitated pulmonary hypertension (rarely).

Therapeutic Nursing Interventions

- Encourage a planned weight loss and exercise program for clients taking amphetamines to reduce weight.
- Weigh clients prior to and weekly throughout the program; obtain height and bone structure measurements.
- Encourage client to maintain a diet history and record of all food and fluid intake.
- Consult a dietitian for developing a well-balanced nutrition plan.
- Persons with anorexia nervosa are at increased risk for substance abuse with non-amphetamine anorexiant drugs.
- Monitor for cardiac symptoms, hyperexcitability, hypertension, and signs of hyperthyroidism throughout the program.

Client Education

- Develop a realistic goal and time frame for losing weight.
- Follow a weight-reduction diet and exercise daily while taking the medication.
- Realize that psychomotor stimulants are a temporary adjunct to diet and exercise.
- Take medication to suppress appetite 30-90 minutes before meals because drug action peaks around an hour following administration.

- Avoid drinking caffeinated drinks and taking other stimulating drugs.
- Avoid taking amphetamines close to bedtime because they cause insomnia.

Drugs That Depress The Central Nervous System

Overview

Sedative, hypnotic, and anxiolytic drugs are classified as central nervous system (CNS) depressants. Sedatives are drugs that produce relaxation and decrease anxiety. Hypnotics are drugs that produce sleep. Hypnotic agents generally have a peak onset of hypnotic effects 15 to 30 minutes after ingestion. Anxiolytics (antianxiety drugs) are used to control anxiety and to relieve apprehension. Sedatives, hypnotics, and anxiolytics have the potential for causing dependence and abuse. These drugs can help to alleviate insomnia and symptoms of anxiety, but they do not alter the life situations and stressors that cause the symptoms. Client should be educated about how CNS depressants can help them cope with life's problems, but they should not rely on these medications to solve their problems. Sedatives and hypnotics can cause hypersensitivity reactions, extreme drowsiness, rebound insomnia, and respiratory depression. Older clients are usually more sensitive to adverse effects from central nervous system depressants and dosages should be adjusted accordingly.

Sedatives and Hypnotics

Overview

The effects of most sedatives and hypnotics are dose-related. In small doses, they induce sedation, while in larger doses they cause drowsiness or sleep. In very large doses, many hypnotics induce general anesthesia. The ideal hypnotic (which has not yet been developed) would:

- Induce sleep soon after administration.
- Promote natural sleep without disrupting normal patterns of sleep stages.
- Allow sleep to end at the usual time of awakening.
- Produce no "hangover."
- Sedatives and hypnotics are usually classified as barbiturates, non-barbiturates, and benzodiazepines.

Barbiturates

Overview

Barbiturates are used for hypnotic and sedative actions. Barbiturates depress the central nervous system, respirations, heart rate, blood pressure, body temperature, and rapid eye movement sleep. Barbiturates are metabolized by the liver and excreted by the kidneys. They do not relieve pain or insomnia caused by pain. Most barbiturates are scheduled drugs. An overdose of barbiturates can produce severe toxicity. Psychological and physical dependence on barbiturates is a serious problem. Withdrawal effects from barbiturates can equal or surpass those of narcotics. Even though barbiturates are considered prototype drugs, they are in limited use today. They have been largely replaced by the benzodiazepines. Two barbiturates still remain in common usage:

- Thiopental (Pentothal) for anesthesia
- Phenobarbital (Nembutal), which is administered for seizures

Uses

- Treat seizures
- Promote anesthesia
- Promote sedation in low doses and sleep in larger doses

Adverse Effects

- Drowsiness, dizziness, and confusion
- Hangover effect
- Anxiety, restlessness, and disorientation
- Sleep disruption due to REM (rapid eye movement) rebound
- Slow respirations proceeding to respiratory depression
- Pinpoint pupils
- Barbiturate poisoning: disorientation, confusion, memory loss, and weight loss

Precautions

- Barbiturates are contraindicated for clients with:
  - Debilitation due to illness
  - Severe respiratory disorders
  - Hypersensitivity reactions
  - History of drug or alcohol abuse
  - Severe liver or kidney disease
  - Intermittent porphyria (a disease of porphyria metabolism)
- Barbiturates should be administered with great caution to pregnant women as they may cause fetal abnormalities and can produce drug dependence in the newborn.
- Barbiturates should not be abruptly discontinued. The client should be weaned from the drug over a period of 2-3 weeks.
- Barbiturates should not be taken at the same time as alcohol or other CNS depressants because sedative effects are dangerously enhanced.
- Barbiturates should be administered cautiously to elderly clients and should be taken early in the evening to prevent drowsiness during the day.

Important Drugs

Thiopental sodium (Pentothal) is administered IV for anesthesia.

Phenobarbital sodium (Luminal, Nembutal) is given for seizures.

Secobarbital sodium (Seconal) is given for preoperative sedation, status epilepticus, acute tetanus convulsions, and the short-term treatment of insomnia.

Amobarbital (Amytal) is administered to produce sleep.

Therapeutic Nursing Interventions

- Take the client's sleep history, inquire about recent sleep patterns, and ask the client if there is a problem that could be causing insomnia.
- Monitor the client during sleep if possible.
- Do not wake the client to administer a sleep medication.
- Provide safety measures to prevent falls, such as placing the client's bed in a low position, putting up the side rails, and accompanying the client to the bathroom. Be sure that the client can always reach the call button.
- Observe the client for adverse effects from barbiturates such as confusion or slurred speech.
- Assess rate and depth of respirations for slowing of rate and shallow respirations.
- Do not administer barbiturates to clients with shallow respirations, or a respiratory rate that is less than 10 breaths per minute.
- Notify the primary care provider if the client requests higher and more frequent doses of a barbiturate.
- Monitor the client carefully for barbiturate overdose, barbiturate dependency and abuse, or suicidal threats. Report adverse findings immediately to the primary care provider.

Client Education

- Recognize barbiturates are habit-forming drugs and should only be taken for a short time period, such as 2-3 weeks.
- Avoid driving vehicles or operating machinery while under the influence of these drugs.
- Abstain from drinking alcohol while taking barbiturates to prevent dangerous over- sedation.
- Never smoke when taking these drugs because of the danger of falling asleep and accidentally starting a fire.
- Take the drug exactly as ordered and do not increase the dosage without first talking with the primary care provider.
- Do not abruptly stop taking the drug. Consult with primary care provider and then gradually wean self off of the drug.

Nonbarbiturates

Overview

Nonbarbiturates are Schedule III or Schedule IV controlled substances. Non-barbiturates are similar to the barbiturates in many ways. Some nonbarbiturates can be purchased over-the-counter for sleep.

Important Drugs and Uses

Buspirone (BuSpar), a prescription drug, is used to manage anxiety.

- Differs chemically and pharmacologically from other anti-anxiety drugs.

Chloral hydrate (Noctec), a prescription drug, is the oldest of the non-barbiturates.

- It is a relatively safe drug, and is available in capsules and syrup.
- It is better suited for putting people to sleep than keeping them asleep.
- Chloral Hydrate is used in pediatrics as a preprocedure drug.

Zolpidem tartrate (Ambien) is a Schedule IV prescription drug used for the short-term management of insomnia.

Paraldehyde (Paral) is a prescription liquid medication used for sedation and to treat alcoholic withdrawal symptoms.

Hydroxyzine (Vistaril) is a prescription antihistamine that is used to induce sleep. It is also used as a pre-and postoperative antiemetic.

Diphenhydramine hydrochloride (Benadryl) is a non-prescription antihistamine used to treat mild insomnia.

Adverse Effects

Buspirone (BuSpar)

- This drug is generally well tolerated.
- The most common side effects include:
  - Light-headedness
  - Headache
  - Nausea
  - Nervousness
- Less commonly, abdominal distress, insomnia, nightmares, and tinnitus

Chloral hydrate (Noctec)

- Common side-effects include:
  - Lethargy
  - Dizziness
  - Confusion
  - Excitability (paradoxical reaction)
  - Hallucination
  - Abdominal distress
- Abrupt withdrawal can lead to delirium and seizures.
  - Without treatment, abstinence syndrome can be fatal.
- This drug is metabolized in the liver; therefore, high doses or long-term treatment can lead to hepatic impairment.

Zolpidem (Ambien)

- Common side effects include:
  - Headache
  - Drowsiness

Hydroxyzine (Vistaril)

- The most common side effect is sedation.
- High doses may cause anticholinergic effects, such as dry mouth.
- Adverse reactions are rare, including skin rash or seizure.

Paraldehyde (Paral)

- Local effects cause irritation to the oral mucosa.
  - Injection may produce tissue necrosis and nerve damage.
- Symptoms of toxicity are serious and potentially life-threatening, including:
  - Hypotension
  - Respiratory depression
  - Liver failure
  - Bleeding gastritis
  - Pulmonary hemorrhage

Therapeutic Nursing Interventions

Buspirone (BuSpar)

- Administer with food to prevent gastric irritation.
- The effects are delayed and make take 2-4 weeks for full effectiveness. Other antidepressant therapy may not be discontinued or tapered slowly until a therapeutic level is achieved.

Chloral hydrate (Noctec)

- This Schedule IV drug has the potential for abuse and addiction.
- Chloral hydrate (Noctec) can interfere with urine glucose testing in diabetics. Those persons should be advised to monitor blood levels while receiving this medication.
- It may be mixed with fruit juice to conceal the flavor and improve compliance with taking the dose, particularly with children. Flavoring from the pharmacy can be added.
- Administer with meals and at least 8 ounces of fluid to decrease gastric irritation.

Zolpidem (Ambien) is a newer drug with no established dose for children under 18 years of age.

Hydroxyzine (Vistaril)

- Monitor vital signs, neuromuscular functioning and anxiety level in clients receiving hydroxyzine (Vistaril).
- Administer into the deep tissue by IM injection only. The Z-track method is preferred. Subcutaneous, intravenous or intra-arterial may cause significant damage.

Paraldehyde (Paral)

- Discard solution after 24 hours because of its rapid decomposition.
- Dilute in milk or juice to mask the flavor.

Client Education

Buspirone (BuSpar)

- Buspirone and hydroxyzine (Vistaril) may cause dry mouth.
  - Take ice chips, gum or hard candy to reduce the side effect.
- The client should be advised to immediately report chest pain, alterations in mentation or sensation to extremities.

- Buspirone is a non-sedative and does not interfere with driving or other activities of daily living.

Chloral hydrate (Noctec)

- Capsules should be swallowed without chewing or crushing. The oral form commonly causes heartburn, nausea and flatulence.
- Chloral hydrate (Noctec) causes sedation. Avoid driving or engaging in activity that requires alertness.
- Do not consume alcohol or other CNS depressant medication while taking this drug.

Zolpidem (Ambien)

- Do not consume alcohol or other CNS depressant medication while taking this drug.
- Take on an empty stomach because food decreases the drug absorption.

Paraldehyde (Paral)

- Do not keep this medication in the home, particularly if small children reside there, because of the potential for poisoning.

Benzodiazepines

Overview

Benzodiazepines have largely replaced the barbiturates as drugs of choice for insomnia because they are safer and have a lower potential for abuse. These agents are classified as Schedule IV controlled substances because of their potential for abuse. Benzodiazepines cause the release of gamma-aminobutyric acid (GABA) substances, which inhibit the transmission of impulses in the CNS.

Uses

- Induce sleep
- Treat insomnia
- Reduce anxiety
- Promote muscle relaxation
- Treat acute alcohol withdrawal
- Promote relaxation prior to surgery or other procedures
- Control seizures
- Treat status epilepticus

Adverse Effects

- Oversedation
- Ataxia
- Memory loss
- Anterograde amnesia (amnesia for events that occurred after the administration of a drug or a particular event)
- Hangover
- Euphoria, excitement, and confusion

- Hypotension
- Respiratory depression
- Gastrointestinal disturbances
- Headache
- Jaundice and rashes
- Withdrawal syndrome characterized by high anxiety
- Benzodiazepine toxicity, due to intentional or accidental overdose

Precautions

- Benzodiazepines should be administered cautiously to the elderly who are at an increased risk of becoming oversedated and falling.
- Benzodiazepines should not be taken with CNS depressants such as alcohol, narcotics, antihistamines, and barbiturates because these substances potentiate the effects.
- These agents should not be abruptly discontinued because of the danger of withdrawal symptoms including anxiety, dysphoria, insomnia, irritability, acute psychosis and seizures. Benzodiazepines should be tapered over a 6-8 week period.
- Benzodiazepines are contraindicated for pregnant women, particularly during the third trimester. The neonate may be born physically dependent and experience withdrawal symptoms.

Important Drugs

Temazepam (Restoril) is used to treat insomnia.

Diazepam (Valium) is used to treat short-term anxiety and seizures.

Clonazepam (Klonopin) is used to treat seizure disorders and panic disorders.

Flurazepam hydrochloride (Dalmane) is used to treat insomnia.

Estazolam (ProSom) is used to treat insomnia.

Quazepam (Doral) is used to treat insomnia.

Triazolam (Halcion) is used for the short-term treatment of insomnia.

Flumazenil (Romazicon) is a benzodiazepine antagonist and the specific antidote for benzodiazepine overdose.

Therapeutic Nursing Interventions

- Provide safety measures to prevent falls: place bed in low position, put up the side rails, and accompany the client to the bathroom. Be sure that the client can always reach the call button.
- Assess for slowing of respiratory rate and shallow respirations.
- Do not administer benzodiazepines to clients with a respiratory rate that is less than 10 breaths per minute, or with shallow respirations.
- Evaluate client carefully for adverse effects from the benzodiazepines.
- Have flumazenil (Romazicon) on hand. It is the specific antidote for benzodiazepine toxicity.
- Monitor elderly clients closely because they are especially sensitive to the hypnotic effects of drugs, and are at greater risk for falls.

Client Education

- Take the medication during or immediately after meals to avoid gastrointestinal symptoms.
- Recognize that benzodiazepines are controlled substances and should be taken only as ordered.
- Avoid driving vehicles or operating machinery while under the influence of these drugs.
- Abstain from drinking alcohol while taking benzodiazepines to prevent dangerous over- sedation.
- Never smoke when taking these drugs because of the danger of falling asleep and starting a fire.
- Immediately report adverse effects to health care provider.
- Never abruptly discontinue these medications because of danger of withdrawal symptoms including sezures, but taper off use over a 6-8 week period.

Anxiolytics (Antianxiety Drugs)

Overview

Although some degree of anxiety is a normal response to episodic stress or situational difficulty, the degree to which anxiety interferes with daily living, decision-making, and the ability to function warrants consideration for treatment. The levels of anxiety may range from mild (tension and worry) to panic (overwhelming state wherein the person can't function independently). If anxiety is severe or prolonged, therapeutic intervention may be indicated, particularly for disorders involving phobias, obsessive-compulsive behaviors, generalized anxiety, or panic disorders.

An anxiolytic drug reduces or relieves anxiety. Increased doses may produce sleep. This classification was previously referred to as tranquilizers. Diazepam (Valium), the prototype for anxiolytic drugs, was developed in the 1960s. It was a landmark drug because it was effective in reducing anxiety. It was thought to be non-addictive; however, the risk for dependency is now well known. Overdose of benzodiazepines is not as toxic as barbiturates. Barbiturates were previously prescribed for anxiety-related symptoms or disorders.

Uses

- Anxiety
- Depression with anxiety
- Muscle tension
- Insomnia
- Symptoms from drug withdrawal
- Preoperative medications

Adverse Effects

- Oversedation
- Ataxia

- Increased risk of falls and accidents
- Hypotension
- Decreased respiratory rate and depth
- Dependence, tolerance, and abuse
- Benzodiazepine toxicity due to intentional or accidental overdose

Precautions

- Many of the precautions for anxiolytic drugs are the same as for the benzodiazepines.
- Anxiolytic drugs should be taken with caution by women who are pregnant or lactating, and by clients with a history of alcoholism or other drug abuse.
- Anxiolytic drugs are contraindicated for clients with severe respiratory disorders because these agents depress the respiratory system.

Important Drugs

Benzodiazepines (used for the purpose of relieving anxiety)

- **Diazepam** (Valium), a long-acting drug (20-50 hours), is the prototype for anxiolytic drugs.
  - Used to treat anxiety, epilepsy, muscle spasm, and panic disorder
  - Also prescribed as a preoperative medication
- May be given orally or by IV, and it can be taken once daily at bedtime
  - Clients should sleep well and benefit from the anxiolytic action throughout the day.
  - The disadvantage of diazepam and other longer-acting benzodiazepines is that the client experiences a more prolonged hangover when the drug is discontinued.
- **Chlordiazepoxide** (Librium) is a long-acting drug (5-30 hours) used to relieve anxiety and anxiety associated with depression.
- Also prescribed as a preoperative medication

Halazepam (Paxipam) is used to treat anxiety.

Lorazepam (Ativan) is used to treat anxiety associated with depression.

- Also prescribed as a preoperative medication

Prazepam (Centrax) is used to treat anxiety associated with depression.

Flumazenil (Romazicon) is a benzodiazepine antagonist and the specific antidote for benzodiazepine overdose.

Diphenhydramine hydrochloride (Benadryl) is a non-prescription antihistamine used to treat mild insomnia.

Buspirone (BuSpar) is used to manage anxiety, but differs chemically and pharmacologically from other antianxiety drugs.

Chloral hydrate (Noctec) is the oldest of the prescription non-barbiturates

Zolpidem tartrate (Ambien) is a Schedule IV prescription drug used for the short-term management of insomnia.

Therapeutic Nursing Interventions

- Assess client for signs and symptoms of severe anxiety or panic.
- Evaluate the client's level of stress and coping skills.
- Evaluate the client's sleep habits, and ask about any problems with insomnia.
- Monitor the client for signs of tolerance and physical dependence on anxiolytic drugs.
- Assess the client's suicide risk from drug overdose, and immediately alert the primary care provider if a risk exists.
- Encourage the client to talk about his or her anxiety and the problems that may be causing it.
    - Acknowledge the client's feelings.
- Provide the client with information that will help to decrease or alleviate anxiety- provoking problems.
- Perform the therapeutic nursing interventions that are appropriate for clients taking benzodiazepines.

Client Education

- Seek professional counseling for anxiety symptoms.
- Learn meditation and guided imagery techniques that can produce calm feelings and reduce anxiety.
- Perform at least 15-30 minutes of physical exercise daily to "work off" anxiety.
- Watch for signs of tolerance and physical dependency (e.g., the amount of medication originally prescribed is no longer adequate to control the anxiety).
- Abrupt discontinuation of the medication can result in withdrawal reaction.
- The medication will affect coordination and motor skills. Do not operate heavy equipment, motor vehicles, or participate in any other activity requiring alertness and coordination.
- Avoid alcohol and other CNS depressants because of the enhanced effects.

Drugs That Treat Mood Disorders

Overview

Mood is a predominant, sustained emotion that affects a person's perception of the world. Moods fluctuate constantly on a continuum between normal/ functional moods and abnormal/dysfunctional moods. Mood disorders are classified as depressive disorders and bipolar disorders. Antidepressants and mood stabilizing agents are the major drug categories used to treat mood disorders.

Antidepressants

Overview

Clinical depression is a mental disorder characterized by an altered, sad mood; a sense of dejection; feelings of worthlessness and hopelessness; loss of appetite; weight loss, or weight gain; insomnia or hypersomnia; loss of energy and profound fatigue; an inability to concentrate; and sometimes, thoughts of death and plans for suicide. The specific cause of depression is unknown, although there are many theories. One theory is that either serotonin, norepinephrine, or both are reduced in depression, while an excess of norepinephrine is produced in mania. Antidepressants may act to alter this biochemical imbalance. In the 1950s, drugs were discovered that could effectively treat depression.

The tricyclic antidepressants (TCAs) and monoamine oxidase (MAO) inhibitors were among the first antidepressants to be developed. The primary clinical indication for antidepressants is major depressive illness. Antidepressants also treat panic disorder as well as enuresis in children. People who respond to the initial course of antidepressant treatment should continue to take the same drugs at the same dosage for 4-9 months. Once clients are symptom free, the drugs can be tapered. Clients with a history of 3 or more episodes of major depression have a 90% chance of having another episode, and, therefore, are candidates for long-term therapy. Antidepressants are classified into the following major groups:

- Cyclic antidepressants (tricyclic and tetracyclic antidepressants)
- Selective serotonin reuptake inhibitors
- MAO inhibitors
- Atypical antidepressants

Cyclic Antidepressants

Overview

Cyclic antidepressants include tricyclic and tetracyclic antidepressants. They are called "cyclic" because the nucleus of these drugs is composed of one or more rings. Cyclic antidepressants prevent the reuptake of norepinephrine and serotonin, thereby increasing concentration levels of these neurotransmitters. The drugs in this group are structurally dissimilar, but they share similar clinical effects and adverse reactions. The long half-life of cyclic antidepressants allows them to be administered once daily. Most cyclic antidepressants cause minor discomfort, but others cause serious illness.

Side effects are usually dose-related. The dosage of these drugs can be gradually increased after the body has had time to adjust. Because of their many adverse effects, cyclic antidepressants are no longer considered the initial drugs of choice for depression. However, they continue to be prescribed for clients who do not respond to other antidepressants. Cyclic antidepressants must be taken for 3-4 weeks or longer before there is a therapeutic response. Plasma levels must be monitored to keep these drugs within the therapeutic range, which ensures that enough medication is available for effectiveness. Cyclic antidepressants have no abuse potential.

Uses

- Short-term depression
- Long-term depression
- Eating disorders
- Chronic headaches
- Insomnia

Adverse Effects

- Dry mouth
- Decreased gastric motility
- Menstrual irregularities
- Blurred vision
- Urinary hesitancy
- Constipation
- Orthostatic hypotension
- Migraine headaches
- Fine tremor
- "Switch process" (depression switches to mania)
- Confusion and delirium in older clients
- Symptoms of acute poisoning include:
    - Cardiac irregularities
    - Hallucinations
    - Bowel or bladder paralysis
    - Respiratory depression

Precautions

- Cyclic antidepressants should be administered with great caution to clients who are at risk of suicide.
    - These drugs are among the most lethal when taken in large doses.
        - 1000-3000 mg can be lethal. This amount of the drug may represent barely a one- week supply.
- These agents should be administered cautiously to clients with panic disorder because cyclic antidepressants have adverse effects that mimic the symptoms of panic (e.g., rapid heart rate, dizziness, nausea, and blurred vision).
- Cyclic antidepressants should be given cautiously to older clients and to clients with a history of heart disease.
- Cyclic antidepressants should not be taken concomitantly with alcohol and other antidepressants because of the potential for overdose or suicide.
- Clients should be withdrawn gradually from these drugs to avoid withdrawal syndrome, which is characterized by malaise, aches, chills, nausea, coryza, and dizziness.

Important Drugs

Imipramine hydrochloride (Tofranil) is the oldest tricyclic antidepressant, and it is the prototype for antidepressants.

Amitriptyline hydrochloride (Elavil) is used to treat depression, often in combination with psychotherapy.

Doxepin hydrochloride (Sinequan) is similar to imipramine in structure and effect. It primarily produces sedation and is useful in the treatment of agitated clients.

Maprotiline (Ludiomil) is a tricyclic antidepressant with anticholinergic properties.

Therapeutic Nursing Interventions

- Administer the drug in a single dose at bedtime to reduce oversedation during the day.
- Draw blood to check plasma level to ensure the drug is circulating within therapeutic levels, and enough of the drug is available for effectiveness.
- Recommend that the client seek mental health counseling in conjunction with taking antidepressant drugs. These drugs help to control the symptoms of depression, but they do not alleviate problems.
- Provide safety measures to prevent falls, such as placing the client's bed in a low position, putting up the side rails, and accompanying the client to the bathroom. Be sure the client can always reach the call button.

Client Education

- Be patient. It takes 1-3 weeks for these drugs to have a therapeutic effect.
- Take drug in one dose at night (per prescription order) to avoid daytime sedation.
- Avoid drinking alcohol or taking other CNS depressants at the same time as cyclic antidepressants to avoid dangerous oversedation.
- See a mental health counselor for help with emotional problems.
- Immediately inform health care provider if depression deepens or suicidal feelings develop.

Selective Serotonin Reuptake Inhibitors (SSRIs)

Overview

The selective serotonin reuptake inhibitors (SSRIs) represent a newer approach to the treatment of clinical depression, and they are generally safer than other antidepressants. SSRIs cause an increase of available serotonin. These drugs have antidepressant effects similar to the cyclic antidepressants, but without the anticholinergic, cardiovascular, and sedative side effects.

Uses

- Depression
- Dysthymia
- Bulimia
- Obsessive-compulsive behavior

Adverse Effects

- Nausea
- Decreased appetite and weight loss
- Diarrhea
- Insomnia or drowsiness
- Headache
- Dry mouth
- Nervousness and anxiety

- Mania
- Male sexual dysfunction
- Dizziness
- Sweating
- Seizures

Precautions

- SSRIs are contraindicated for clients who are taking MAO inhibitors because this drug combination can cause serious and even fatal results. At least 5 weeks should pass following discontinuation of MAO inhibitors before taking SSRIs.
- SSRIs should be administered with caution to clients with anxiety disorders or mania.
- These agents should be administered with caution to clients with severe kidney or liver disease. The primary care provider should reduce the dosage for these clients.
- SSRIs should be administered with caution to clients who are taking anticoagulants because both categories of drugs are protein-bound.
- Clients taking SSRIs should be closely supervised because of the risk of suicide due to depression.

Important Drugs

Fluoxetine (Prozac) was the first SSRI on the market. It has few side effects compared with other antidepressants.

Sertraline (Zoloft) is used to treat:

- Depression (in association with psychotherapy)
- Panic disorder
- Obsessive-compulsive disorder (OCD)
- Post-traumatic stress disorder (PTSD)

Paroxetine (Paxil) is used to treat:

- Depression
- Panic disorder
- OCD
- Social anxiety disease

Therapeutic Nursing Interventions

- Recommend that the client seek mental health counseling in conjunction with taking SSRIs.
- Administer drug with meals to prevent gastrointestinal symptoms.
- Monitor client for improved mood, or for increased depression and suicidal tendencies.
- Weigh client weekly and observe for weight loss, which is a side effect of the drug.
- Provide safety measures to prevent falls such as placing the client's bed in a low position, putting up the side rails, and accompanying the client to the bathroom.
    - Be sure the client can always reach the call button.

Client Education

- It takes 1-3 weeks for drugs to have a therapeutic effect.
- Take medication early in the day to prevent insomnia.
- Take medication at bedtime if daytime drowsiness is a problem.
- Suck on hard candy to relieve dry mouth.
- Eat a bland diet to prevent diarrhea.
- Perform relaxation techniques to relieve nervousness.
- Take a mild non-opioid analgesic to relieve headache.
- Take medication following sexual relations to prevent male sexual dysfunction.
- Perform good hygiene if sweating is a side effect.
- Never abruptly stop taking this medication without first consulting with the primary care provider.

Monoamine Oxidase (MAO) Inhibitors

Overview

MAO inhibitors block the action of monoamine oxidase, which are a group of enzymes present in brain, liver, kidney, spleen cells and blood platelets.

- These enzymes are able to metabolize epinephrine, norepinephrine, and serotonin, which are neurotransmitters.
- By inhibiting the action of monoamine oxidase, MAO inhibitors interfere with the degradation of epinephrine, norepinephrine and serotonin, and increase the levels of these neurotransmitters.
- The therapeutic effect of monoamine oxidase (MAO) inhibitors on depression supports the theory that depression is caused by low levels of norepinephrine and/or serotonin.

MAO inhibitors generally have fewer anticholinergic, cardiovascular, and sedative effects than other antidepressants. These agents are nonaddicting and clients do not develop tolerance. Clients should be on appropriate dietary restrictions several days before starting the drug, and for two weeks after the drug has been discontinued.

Uses

Depression that does not respond to:

- Other antidepressant drugs
- Psychotherapy
- Electroconvulsive shock therapy (EST)

Adverse Effects

- Orthostatic hypotension
- Weight gain
- Sexual dysfunction
- Edema

- Toxicity from overdose: insomnia, agitation, confusion, and convulsions
- Hypertensive crisis when taken with foods that contain tyramine
  - Tyramine is an amino acid released from proteins in foods when they undergo hydrolysis by fermenting, aging, smoking, pickling, or spoiling.
  - Tyramine is deactivated by MAO in the gut wall and liver.
  - When MAO enzymes are inhibited, tyramine may cause the release of large amounts of norepinephrine and cause a hypertensive crisis.
  - Hypertensive crisis may be fatal.

Precautions

- MAO inhibitors must be taken in conjunction with special dietary restrictions that reduce the ingestion of tyramine and caffeine.
- MAO inhibitors should not be taken concomitantly with other prescription or OTC medications without the primary care provider's permission, because of the possibility of severe drug interactions.
- These agents should be administered with caution to clients with cardiovascular disease, liver disease, kidney disease, hypertension, pheochromocytoma, or an inability to comply with dietary restrictions.
- MAO inhibitors should not be given concomitantly with meperidine (Demerol) because the combination could cause a hypertensive crisis. Meperidine is contraindicated for 21 days following cessation of MAO inhibitors.

Important Drugs

- Phenelzine sulfate (Nardil) is used to treat neurotic depression associated with anxiety when client has been unresponsive to other antidepressants.
- Tranylcypromine sulfate (Parnate) is used to treat severe depression in hospitalized clients.

Therapeutic Nursing Interventions

- Provide client with a list of foods that should be avoided because they contain tyramine, which could precipitate a hypertensive crisis.
- Weigh the client upon starting drug therapy and throughout the course of therapy. Document weight gain.
- Educate client's family members and friends about depression and its therapy.

Client Education

- Comply with dietary restrictions, and avoid these foods that are high in tyramine:
  - Cheese, except for cottage cheese
  - Pizza with cheese
  - Fermented or pickled foods
  - Beer or red wine
  - Chocolate
  - Yogurt
  - Meat extracts
  - Avocados, raisins, figs
- Avoid alcohol while taking this medication because of sedating effects.

- Avoid any medications that might contain tyramine during and for at least two weeks following cessation of drug therapy.
- Consult with the primary care provider before taking any other medications, including OTC medications.
- Avoid caffeinated drinks and medications containing caffeine because of the risk of hypertensive crisis.
- Change positions gradually to avoid orthostatic hypotension.
- Notify health care provider immediately if any adverse effects develop.
- Carry an identification card that provides information about the MAO inhibitor drug regime and dietary restrictions.

Mood Stabilizing Drugs

Overview

Lithium is the drug of choice for the long-term management of bipolar disorder (also called manic-depression). Bipolar disorder is characterized by mood swings or cycles of acute mania, followed by acute depression, with periods of normalcy. The manic phase is characterized by an elevated and expansive mood and irritability. The exact mechanism by which lithium stabilizes mood swings is not clear.

Lithium appears to inhibit the release of both norepinephrine and dopamine, and it also increases reuptake of catecholamine transmitters. This action corrects the catecholamine response for clients with bipolar disease. There is a direct relationship between sodium intake and lithium excretion. A lowered sodium intake slows the excretion of lithium and results in accumulation. The body does not metabolize lithium. Lithium is excreted entirely by the kidneys. Thus, it is essential for the client to have functioning kidneys. The onset of acute antimanic effects of lithium usually occurs within 5-7 days.

Until therapeutic levels (0.6 to 1.2 mEq/L) are attained, symptoms of agitation may be controlled with haloperidol (Haldol) or chlorpromazine hydrochloride (Thorazine). The client may report slight nausea, thirst, weakness, tiredness, and loose stools during the first week of therapy. A complete therapeutic response usually occurs in about 3 weeks. Usually, the client must continue lithium therapy for years.

Uses

- Lithium salts are used to treat bipolar disease.

Adverse Effects

- Muscle twitching
- Diarrhea
- Loss of appetite
- Weight gain
- Dizziness
- Visual disturbances
- Severe thirst

- Metallic taste in mouth
- Oliguria
- Convulsions and death
- Hyperthyroidism (long-term lithium therapy)

Precautions

- Lithium is contraindicated for clients who have had leukemia because the leukemia may be reactivated by taking lithium.
- Lithium should be administered with caution to pregnant women, and to clients with renal or cardiovascular disease, severe dehydration, or sodium depletion, or who are taking diuretics or nonsteroidal anti-inflammatory agents.
- Dosages of lithium should be lowered for elderly clients because of their decreased renal and cardiovascular function.

Important Drugs

Lithium carbonate (Eskalith, Lithane, Lithonate) tablets or capsules

Lithium citrate syrup (Cibalith-S)

Therapeutic Nursing Interventions

- Assess client's mood and behavior before starting lithium therapy and monitor mood changes throughout the course of therapy.
- If the client is highly agitated, administer haloperidol (Haldol) or chlorpromazine hydrochloride (Thorazine) during the initial 6-10 days after starting lithium therapy.
- Monitor serum lithium levels 2-3 times per week for at least 2 months, to ensure lithium levels have not exceeded the therapeutic range.
- Monitor input and output (I & O) and encourage a fluid intake of at least 2000-3000 mL per day to prevent drug toxicity.
- Assess for signs of urinary tract dysfunction and monitor for serum creatinine levels > 1.2 mg/dL.
- Monitor client for signs and symptoms of lithium overdose or toxicity, and immediately report manifestations to the primary care provider.
- Weigh client at least every 3 months and monitor for weight gain.

Client Education

- Closely follow the prescribed dosage schedule because the range of therapeutic effectiveness for this drug is very narrow.
- Never double the dosage if a dose is missed. Contact the primary care provider immediately for instructions.
- Expect slight nausea, thirst, weakness, tiredness, loose stools, and frequent urination during the first week of therapy. If symptoms continue after the first week, notify the health care provider.
- Expect that it will take at least 1 or 2 weeks of drug therapy before symptoms improve.
- Take lithium with food or milk to lessen gastrointestinal symptoms.

- Drink at least 2-3 quarts of water a day to prevent dehydration, which can precipitate drug toxicity.
- Avoid increasing or decreasing the amount of salt intake per day without talking with the primary care provider. A lowered sodium intake slows the excretion of lithium and results in accumulation of the drug.
- Carry an identification card that states that you are taking lithium medication.

Drugs That Treat Psychiatric Disorders

Overview

Antipsychotic drugs are also called psychotropic drugs, psychoactive drugs, or neuroleptic drugs. Psychosis is the major indication for the use of these drugs. Schizophrenia is the most common functional psychosis. Schizophrenia is not a single disease but a group of psychiatric alterations. Antipsychotic drugs are also used to treat visual, auditory, or olfactory hallucinations, delusions, and extreme agitation. Antipsychotic drugs do not cure psychosis. However, they do help clients maintain their lives outside of mental institutions, and they increase clients' abilities to cope with stressors in the environment. When used in conjunction with other therapies, antipsychotic drugs are a valuable part of the client's total care.

There is no "perfect" antipsychotic drug, because all of these medications produce severe adverse effects. High-potency drugs are more likely to produce extrapyramidal adverse effects, while low-potency agents produce sedation and hypotension. Most antipsychotic drugs are equally effective in equivalent doses. The drug of choice is usually the one the client can best tolerate. The oral or intramuscular route may be chosen, although the oral route is used more frequently. There are two major categories of antipsychotic drugs: phenothiazines and non-phenothiazines.

Phenothiazines

Overview

Most of the currently used antipsychotic drugs are in the phenothiazine class. The prototype for the phenothiazines is chlorpromazine (Thorazine). The action of the phenothiazines is not clearly understood. These drugs apparently block dopamine receptors in the limbic system of the brain. Dopamine is a neurotransmitter that carries signals between nerve cells. The limbic system is the major system for regulating emotion and controlling patterns of behavior. Drugs that increase dopamine levels, such as the amphetamines, can cause schizophrenic symptoms: delusions, hallucinations, inappropriate affect, and social isolation. Approximately one-third to as many as one- half of all clients experience some type of extrapyramidal adverse effect from taking antipsychotic drugs.

Phenothiazines are not addictive. Optimum therapeutic effects for psychoactive drugs may take up to 6-7 weeks. Antipsychotics are highly lipophilic and protein bound, so they accumulate in body tissues. Drug effects continue for weeks or even months after the last dose.

Uses

- Psychiatric disorders:
  - Schizophrenia
  - Acute mania
  - Psychotic depressions
- Nausea and vomiting
- Intractable hiccups

Adverse Effects

Extrapyramidal reactions can appear after one or more doses, and they are common responses to antipsychotic drug therapy:

Parkinsonism

- Mask-like facial expression
- Muscular rigidity and tremors
- Drooling and restlessness
- Decrease in reciprocal arm movements when walking
- Pin-rolling motion of the fingers

Akathisia

- Extreme restlessness occurs weeks to months into treatment
- Involuntary motor restlessness (moves lips and taps feet)
- Compulsion to walk

Acute dystonia

- Disordered muscle tonicity
- Uncoordinated jerking
- Spastic movements of face, neck, eyes, tongue, and limbs
- Respiratory distress
- Facial grimacing and frequent blinking
- Torticollis or opisthotonus
- Oculogyric crisis (eyes roll back)

Tardive dyskinesia

- Abnormal muscle movements around the mouth
- Lip smacking
- Tongue darting
- Constant chewing
  - This is the most serious extrapyramidal side effect.
  - In 10-20% of clients receiving long-term therapy, some symptoms are late to develop.
  - Symptoms are generally irreversible.

Perioral tremor (rabbit syndrome)

- Tremor similar to Parkinsonism

Neuroleptic malignant syndrome

- Catatonia
- Fever
- Erratic blood pressure

Anticholinergic adverse effects

- Dry mouth
- Blurred vision
- Constipation
- Urinary retention
- Edema and weight gain

- Postural hypotension
- Tachycardia as compensatory for decreased blood pressure
- Agranulocytosis and reduction in the number of circulating neutrophils
- Cholestatic hepatitis (edema of bile ducts)
- Menstrual irregularities
- Decreased libido
- Lowering of seizure threshold
- Excessive sedation (most likely during first few days of treatment, tends to decrease over time)
- Hypo/hyperthermia (due to CNS effects); client may be unaware of potentially dangerous body temperature changes
- Jaundice, which may indicate severe hepatotoxic hypersensitivity reaction
- Photosensitivity

Precautions

- Phenothiazines should be administered with caution to elderly clients because they are at greater risk of developing adverse effects.
- These agents should be administered with caution to clients with bone marrow depression, cardiovascular disease, alcoholism, liver disease, Parkinson's disease, glaucoma, peptic ulcer, and respiratory disorders.
- Phenothiazines are contraindicated for clients who are hypersensitive to these drugs.
- Clients taking phenothiazines should avoid alcohol due to additive sedative effects.

Important Drugs

Chlorpromazine (Thorazine, Ormazine) is the prototype for the phenothiazines. This drug is usually administered intramuscularly in an emergency situation because it rapidly calms the client who is extremely agitated.

Fluphenazine (Permitil, Prolixin) is used to manage psychotic disorders and neurogenic pain.

Trifluoperazine (Stelazine, Suprazine) produces less sedation but more extrapyramidal side effects.

Therapeutic Nursing Interventions

- Obtain the client's psychiatric history, and assess client's behavior before starting antipsychotic drug therapy.
- Monitor psychiatric changes throughout the course of therapy. Observe for presence or absence of hallucinations, delusions, sleep disturbances, and paranoia. Look for subtle clues that suggest a client is responding to the medication.
- Distinguish between akathisia (an adverse effect of the drug) and agitation due to psychosis.
- Avoid extrapyramidal effects by giving the smallest possible dose, as ordered.
- Administer medication either by mouth or by intramuscular injection. Administer IM injections slowly and deeply into the tissue. Massage the injection site to reduce pain.
- When giving medication orally, make certain that the client swallows the medication.
- When giving medication IV, monitor for hypotension. Also, take care to avoid extravasation because of tissue irritation.
- Administer prophylactic anticonvulsant medications, if ordered, to raise or increase the seizure threshold.
- Monitor blood pressure and observe for hypotension.
- Because client compliance is very important, take additional time to teach clients and their families about antipsychotic medications.

Client Education

- Be patient because sedative effects are prominent during the first week of therapy, and therapeutic effects may take from several days to 6 or 7 weeks to develop. Full improvement could take up to 6 months.
- Wear protective clothing when out in the sun because these drugs cause photosensitivity.
- Report adverse effects to health care provider.
- Take care when driving or operating machinery because of sedative effects of drugs.
- Take medication exactly as ordered.

Non-phenothiazines

Overview

While most antipsychotic drugs are classified as phenothiazines, there are a number of non-phenothiazines. Non-phenothiazines are atypical antipsychotics that control the negative symptoms of psychosis (e.g., flat affect), as well as the positive symptoms (e.g., hallucinations), whereas traditional antipsychotic drugs reduce only the positive symptoms. Non-phenothiazines are also useful for clients who do not tolerate traditional agents. They reduce symptoms not responsive to traditional antipsychotic agents and produce less:

Extrapyramidal symptoms: Involuntary movements, including tremors, athetoid movement, motor restlessness, apprehension and irritability, facial movements and tongue thrusting, shuffling gait, drooling, cogwheel movement with rigidity, and slow movement

Tardive dyskinesia: Involuntary movements marked by rhythmic, wormlike motion involving the tongue, facial muscles, fingers and toes, often in the form of chewing, lip smacking, facial tics, and rocking

Uses

- Schizophrenia
- Depression with psychotic features
- Organic brain syndrome
- Drug-related psychosis
- Delirium
- Dementia
- Acute and chronic psychosis
- Tourette's syndrome
- Severe behavioral problems in children

Adverse Effects

Clozapine (Clozaril)

- The most significant side effects are:
  - Life-threatening agranulocytosis (a significant decrease in the number of neutrophils)
  - Neuroleptic malignant syndrome (fever, tachycardia, respiratory distress, seizure, pallor, diaphoresis, incontinence, and muscle rigidity)
  - Lowered seizure threshold
- Other effects include:
  - Transient fever during the first few weeks of therapy
  - Constipation
  - Hypotension
  - Tachycardia
  - Dizziness
  - Sedation

Haloperidol (Haldol)

- Seizures
- Neuroleptic malignant syndrome
- Blurred vision
- Dry conjunctival and buccal membranes
- Constipation
- Extrapyramidal symptoms

Precautions

- Contraindicated for clients with:
  - Bleeding disorders
  - History of bone marrow depression
  - Pregnancy and lactation
- Cautious use for clients with:
  - Narrow-angle glaucoma
  - Benign prostatic hypertrophy
  - Seizure disorder
- Cautious use for children (safety not established)

Important Drugs

Thiothixene (Navane) is used to treat clients with chronic schizophrenia who are unresponsive to other antipsychotic agents.

Haloperidol (Haldol) is prescribed for acute and chronic psychoses, Tourette's syndrome, and severe childhood behavioral disorders. This drug is contraindicated for clients with Parkinson's disease because it causes severe extrapyramidal effects.

Clozapine (Clozaril) is used for clients with schizophrenia who are unresponsive to other antipsychotic agents. Because clozapine may cause agranulocytosis (a significant decrease in the number of neutrophils), it is important for the client to undergo weekly blood tests. Drug therapy should be discontinued at the first sign of bone marrow failure.

Molindone (Moban) causes less weight gain than other antipsychotic drugs.

Loxapine (Loxitane) is similar to haloperidol. It causes a moderate degree of sedation and few anticholinergic effects, but frequently leads to extrapyramidal effects.

Risperidone (Risperdal) helps to control the symptoms of psychotic disorders.

Olanzapine (Zyprexa) helps to control the symptoms of psychotic disorders.

Therapeutic Nursing Interventions

- For a client taking clozapine (Clozaril), determine the baseline white blood cell (WBC) count prior to start of treatment, and then weekly for the first four weeks of treatment. Report neutropenia to the prescribing provider.
- Monitor blood pressure and pulse prior to administration.
- Monitor for tachycardia and hypotension, particularly if the client is taking higher doses.
- Assess for signs of tardive dyskinesia or extrapyramidal symptoms. Report finding to health care provider. Reduction in dose or change to another medication may be necessary.
- Provide safety precautions for the client with seizure risk. Clozapine lowers the seizure threshold.
- Assess for signs of dehydration, particularly in elderly persons. Provide fluids as needed.

- High-fiber diet with liberal fluid intake may be needed for constipation effects of the drug.
- After injection of the medication, the client should maintain a recumbent position for 30 minutes.
- Carefully assess the mental status and responsiveness to therapy.
- Assess for signs of neuroleptic malignant syndrome. Report symptoms immediately.
- Electrocardiogram (ECG) may be necessary for the client taking haloperidol (Haldol).
    - Can cause QT-interval changes in some persons.

Client Education

- Consume a high-fiber diet and increase fluid intake to prevent constipation.
- Administer with food or liquids to minimize gastric irritation. Do not take with coffee or tea.
- Take any missed dose as soon as it is remembered. Do not skip doses.
- Avoid driving and any other activity requiring mental alertness while taking the drug, particularly in the first few weeks until a stable, therapeutic effect is achieved.
- Use sunscreens, sunglasses and protective clothing when exposed to the sun to prevent photosensitivity reactions.
- Consult with health care provider before taking any OTC medication, particularly cough suppressants.
- Avoid alcohol and other CNS depressants during treatment.

Drugs That Treat Seizures

Overview

Drugs that are prescribed to treat epilepsy and other seizure disorders are called antiseizure medications or anticonvulsants. A **seizure** is a sudden, uncontrolled episode during which there is a paroxysmal discharge of neurons in the brain. **Epilepsy** is a chronic disorder characterized by sporadic recurrent seizures resulting from a brain dysfunction or an abnormal discharge of neurons. About 1% of the population has epilepsy. About 70% of seizures do not have an identifiable cause; these are called idiopathic or primary seizures.

Other causes of seizures are:

- Head injury
- Cerebral vascular accident (CVA)
- Brain tumors
- Drug toxicity
- Metabolic imbalances

The most common types of seizures are:

- Simple partial or focal seizures, which usually do not involve a loss of consciousness.

- Complex partial seizures (temporal lobe seizures or psychomotor seizures), which impair consciousness.
- Absence seizures (formerly called petit mal), which are characterized by a very brief loss of consciousness.
- Generalized seizures are bilaterally symmetric and do not have a local onset. These include tonic seizures, clonic seizures, tonic-clonic (grand mal) seizures, and atonic seizures (drop attacks).
- Status epilepticus is a life-threatening emergency characterized by generalized tonic-clonic convulsions, which last for 30 minutes or more without the client regaining consciousness.

Antiseizure drugs act to depress abnormal electrical activity in the brain, control seizure activity, and allow the client to live a normal life. The principles of anticonvulsant therapy include the following:

- Start with a single drug, and increase the dosage until the seizures have stopped.
- If the first drug fails to stop the seizures, try a second drug.
- To guide dosage, the primary care provider should use the drug's therapeutic range. The therapeutic range is the drug serum level below which seizures continue, and above which the drug produces toxic effects.
- Use two drugs if necessary to control seizures.

Noncompliance with the drug regime is the major reason for the failure of seizure control. Seizures may result from the abrupt discontinuation of antiseizure drugs. Thus, drugs should be discontinued gradually. Major classifications of antiseizure drugs are barbiturates, hydantoins, and benzodiazepines.

Barbiturates

Overview

Barbiturates control seizures by increasing the threshold for seizures. To be effective in controlling seizures, the client may require a loading dose of barbiturates.

Uses

- All types of seizures except for absence seizures.
- Status epilepticus, for which barbiturates are considered secondary drugs.
- Treatment and prevention of recurrent seizures in infants and young children, especially for the prevention of febrile seizures. Barbiturates are often administered concomitantly with phenytoin.

Adverse Effects

Most common

- Ataxia
- Dizziness
- Hangover effect and drowsiness
- Hypersensitivity reaction

Less common

- Constipation
- Nausea and vomiting
- Insomnia and restlessness
- Night terrors
- Stevens-Johnson Syndrome (also called erythema multiforme major), a severe inflammatory disease mostly occurring in persons ages 20-40 that can result in death. Symptoms include:
    - Skin rash (usually on the legs, feet, arms and hands)
    - Fever
    - Extreme fatigue
    - Joint pains
    - Vision abnormalities (bloodshot eyes, eye pain, burning, itching)
    - Respiratory infection
    - Vomiting or diarrhea

Precautions

- Barbiturates are contraindicated for clients with:
    - Debilitation
    - Severe respiratory disorders
    - Hypersensitivity reactions
    - History of alcohol or drug abuse
    - Severe liver or kidney impairment
- Use cautiously with elderly persons to prevent drowsiness during the day or increased confusion. Measures to ensure safety are especially important for these clients.
- A paradoxical reaction can occur, resulting in CNS excitation (restlessness, anxiety, irritability, tachycardia, and insomnia).
- Acute toxic effects can be potentially lethal. Symptoms include bradycardia, respiratory distress, ataxia, and extreme weakness.

Important Drugs

Phenobarbital sodium (Luminal) is a long-acting barbiturate.

- Phenobarbital is used for generalized and tonic-clonic partial seizures.
- It also effective for status epilepticus, and is used to treat febrile seizures in children.
- The half-life of barbiturates is long (60-120 hours).
- CNS depression is a major adverse effect of phenobarbital.

Primidone (Mysoline) is a barbiturate used in the management of psychomotor seizures and generalized tonic-clonic (grand mal) seizures. It is also used to treat essential tremor.

Therapeutic Nursing Interventions

- Take the client's history of seizures. Inquire about the events and client behaviors prior to, during, and after a seizure. Assess the duration and characteristics of the seizures.
- Record the medications the client has been taking to control seizures.
- Evaluate the impact of seizures on the client's mental health and life.
- Assess the client's sleep patterns prior to starting medication, and throughout course of therapy.
- Evaluate the client's response to the drug dosage. Report if the client is continuing to have seizures or if the person is experiencing adverse effects.
- Have primary care provider adjust the dosage for better control of seizures and adverse effects.
- Provide safety measures to prevent falls, such as placing the client's bed in a low position, putting up the side rails, and accompanying the client to the bathroom. Be sure that the client can always reach the call button.
- Observe the client for adverse effects from barbiturates such as confusion or slurred speech.
- Do not administer barbiturates in persons with respiratory rates less than 10 breaths/minute.
- Pregnant clients receiving barbiturates in the last month prior to delivery may need exogenous vitamin K injections to prevent hemorrhagic complications. Inform primary care provider of the client's medication history.

Client Education

- Take the drug exactly as ordered, and abide by drug regime completely.
- Follow list of written instructions on how to take anticonvulsant drugs.
- Mark each dose down on a calendar or in a date book.
- Use a pill box or container compartmentalized by day to keep track of daily medications.
- Use daily routines, such as meals or watching a special news program, as reminders to take medications.
- Avoid driving or operating machinery until response to the drug is known.
- Avoid drinking alcohol or using products that contain alcohol, such as mouthwash and certain OTC medications.
- Avoid taking any other medications without first consulting with the primary care provider.
- Carry an identification card that states you are on anticonvulsant therapy.
- Do not abruptly stop taking the drug without consulting with primary care provider. Usually the medication is weaned slowly with seizure precautions.
- Clients taking oral contraceptives should be advised to use a non-hormonal method of pregnancy prevention with concurrent use of barbiturates.

Hydantoins

Overview

Hydantoins are antiseizure drugs that reduce seizure focal activity, and thus the spread of abnormal electrical discharges to other areas of the brain. Hydantoins do not produce serious adverse effects at therapeutic levels.

Uses

- Hydantoins are prescribed for all types of seizures except absence seizures.

Adverse Effects

- Gingival hyperplasia, which is an overgrowth of gum tissue due to altered collagen metabolism. It may develop during long-term therapy, and it is a common sign of toxicity in children and adolescents.
- Nausea and vomiting
- Sedation
- Blood dyscrasias
- Rashes
- Dysrhythmias
- Hypotension

Precautions

- Hydantoins are contraindicated for clients who are hypersensitive to these drugs.
- Hydantoins are also contraindicated for clients with severe liver, kidney, or thyroid disorders, alcoholism, blood dyscrasias, diabetes mellitus, and cardiac impairment.
- Hydantoins should be administered with caution to elderly clients, debilitated clients, and pregnant women because of the danger of fetal abnormalities.
- Osteomalacia has been associated with phenytoin therapy and appears to be caused by the interference of phenytoin with vitamin D metabolism. Clients with osteoporosis, rickets, osteogenesis imperfecta, or disorders of vitamin D metabolism should take phenytoin with caution and for short-term use only.

Important Drugs

Phenytoin (Dilantin) is usually the initial drug of choice for seizure control.

- It is used for tonic-clonic and some psychomotor seizures.
- Phenytoin is only soluble in alkaline solutions, and thus it must be given in NS solution.
- Rapid IV infusion of phenytoin can produce cardiovascular collapse.
- Adverse effects are gastric irritation, gingival hypertrophy, and skin rash.
- Phenytoin may increase the incidence of congenital defects in the newborn.

Fosphenytoin (Cerebyx) can be given IV or IM to clients who cannot take oral phenytoin. It may be mixed in either normal saline solution or D5W, and it can be given IV more rapidly than phenytoin.

Mephenytoin (Mesantoin) is not as effective a drug as other hydantoins, and it produces a higher incidence of blood dyscrasias and skin rashes.

Therapeutic Nursing Interventions

- Obtain client's history of seizures.
- Monitor laboratory studies to make certain the client is maintaining a therapeutic serum level of the drug. Therapeutic serum concentrations of phenytoin (Dilantin) are 10-20 mcg/mL.
- Administer medication with food if client experiences gastric distress.
- When giving these agents per IV, check the rate every minute to detect dangerous toxic effects.
- Check the IV site for extravasation of the solution, which can cause tissue sloughing.
- If the IV fluid is infiltrating, stop the infusion immediately and call the primary care provider.
- Assess the client's mouth and gums for gingival hyperplasia.
- Monitor laboratory tests for signs of blood dyscrasia, liver dysfunction, and renal dysfunction.

Client Education

- Take medication exactly as ordered and comply with the therapeutic program.
- Observe for gum changes or bleeding, and use good oral hygiene.
- See the dentist on a regular schedule for oral examinations and teeth cleaning.
- Take medication with food to minimize gastric irritation.

Benzodiazepines

Overview

Benzodiazepines are used to suppress seizure activity by causing the release of a substance called gamma-aminobutyric acid (GABA), which inhibits nerve transmission.

Uses

- Anticonvulsant therapy for status epilepticus or severe, recurrent seizures
- Sedative or hypnotic uses (preoperative sedation)
- Alcohol withdrawal
- Sleep disorders
- Neuromuscular disease

Important Drugs

Clonazepam (Klonopin) is used to treat absence seizures and myotonic seizures.

Diazepam (Valium) is the drug of choice for the treatment of status epilepticus.

Lorazepam (Ativan, Alzapam) is used to treat status epilepticus.

Clorazepate (Tranxene) is used to treat absence seizures and myotonic seizures.

Adverse Effects

- Drowsiness, fatigue, and lethargy
- Muscular incoordination
- Ataxia
- Hypotension
- Dizziness
- Anorexia

Therapeutic Nursing Interventions

- Provide safety measures to prevent falls: place bed in low position, put up the side rails, and accompany the client to the bathroom. Be sure that the client can always reach the call button.
- Assess for slowing of respiratory rate and shallow respirations.
- Do not administer benzodiazepines to clients with a respiratory rate that is less than 10 breaths per minute, or with shallow respirations.
- Evaluate client carefully for adverse effects from the benzodiazepines.
- Have flumazenil (Romazicon) on hand. It is the specific antidote for benzodiazepine toxicity.
- Monitor elderly clients closely because they are especially sensitive to the hypnotic effects of drugs. Also, the elderly are at greater risk for falls.
- For long-term therapy, monitor laboratory findings and report abnormalities indicating liver or renal impairment.

Client Education

- Take the medication during or immediately after meals to avoid gastrointestinal symptoms.
- Recognize that benzodiazepines are controlled substances and should be taken only as ordered.
- Avoid driving vehicles or operating machinery while under the influence of these drugs.
- Abstain from drinking alcohol while taking benzodiazepines to prevent dangerous over-sedation.
- Never smoke when taking these drugs because of the danger of falling asleep and starting a fire.
- Immediately report adverse effects to health care provider.
- Never abruptly discontinue these medications because of the danger of withdrawal symptoms, but taper off use over a 6-8 week period.

Other Anticonvulsants

Important Drugs

Carbamazepine (Tegretol) is used to treat absence and mixed seizures.

Ethosuximide (Zarontin) is the drug of choice for absence seizures.

- Gastric irritation is the most common side effect.

- More serious side effects are blood dyscrasias, hepatic damage, and renal damage.

Felbamate (Felbatol) has a structure similar to meprobamate (Equanil) and is primarily used for partial seizures.

Gabapentin (Neurontin) is used to treat clients with partial seizures.

- Clients with renal disorders may require a reduced dosage because gabapentin is excreted entirely by the kidneys.
- Antacids are not given within 2 hours of administering gabapentin because they reduce the usefulness of the drug by 20%.

Lamotrigine (Lamictal) is used to treat clients with partial seizures. This medication can cause Stevens-Johnson syndrome, which is characterized by a fever and a widespread, severe cutaneous rash.

Phensuximide (Milontin) is used primarily for absence seizures.

Primidone (Mysoline) is used to treat all seizure disorders except for absence seizures. This drug can be substituted for phenobarbital in the treatment of seizures.

Trimethadione (Tridione) is used to treat refractory absence seizures. Originally the drug of choice for absence seizures, trimethadione has been largely replaced by the newer valproic acid.

Valproic acid (Depakene) is the drug of choice for absence seizures.

- It is also used to treat myoclonic seizures, generalized tonic-clonic seizures, and atonic attacks.
- This medication is also prescribed to prevent migraine headaches.

Drugs That Treat Common Neurological Disorders

Drugs That Treat Parkinson's Disease

Overview

Parkinson's disease is a progressive, idiopathic neurologic disorder caused by depletion, degeneration, or destruction of dopamine in neurons located in the basal ganglia of the brain. Parkinsonism is an involuntary movement characterized by four cardinal features:

- Tremor at rest (usually begins with the hands and may also involve the head and the neck)
- Akinesia (complete or partial loss of muscle movements)
- Rigidity (increased muscle tone)
- Disturbance of posture and equilibrium

Clients with Parkinson's disease have symptoms such as shuffling gait, non-intentional tremor, mask-like facial expression, and weakness. Drugs, encephalitis, trauma, neurotoxins, and arteriosclerosis are the cause of 15% of Parkinson's diagnoses, while 85% of Parkinson's diagnoses are idiopathic (no apparent cause). There is no cure for Parkinson's disease. The goal for clients with Parkinson's disease is to allay the symptoms and help the client live as normal a life as possible. The pharmacologic goal of antiparkinsonism drugs is to strengthen dopaminergic action with dopaminergic drugs, or to reduce cholinergic action with anticholinergic drugs. The two major categories of antiparkinsonism drugs are dopaminergic drugs and anticholinergic drugs (antimuscarinics).

Dopaminergic Drugs

Overview

Dopaminergic drugs act in the brain to improve motor function by increasing the amount of dopamine concentration and enhancing neurotransmission of dopamine. There are six chemically unrelated drugs that act as dopaminergics.

Uses

- Control the symptoms of Parkinson's disease
- Do not help to control drug-induced extrapyramidal reactions

Adverse Effects

Early symptoms (to which client may become tolerant)

- Nausea and vomiting
- Anorexia
- Orthostatic hypotension
- Dizziness
- Dysrhythmias

Late symptoms that occur after long-term therapy

- **Involuntary movements** (dyskinesias)
  - May develop during the time of peak drug action
  - May develop at the end of period of drug action ("end-of-dose" failure)
  - Symptoms include facial grimacing, head bobbing, and rocking movements of the extremities and trunk
  - Symptoms affect approximately 15-40% of clients after 2-3 years of drug therapy, with frequency increasing after 5 years.
- **Akinetic spells**
  - Client becomes immobilized for periods. This is part of the "on/off" phenomenon during which clients has functional periods followed by dysfunctional periods.
- Severe anxiety
- Nightmares
- Depression
- Hallucinations
- Memory loss
- Psychotic behavior

Precautions

- Dopaminergic drugs are contraindicated for clients with narrow-angle glaucoma because it can cause mydriasis, which worsen the glaucoma.
- These drugs are also contraindicated for clients with a history of melanoma. Levodopa is suspected to be a precursor of melanin, a pigment that provides color to the skin and hair. Melanin stimulates melanomas to develop and grow.
- Dopaminergic drugs should be used with caution in clients with a history of gastrointestinal disease, heart disease, or psychiatric disorders.

Important Drugs

Levodopa or L-dopa (Dopar, Larodopa) is the most effective drug for Parkinson's disease.

- **Levodopa** is the immediate precursor to dopamine.
    - Dopamine cannot be used for replacement therapy because it does not enter the brain in sufficient amounts.
    - A small portion of levodopa enters the brain and is converted to dopamine.
- Levodopa is used to treat idiopathic types of Parkinson's disease. It is ineffective against drug-induced extrapyramidal reactions.
- Levodopa improves the functional capacity in about 75% of clients.
- The most distressing problem with levodopa is loss of effectiveness after 3-5 years. This problem takes one of two forms:
    - "On-off" phenomenon characterized by sharp fluctuations in the client's mobility/immobility
    - End of dose deterioration (a progressive decline in the duration of beneficial effects)
- Abrupt discontinuation of levodopa can cause neuroleptic malignant syndrome, which is a side effect of antipsychotic drugs.
    - This syndrome is caused by a rapid fall in brain dopamine levels.
    - It is characterized by high fever and muscle rigidity.
- The most common adverse effects of levodopa are nausea and vomiting, although some clients also develop anorexia.
- Tolerance to levodopa occurs in a few weeks, and may cause or worsen psychotic behavior and orthostatic hypotension.
- An early sign of drug toxicity is twitching of the eyelids.

Carbidopa-levodopa (Sinemet) allows more levodopa to be converted to dopamine in the brain by inhibiting peripheral conversion of levodopa to dopamine.

Therapeutic Nursing Interventions

- Assess client for symptoms of Parkinson's disease before and throughout drug therapy.
- Monitor client for early and late adverse effects produced by dopaminergic drugs.
- Assess client for depression, hallucinations, confusion, and other psychiatric problems.

- Assess client's skin on a routine basis for skin lesions, which could indicate drug- induced malignant melanoma.
- Assist the client with a "drug holiday" if prescribed by the primary care provider. The drug holiday may last as long as 14 days, depending on the client's reaction.
    - Taper off the medication over a three-day period and then discontinue as ordered.
    - Throughout the drug holiday, assess client's mobility, functional abilities, mental status, sleep patterns, respiratory function, speech, swallowing, and circulation. Observe for dyskinesia/dystonia.
    - During the "drug holiday," provide the client with physical therapy, diet therapy, elastic stockings, a water mattress, and turning assistance as needed.
    - Once the drug holiday is over, restart the medication and carefully assess the client's reaction.
    - Administer maintenance doses of the medication as prescribed and continue to assess client. Client's reaction to the medication should have improved.

Client Education

- Eat food shortly after taking the drug to reduce gastric irritation.
- Divide foods high in protein into several meals, because too much protein intake at one time may impair the action of the dopaminergic drugs.
- Avoid driving or operating machinery until action of the drug is known. These drugs can cause dizziness and confusion.
- Contact primary care provider before taking any OTC drugs, cold medications, or multivitamin preparations that may contain pyridoxine (vitamin B6) which can reverse the effects of levodopa.
- Expect harmless darkening of the sweat or urine.
- Stand up slowly from a lying position to avoid orthostatic hypotension.
- Report skin lesions immediately to the health care provider.

Anticholinergics (Antimuscarinics)

Overview

Anticholinergic drugs counteract the cholinergic activity in the brain that is believed to be present in Parkinson's disease. Only anticholinergics that are centrally active and cross the blood-brain barrier are used in the treatment of Parkinson's disease. Anticholinergics may be used alone or with amantadine (Symmetrel) in the early stages of Parkinson's disease, or they may be given with levodopa in the later stages.

Anticholinergics are not effective when used alone as the disease advances. Abrupt withdrawal of these agents can cause confusion, exhaustion, and exacerbation of symptoms. Atropine and scopolamine were the first anticholinergic agents to be used to treat Parkinson's disease. Synthetic drugs such as trihexyphenidyl (Artane) and benztropine (Cogentin) have now replaced these agents.

Uses

- Clients in the early stages of Parkinson's disease
- Younger clients who will need long-term therapy
- Clients with tremor and rigidity
- Drug-induced Parkinsonism

Adverse Effects

- Dry mouth
- Mydriasis
- Constipation
- Urinary retention
- Tachycardia
- Mental confusion and hallucinations

Precautions

- Anticholinergic agents should be administered with caution to very young or elderly clients because these individuals are more susceptible to toxic effects than adults.
- Anticholinergic agents are contraindicated for clients who are hypersensitive to these drugs, or who have narrow-angle glaucoma.
- These agents should be administered with caution to clients with prostatic hypertrophy or clients who may develop urinary retention as a side effect.
- Anticholinergic agents should be administered with caution to clients taking antihistamines, phenothiazines, tricyclic antidepressants, or digoxin because of adverse effects.

Important Drugs

Trihexyphenidyl (Artane) is the most frequently used anticholinergic.

- Prescribed for initial or adjunct treatment of all forms of Parkinsonism, including drug- induced disease.

Benztropine (Cogentin) may be useful in treating elderly clients who cannot tolerate the CNS stimulating properties of trihexyphenidyl (Artane).

Therapeutic Nursing Interventions

- Assess client for symptoms of Parkinson's disease before and throughout drug therapy.
- Monitor input and output (I & O) and assess for urinary retention.
- Assess client for nervousness, agitation, and other signs of psychiatric disturbances.
- If client cannot tolerate anticholinergic therapy, taper off the medication slowly as ordered to prevent a withdrawal reaction (insomnia, extrapyramidal symptoms, anxiety).

Client Education

- Sit up or stand up slowly to reduce orthostatic hypotension.
- Use mouthwash and chew sugarless gum to reduce dry mouth.

- Avoid becoming overheated during hot weather as anticholinergics reduce capacity to perspire. Remain in an air-conditioned environment.
- Eat high-fiber foods and drink at least eight 8-ounce servings of water daily to prevent constipation, a side effect of anticholinergics.
- Report adverse effects to the health care provider.

Other Antiparkinson Drugs

Amantadine (Symmetrel) is a dopamine receptor agonist and a synthetic antiviral agent used to prevent influenza A virus infection. It causes release of dopamine in the brain.

- This agent is prescribed during the early phases of Parkinson's disease when the client does not yet have tremor.
- During the later stages of the disease, the agent may be administered concurrently with an anticholinergic drug.
- Amantadine loses its effectiveness after several months. Thus it is necessary to interrupt treatment for several months, and then restart therapy.
- Adverse effects from amantadine are mottled purple-colored skin, edema, drowsiness, and confusion.
- These adverse effects are reversible within 2-6 weeks after discontinuing the drug.

Pergolide (Permax) is a dopamine receptor agonist that directly stimulates postsynaptic dopamine receptors.

- Pergolide helps to reduce tremor and improve posture, akinesia, rigidity, and equilibrium problems.
- The most frequent side effects include nausea, constipation, orthostatic hypotension, hallucinations, dyskinesia, somnolence, and rhinitis.

Pramipexole (Mirapex) is a nonergot dopamine receptor agonist, which is used to control the signs and symptoms of Parkinson's disease.

Ropinirole hydrochloride (Requip) is a nonergot dopamine agonist used to relieve the signs and symptoms of Parkinson's disease.

Bromocriptine (Parlodel), a dopamine receptor agonist, is more effective for treating Parkinson's disease than amantadine and anticholinergic drugs.

Selegiline hydrochloride (Eldepryl) is a monoamine oxidase type B inhibitor, which is prescribed as an adjuvant agent to levodopa/carbidopa to treat Parkinson's disease.

Entacapone (Comtan) inhibits the enzyme that breaks down levodopa, thereby enhancing its effects and increasing its duration of action.

Drugs That Treat Myasthenia Gravis

Overview

Myasthenia gravis is an autoimmune neuromuscular disease characterized by muscle weakness and abnormal fatigue that is relieved by rest. Other symptoms include:

- Drooping of the upper eyelid (ptosis) with a sustained gaze.

- Muscle weakness of the face resulting in an expressionless face, droopy eyelids, and a mouth that hangs open.
- Limb weakness.
- Extreme fatigue.

Exacerbations are precipitated by stress, hormonal changes, and the use of alcohol or other drugs, which include mycin antibiotics, quinidine, morphine, barbiturates, phenothiazines, and tranquilizers. Antimyasthenic agents treat myasthenia gravis, but they do not cure this disease. The goal of antimyasthenic therapy is to help the client maintain as normal a lifestyle as possible.

Antimyasthenic Drugs

Overview

Cholinesterase inhibitors comprise the major group of antimyasthenics. Immunosuppressant agents may also be used to repair the immunologic problem causing the disease. The dosage of cholinesterase inhibitors is individualized to the client's needs. The client usually begins drug therapy with a small dose of a cholinesterase inhibitor, and then progresses to 3 or 4 doses per day. Dosage requirements may change if the client develops any complications such as a respiratory infection, or is faced with increased emotional stress. Over time, antimyasthenic drugs may become less effective. "Drug holidays" are then used to restore their effectiveness.

Uses

- Enhance and prolong cholinergic nerve transmission, which helps to control the symptoms of myasthenia gravis
- Reverse the action of neuromuscular blockers, which are used during surgical anesthesia, electroconvulsive therapy, and intubation of clients

Adverse Effects

- General muscle weakness
- Increased bronchial secretions
- Weakness of respiratory muscles progressing to respiratory muscle paralysis
- Increased salivation and sweating
- Nausea and vomiting
- Bradycardia and decreased cardiac output progressing to cardiovascular collapse
- Hypotension
- Tremor
- Anxiety, confusion, and restlessness
- Convulsions and coma

Precautions

- Cholinesterase inhibitors are contraindicated for clients who are hypersensitive to these agents.
- These agents should be not be given with ganglionic blocking agents because this combination of drugs can cause severe hypotension.

- Cholinesterase inhibitors should be administered very cautiously with drugs that cause anticholinergic effects such as antihistamines, antidepressants, atropine, haloperidol, phenothiazines, and quinidine.
- Administration of too low a dose of cholinesterase inhibitors may result in myasthenic crisis, which is characterized by a sudden worsening of the symptoms, severe muscle weakness, and respiratory paralysis.
- Administration of an overdose of cholinesterase inhibitors may result in cholinergic crisis, which is characterized by abdominal cramps, diarrhea, dyspnea, and excessive pulmonary secretions.

Important Drugs

Neostigmine bromide (Prostigmin) is used in the diagnosis and treatment of myasthenia gravis. It blocks acetylcholinesterase, an enzyme that destroys acetylcholine.

Edrophonium chloride (Tensilon)

- Edrophonium is used to diagnose myasthenia gravis.
- It is also used to differentiate between myasthenia crisis (not enough medication is being administered) and cholinergic crisis (too much medication is being administered).

Pyridostigmine bromide (Mestinon) is the maintenance drug of choice for myasthenia gravis.

Atropine sulfate, an anticholinergic agent, is used as an antidote to counteract the severe adverse effects of cholinesterase inhibitors.

Therapeutic Nursing Interventions

- Assess for signs and symptoms of myasthenia gravis (drooping of the upper eyelid, double vision, and difficulty chewing and swallowing). Monitor for improvement in symptoms or increased symptoms.
- Assess for adverse effects of antimyasthenic medications.
- Assess respiratory rate and quality of respirations. Listen for increased bronchial secretions and diminished breath sounds.
- Administer the dosage of medication exactly as ordered and at the correct time in order to prevent myasthenic crisis or cholinergic crisis.

Client Education

- Plan on taking the medication for the rest of life.
- Take the correct dosage of the medication exactly on time to prevent myasthenic crisis or cholinergic crisis.
- Take the medication with food to decrease gastrointestinal adverse effects.
- Take the medication 30-60 minutes prior to meals to increase the muscle strength required to eat.
- Report adverse effects of drugs to health care provider.
- Carry an identification card at all times that details the medication regimen for myasthenia gravis.

Drugs That Promote Anesthesia

Overview

Anesthetic agents cause partial or complete loss of sensation with or without loss of consciousness. Anesthetics are usually administered by injection or inhalation. Only nurses who are trained as certified registered nurse anesthetists (CRNA) are allowed to give anesthetics. However, nurses need to be knowledgeable about anesthesia because they play active roles in all phases of perioperative care. The major types of anesthetic agents are general anesthetics and local/regional anesthetics.

General Anesthesia

Overview

General anesthesia is the administration of drugs that produce progressive, reversible central nervous system depression accompanied by a loss of consciousness. The three stages of general anesthesia are:

Induction: The administration of a sufficient amount of anesthetic to produce a loss of consciousness and the loss of response to sensations of pain, touch, taste, and temperature.

Maintenance: Maintaining the client at the desired level of anesthesia. During the maintenance stage, the anesthesiologist continually monitors the client's blood pressure, respirations, pulse, pupil response, reflexes, and eye movements.

Recovery: Reversal of anesthesia by either stopping the administration of the anesthetic or giving the client an antidote to the type of anesthetic agent administered.

Balanced anesthesia is the use of combinations of drugs to produce anesthesia. Drugs include sedative-hypnotics, antianxiety agents, analgesics, anticholinergics, and neuromuscular blocking agents. Sedative-hypnotics and antianxiety agents may be given either the night before surgery or a few hours before the surgery is scheduled. These agents decrease anxiety and generally make the administration of anesthesia easier for the client. Benzodiazepines such as diazepam (Valium) are used. Anticholinergics are given to prevent the vagal stimulation associated with general surgery and to reverse the effects of anesthesia after surgery. Analgesics potentiate the CNS depression produced by other drugs, and thus, fewer anesthetics may be required. Analgesics also make the client more comfortable during the perioperative period. Neuromuscular blocking agents are used to produce muscle paralysis. These drugs do not cause sedation, thus the client remains fully awake. These agents are prescribed for clients who are on ventilators. Succinylcholine (Anectine) is a commonly used neuromuscular blocking agent. Inhalation or intravenous routes are used for general anesthesia.

Inhalation Anesthesia

Overview

Inhalation anesthesia given in hospitals is usually administered with volatile liquid anesthetics, such as halothane. Gases such as nitrous oxide are used extensively in dental offices. Inhalation anesthesia is usually administered by means of a non- rebreathing valve-type delivery system. Other delivery systems (which are seldom used today) are the open system and closed system. Ideally, general inhalation anesthesia should induce unconsciousness and provide analgesia, muscle relaxation, and amnesia without adverse effects. However, because the ideal inhalation anesthetic does not yet exist, the following drugs are combined to produce the best anesthesia results:

- **Short-acting barbiturates** to induce anesthesia
- **Neuromuscular blocking agents** to promote muscle relaxation
- **Opioid analgesics** to provide analgesia
- **N_2O** (nitrous oxide) to provide analgesia

Uses

- General inhalation anesthetics are given to provide rapid and safe anesthesia while the client undergoes surgery or other major procedures.

Adverse Effects

- Respiratory depression
- Dysrhythmias
- Hypotension
- Cardiovascular depression and failure
- Nausea and vomiting
- Hypothermia
- Malignant hyperthermia (rapid body temperature increase accompanied by hypertension, tachycardia, and muscle rigidity)
- Aspiration pneumonia
- Nephrotoxicity
- Hepatotoxicity

Precautions

- Specific inhalation anesthetics are contraindicated for clients who have experienced hypersensitivity reactions to those anesthetics in the past.
- Inhalation anesthetics should be administered with caution to clients with chronic obstructive pulmonary disease (COPD), asthma, emphysema, or CHF (congestive heart failure (CHF).
- Inhalation anesthetics should be administered with caution to elderly clients because they may have pre-existing disorders that complicate recovery from anesthesia and surgery.
- Elderly clients may also have adverse reactions to the short-acting barbiturates, neuromuscular blocking agents, and opioid analgesics that are administered with the inhalation anesthetic.

Important Drugs

Nitrous oxide (N_2O)

- The first of the modern anesthetics
- This anesthetic is often called "laughing gas" because clients who inhale it act like they are intoxicated.
- Produces relatively light anesthesia
- Seldom used alone except for dental work and minor surgical procedures
- May also be administered during the second stage of labor
- Has relatively few major adverse effects, but has limited use

Halothane (Fluothane) is frequently used, especially for children. Unfortunately, halothane has a narrow safety range and it can severely depress the cardiovascular and respiratory systems.

Methoxyflurane (Penthrane) is the most powerful inhalation anesthetic available. Methoxyflurane is not often used because it produces many adverse effects and has a narrow safety range.

Enflurane (Ethrane) has effects that are similar to halothane. This anesthetic is administered to adults only.

Therapeutic Nursing Interventions

- Conduct a thorough preoperative physical assessment of the client, and obtain a complete medical history.
    - Note any risk factors that could cause adverse reactions to inhalation anesthesia such as COPD, asthma, emphysema, or heart disease.
    - Note if the client has any drug allergies, or has had any prior adverse reactions to anesthetics.
    - If so, notify the surgeon at once.
    - Ask when the client last ate solid food or drank any fluids. The client should not eat within 8 hours of the surgery, or ingest any fluids 4-6 hours prior to surgery.
    - Inquire about any prescribed, OTC, or recreational drugs that the client has taken within the last 72 hours. Recently ingested drugs may influence the choice of anesthetic.
    - Check with the client's primary care provider to determine if the dosage or schedule for regularly prescribed drugs should be altered due to the surgery.
    - Assess the client's psychological status. Report to the surgeon if the client is agitated, fearful of surgery, or is anxious about the anesthetic.
- Administer preoperative medications as ordered.
- Review and check-off each item on the preoperative checklist before transporting the client to the preanesthesia care unit. Make certain side rails are raised on the stretcher.
- Provide emotional reassurance if the client appears anxious or fearful.
- Provide the client's records and give a complete report to the preanesthesia staff.
- If possible, arrange for the anesthesiologist to visit with the client prior to surgery.

- During the immediate postoperative period, obtain information about the anesthesia the client received during surgery, as well as any adjunctive drugs.
- Place the client in a side-lying position or with the head to the side to prevent aspiration of fluids into the lungs. Protect the client from falls with raised side rails and safety straps.
- Provide postanesthesia care by continually assessing the client's:
  - Vital signs
  - Airway patency and ventilation
  - Body temperature
  - Level of consciousness
  - Skin color and condition
  - Blood oxygen levels
  - Mucous membranes, gums, and nail beds for cyanosis
  - Electrocardiogram (ECG) readings
  - Intake and output
  - Neuromuscular function
  - Movement of extremities
  - Pain level
- During the postanesthesia period, assess the client for the after-effects of anesthesia such as extreme drowsiness, retching and vomiting, irregular respiratory patterns, restlessness, or excitation.
- Notify the anesthetist if the client does not have a satisfactory return of sensation, grip, or gag reflex.
- Administer analgesics as ordered once the client starts to recover from the effects of the anesthesia and begins to experience pain.
- Administer antiemetic medications if the client develops nausea and vomiting, a common adverse effect from anesthetics.
- Ask the client to turn, breathe deeply, and cough in order to expel anesthetic gases and stop secretions from pooling.
- Ensure that the client who does not have a catheter voids at least 200 mL of urine within 6 hours after surgery. Anesthesia can temporary depress bladder function and suppress the urge to void. Palpate the bladder following voiding to assess for bladder distention.
- Mobilize the client as soon as possible after surgery to relieve abdominal distention and discomfort. Anesthetics and muscle relaxants decrease intestinal mobility and cause abdominal symptoms.
- Document all assessment and client reactions as well as nursing interventions.

Client Education

- Avoid eating for at least 8 hours prior to surgery, or drinking fluids for at least 4-6 hours prior to surgery to prevent aspiration during surgery.
- Remain in bed to prevent falls once preoperative medications have been administered. Preoperative medications are usually given 30-60 minutes prior to surgery.

- Following surgery, notify the nurse of nausea; an antiemetic can be given for relief.
- Ask the nurse for pain medication as soon as pain is felt.
- After being discharged home, notify the health care provider if unable to void or if only voiding small amounts of urine.
- Take postoperative medications exactly as ordered, and carefully follow postoperative instructions for wound care.
- Call health care provider with any questions or concerns.
- Schedule follow-up appointments with the surgeon for postoperative evaluation.

Intravenous Anesthesia

Overview

Intravenous anesthesia agents are used for the induction or maintenance of general anesthesia, and also to produce amnesia. The primary use for amnesic agents is to prevent memory and to reduce the emotional distress of the event. The drugs most commonly used for intravenous anesthesia are the ultra-short-acting barbiturates and the neuroleptics. Intravenous conscious sedation may be used for local, regional, and intravenous anesthesia. IV conscious sedation reduces the level of consciousness, but allows clients to maintain their airway independently and respond to verbal commands and physical stimulation. Conscious sedation has no effect on pain reduction, and thus clients do require medication for pain. To provide conscious sedation, nurses must receive special training and be certified by state laws to perform the procedure.

Uses

- Prior to the administration of general inhalation anesthesia
- Promote conscious sedation
- Promote amnesia concerning surgery
- Lessen anxiety concerning surgery

Adverse Effects

- Bronchospasm
- Apnea
- Laryngospasm
- Respiratory depression
- Cardiovascular depression
- Hypotension

Precautions

- Intravenous anesthetics are contraindicated for clients who have experienced hypersensitivity reactions to these anesthetics in the past.
- Intravenous anesthetics should be administered with caution to the elderly and clients with a history of cardiac, respiratory, or renal disease.

Important Drugs

Fentanyl citrate (Sublimaze) is an opioid narcotic that is used to produce a state of reduced awareness and reduced sensory perception.

Thiopental sodium (Pentothal) is a very short-acting barbiturate with a rapid onset. It has a duration of action of 15 minutes or less. This agent is one of the most popular barbiturate anesthetics. It is primarily used during the induction phase of anesthesia.

Methohexital sodium (Brevital) is a very short-acting barbiturate that is 5 times as strong as thiopental sodium. This agent may be employed during outpatient procedures or electroconvulsive therapy.

Ketamine (Ketalar) is a rapid-acting non-barbiturate best suited for short diagnostic or surgical procedures. It produces analgesia and amnesia, but not muscular relaxation. Ketamine is usually used to induce anesthesia or as an adjunct to it.

Propofol (Diprivan) is an intravenous sedative-hypnotic agent used for induction and/or maintenance of anesthesia or sedation as part of a balanced anesthetic technique.

- Not recommended for induction of anesthesia in clients less than 3 years of age or obstetric clients
- Not recommended for maintenance of anesthesia in clients less than 2 months of age

Therapeutic Nursing Interventions

- Instruct client concerning the effects of intravenous anesthetics and conscious sedation.
- Have emergency equipment available, such as suction, crash cart with a defibrillator, and positive pressure oxygen device.
- Protect client from injury or falls.
- Provide medication as ordered for pain relief following procedure.
- Monitor client following procedure for any adverse reactions or complications.
- Document all assessment and client reactions as well as nursing interventions.
- Approximately half of all persons receiving Ketamine (Ketalar) experience hallucinations. Premedication with diazepam (Valium) may alleviate the related anxiety.
- Keep environmental stimulation to a minimum during the recovery.
- Move and position the client slowly in the immediate recovery phase to prevent hypotension. Fluid or vasopressors may be necessary for the stabilization of blood pressure.
- Help the client to assume recumbent position if experiencing nausea and vomiting, dizziness, or syncope.
- Intravenous anesthetics are incompatible with a wide range of solutions. The nurse should consult with the pharmacist and drug formulary for any questions of compatibility. Any solution that is cloudy or contains precipitate should be discarded and reported to the pharmacist or prescribing practitioner.

Client Education

- Avoid eating for at least 8 hours prior to surgery, or drinking fluids for at least 4-6 hours prior to surgery to prevent aspiration during surgery.
- Remain in bed to prevent falls once preoperative medications have been administered. Preoperative medications are usually given 30-60 minutes prior to surgery.
- Following surgery, notify the nurse of nausea; an antiemetic can be given for relief.
- Ask the nurse for pain medication as soon as pain is felt.
- After being discharged home, notify the health care provider if unable to void or if only voiding small amounts of urine. Take postoperative medications exactly as ordered, carefully following postoperative instructions for wound care. Call health care provider with questions or concerns.
- Do not drive or ingest alcohol for 24 hours after recovery.
- Schedule follow-up appointments with the surgeon for postoperative evaluation.

Local/Regional Anesthesia

Overview

Local and regional anesthetics are administered to anesthetize small areas or larger areas of the body by acting on nerves or nerve tracts. The two major types of local anesthetics are amides and esters. To administer local anesthetics, nurses must receive special training and be certified by state laws. However, nurses are responsible for monitoring the client who is receiving local or regional anesthesia. Local and regional anesthetics may be classified as follows:

Surface or **topical anesthetics** may be in the form of an ointment, a solution, or a powder. They do not penetrate the skin.

Freezing is also used to provide local anesthesia.

Injectable local anesthetics block pain at the site into which they are administered. These agents are used for dental procedures and minor surgical procedures. Often epinephrine is included with the agent to constrict local vessels.

Spinal anesthesia is accomplished by injection of anesthetic either into the spinal canal or into the epidural space. Postoperatively, headache is the most common complaint by clients receiving spinal anesthesia.

A **caudal block** is placed near the sacrum, and a saddle block is given in the lower end of the spinal column to block the perineal area.

Intravenous regional anesthesia is anesthesia of an entire area of the body.

Uses

- Dental procedures
- Labor and delivery
- Minor surgical procedures
- Diagnostic procedures

Adverse Effects

- Hypersensitivity reactions (rash, hives, itching, edema)
- Skin irritation
- Anaphylactic reactions (very rare)
- Headache (spinal anesthesia)
- Cardiac and respiratory depression

Precautions

- Specific local/regional anesthetics are contraindicated for clients who have experienced a hypersensitivity reaction to those anesthetics in the past.
- Local/regional anesthetics should be administered with caution to clients with:
  - Cardiovascular disorders
  - Coagulation problems due to blood diseases or anticoagulant therapy
  - Inflammation or infection in the area of the injection

Important Drugs

Esters

Procaine (Novocaine) is the prototype for local anesthetics. It is primarily used for nerve blocks.

Benzocaine is a topical anesthetic used on the skin and mucous membranes.

Tetracaine hydrochloride (Pontocaine) is used for nerve blocks. It is also available in ointment form as a topical anesthetic for the eye.

Amides

Lidocaine (Xylocaine) is used for nerve blocks and for topical anesthesia.

Prilocaine (Citanest) is used for nerve blocks. It produces around 40% fewer toxic effects than lidocaine. It is not used for topical anesthesia.

Mepivacaine (Carbocaine) is used for nerve blocks.

Therapeutic Nursing Interventions

- Assess if the client has any drug allergies, or has had any prior adverse reactions to local or regional anesthetics. If so, notify the primary care provider at once.
- Monitor blood pressure, pulse, and respirations prior to, during, and following the procedure.
- Ensure safety measures and protect the client from falls.
- Position the client properly for local, regional, or spinal anesthesia.
- Following the procedure, monitor the site that was anesthetized for a return to normal appearance and function.
- Discharge the client with clear instructions for self-care, and an appointment with the health care provider for a postoperative evaluation.

Client Education

- Report to the health care provider if motor function and sensation fail to return following the procedure.

- If the procedure involved the throat, avoid eating or drinking until motor function and sensation in the throat has returned.
- When a local anesthetic has been used for a dental procedure, avoid chewing solid food until sensation returns. The client could accidentally bite the tongue or cheek.
- Carefully follow instructions for home care of the dental or surgical site, and schedule a follow-up appointment with the health care provider.

Critical Thinking Exercise: Drugs Affecting the Nervous System

Note: *It is recommended that the following exercises be reviewed with a partner or in a small group to achieve maximum student interaction and to enhance critical thinking skills.*

Situation: M.M., a 32-year-old mother of three, was brought to the hospital by her husband for increasingly erratic behavior. She has been staying up nights "cleaning the house," sleeping only a few hours a day for the last four days. Her husband informs you she has been eating very little, stating she doesn't have time, yet she spends many hours shopping during the day and has spent large amounts of money. More seriously, she has left the children, ages 3, 5, and 8, alone several times stating, "I have important work to do." You do a quick head-to-toe assessment and note the following: She is unkempt, dressed inappropriately with multiple layers of clothes of differing fabrics and patterns. She is wearing a pair of old tennis shoes with mismatched socks. Her mood is euphoric, her speech pressured, and you note she does not seem to be able to stay on topic as you interview her. When she does answer, she demonstrates flight of ideas and erratic thinking patterns. She can't understand what "the fuss" is all about and sees no reason to come to the hospital.

Her husband tells the doctor that M.M. has a long history of manic and depressive episodes, but it was only during this last year that she was formally diagnosed with bipolar disorder and started on lithium. Since then, her mood has been relatively stable and she has been able to function normally.

You learn M.M.'s current dose of lithium carbonate (Lithobid) is 200 mg po tid and she has been taking it regularly and tolerating it well until this last week. The physician orders stat lithium levels and admits M.M. for further evaluation.

1. Based on your nursing knowledge, what information do you know about lithium that is pertinent to this client?

2. The lithium levels come back and are found to be 0.45 mEq/L. The physician views the lab results and writes an order for chlorpromazine hydrochloride (Thorazine) IM stat and prn q 6-8 hours for agitation, and increases the lithium to 300 mg of lithium po tid. Why do you think Thorazine has been ordered? What are some of the most important nursing considerations involved in administering this drug?

3. After four days, M.M.'s condition stabilizes and she is being prepared for discharge home on 300 mg lithium po tid. What discharge teaching is most important for this client and her family?

4. **Exercise**: In the table below, match the drug in the left-hand column to its appropriate category or classification in the right-hand column.

Drug	Classification
Chlorpromazine	Cholinergic
Lithium	Anti-adrenergic
Metoclopramide	Skeletal muscle relaxant
Epinephrine HCL	Barbiturate
Ergotamine tartrate	Antidepressant
Baclofen	Barbiturate
Nembutal	Benzodiazapine
Xanax	Antipsychotic
Fluoxetine	Mood stabilizer
Phenobarbital	Adrenergic

CHAPTER 6

Drugs Affecting the Cardiovascular System

Key Points

- Heart failure develops when the heart muscle fails to pump effectively and sufficient blood does not circulate to the lungs and body tissues.
- Heart failure may be right-sided or left-sided.
- Cardiotonic-inotropic agents are the major drugs used to treat heart failure.
- These agents increase the tonicity of the heart and the force of myocardial contraction, thereby improving the heart's pumping action.
- Digoxin is the most frequently prescribed digitalis preparation in the U.S.
- A larger dose called a "digitalizing dose" may be given initially to achieve more rapid therapeutic drug effects.
- Because digitalis has a low therapeutic index, even a therapeutic dose of a digitalis glycoside can produce digitalis toxicity.
- Digoxin Immune Fab (fragment antigen binding) (Digibind) is used to treat life-threatening digitalis toxicity.
- There are four major types of angina: stable angina, unstable angina, variant (**Prinzmetal's angina**), and refractory angina.
- Organic nitrates such as nitroglycerin (NTG) are the first-line drugs to treat and prevent anginal attacks.
- NTG is administered by:
    - Tablets that are placed under the tongue
    - Skin patches
    - Metered aerosol sprays
    - Sustained release tablets
    - Ointments
    - IV solution
- Beta-adrenergic blockers and calcium channel blockers are also used to treat angina.
- Beta blockers are the mainstay of prophylactic treatment for chronic stable angina. These agents should never be discontinued abruptly because of the risk of anginal attack or myocardial infarction.
- Calcium channel blockers are as effective as nitrates, and may be more therapeutic than beta blockers in the treatment of unstable and variant angina.
- Hyperlipidemias are disorders characterized by abnormally elevated serum levels of cholesterol or triglycerides.
- Antihyperlipidemic drugs are prescribed to reduce serum lipids or improve their ratios when a low cholesterol diet has failed to control lipid levels.
- Lipid-lowering medications that are used to treat hyperlipidemias include bile acid sequestrants, HMG-CoA reductase inhibitors, and fibric acid derivatives.

- A **positive inotropic** effect produces increased strength of myocardial contraction.
  - Clients with pump failure respond to drugs with this action.
- A **positive chronotropic** effect refers to increased cardiac rate.
  - Clients with bradyarrhythmias respond to drugs with this action.
- A **negative chronotropic** drug is used to treat clients with tachyarrhythmias (e.g., supraventricular tachycardia).
- A **positive dromotropic** effect refers to increased atrioventricular conduction.
  - Drugs with this action may be used for clients with heart block.
- A **negative dromotropic** drug blocks conduction for clients with conduction disorders, such as atrial fibrillation.
- Dysrhythmias:
  - Are disturbances in the electrical conduction system of the heart
  - May be benign or life-threatening
  - May or may not require drug therapy
- Major groups of antidysrhythmic drugs include:
  - Group I (sodium channel blockers)
    - IA
    - IB
    - IC
  - Group II (beta-adrenergic blockers)
  - Group III (potassium channel blockers)
  - Group IV (calcium channel blockers)
  - Hypertension is usually defined as a systolic blood pressure > 140 mmHg or a diastolic blood pressure > 90 mmHg.
  - Drugs that lower blood pressure reduce either cardiac output and/or peripheral vascular resistance.
- The major goals of antihypertensive therapy are to lower blood pressure to the lowest reading that can be tolerated by the client (usually < 90 mmHg diastolic), and prevent the complications of hypertension.
- Major types of antihypertensive agents include:
  - Diuretics
  - Angiotensin-converting enzyme (ACE) inhibitors
  - Angiotensin-II receptor antagonists
  - Antiadrenergics/sympatholytics
  - Beta-adrenergic blockers
  - Calcium channel blockers
  - Direct-acting vasodilators
- The antihypertensive drug regimen needs to be individualized for each client for optimum compliance.
- Shock is a condition caused by acute peripheral circulatory failure. It is characterized by severe hypotension, oliguria, pallor, and poor perfusion.
- The goal of therapy for all forms of shock is to increase blood flow through the coronary and cerebral vessels, and to correct the hypoperfusion of vital organs.
- The adrenergics are the major drugs used to treat shock.

Drugs That Treat Heart Failure

Adrenergic (Sympathomimetic) Drugs

Overview

Cardiotonic-inotropic agents are the major drugs used to treat heart failure. Cardiotonic-inotropic agents increase the tonicity of the heart and the force of myocardial contraction, thereby improving the heart's pumping action. For instance, digitalis strengthens the heart. Inotropic agents do not increase the rate of contraction. Chronotropic drugs affect the rate of contraction.

Heart failure is classified as follows:

- **Left-sided failure**: Is due to ventricular muscle damage or fluid overload that reduces cardiac output; the heart is unable to pump blood returned from the lungs, resulting in dyspnea and orthopnea.
- **Right-sided failure**: Is due to pulmonary hypertension; the heart is unable to accommodate blood returned to it from the systemic veins. Right-sided pump failure results in dependent edema and systemic venous distension.

Most clients have both forms of heart failure. It is possible for clients to have right-sided failure and not left-sided failure, but not the other way around. The body attempts to compensate for a failing heart by increasing sympathetic nervous system activity, heart size, and renin-angiotensin, which results in increased sodium and water retention.

The overall therapeutic drug therapy program for heart failure is aimed at altering and controlling compensatory mechanisms:

- Diuretics reduce blood volume.
- Cardiotonic-inotropic agents, such as the digitalis glycosides and bipyridine derivatives, strengthen the failing heart.
- Vasodilators decrease peripheral resistance.
- Angiotensin-converting enzyme (ACE) inhibitors dilate both veins and arteries, decrease preload and afterload, and decrease the workload of the heart.

Digitalis Glycosides

Overview

Digitalis glycosides are also called cardiac glycosides. Digitalis is produced from plants. These drugs are called glycosides because they contain a sugar molecule, which is attached to a steroid nucleus. In addition to their use in the treatment of heart failure, digitalis preparations are used to treat dysrhythmias. Digitalis slows the rate of ventricular contraction, which increases the force of contraction, increasing stroke volume and cardiac output. These factors help to decrease the workload of the failing heart. In order to achieve more rapid drug effects, a larger dose of digitalis may be given initially. This is called a "digitalizing dose" or a "loading dose." A "loading dose" of digitalis is a large enough dose of digitalis to quickly reach therapeutic blood levels of the drug, and control the manifestations of heart failure with minimal adverse effects. Digitalis has a low therapeutic index, and thus a therapeutic dose of digitalis may still produce signs of toxicity. Hypokalemia is an important contributing factor to toxicity. Many clients with heart failure also receive furosemide (Lasix), which is a potassium-wasting diuretic. Age extremes and renal damage also raise the risk of digitalis toxicity.

Uses

- Congestive heart failure (CHF)
- Atrial fibrillation
- Atrial flutter
- Supraventricular tachycardia
- Paroxysmal atrial tachycardia

Adverse Effects

Cardiac symptoms

- Ventricular bigeminy or trigeminy: Initial signs of digitalis toxicity in adults
- Atrial tachycardia with varying heart block
- Second-degree (intermittent conduction failure) atrioventricular (AV) heart block (Wenckebach): Initial sign of toxicity in children
- AV dissociation
- Complete heart block due to slowing of conduction through the AV junction
- Sinus bradycardia
- Edema, sudden weight gain
- Difficulty breathing

Gastrointestinal symptoms

- Anorexia: Initial sign of digitalis toxicity in adults
- Nausea and vomiting
- Abdominal discomfort
- Diarrhea
- Upset stomach: Initial signs of digitalis toxicity in children

Neurologic symptoms

- Headache
- Drowsiness
- Blurred vision
- Dizziness
- Extreme fatigue
- Confusion and disorientation
- Psychosis
- Convulsions
- Coma
- Visual Disturbances

- Blurred or yellow vision (hallmark sign)
- Halos and colored dots (hallmark sign)
- Double vision

Life-threatening digitalis toxicity is indicated by:

- Shock
- Cardiac arrest
- Severe ventricular dysrhythmias
- Bradycardia
- Hypokalemia

Precautions

- Digitalis preparations should be administered with caution to:
  - Elderly clients who tend to be more susceptible to toxicity, due to renal insufficiency
  - Clients who are also taking quinidine (an antidysrhythmic drug), or verapamil (Calan, Isoptin), or clients taking erythromycin or clarithromycin
- Intravenous digitalis should be administered cautiously because too rapid an infusion can precipitate toxicity.
- Digitalis preparations are contraindicated for clients with:
  - Heart block
  - Cardiomyopathy
  - Wolf-Parkinson-White syndrome (also called atrioventricular nodal reentrant tachycardia). The electrical impulse may return to the upper chamber over an abnormal extra connection that typically has been present since birth. The returning electrical impulse may once again go down the "normal" conduction system, creating an additional heartbeat. Each time this cycle repeats itself, the heart beats. Rapid heart beating is simply the repeating of this kind of cycle many times. This process is the most common mechanism of an arrhythmia in clients with extra connections.
- Predisposing factors for the development of digitalis toxicity include the following:
  - Electrolyte imbalances:
    - Hypokalemia
    - Hypomagnesemia
    - Hypercalcemia
  - Acid-base imbalances
  - Hypothyroidism
  - Renal or hepatic disease
  - Dehydration

Important Drugs

Digoxin

- Digoxin is the most frequently prescribed digitalis preparation in the United States.

- Digoxin and the other cardiac glycosides are unique in their ability to increase contractility without elevating the oxygen requirement of the myocardium.
    - It is this property that makes this group of drugs so valuable.
- By increasing contractility and decreasing the heart rate, digoxin helps the failing heart meet the oxygen needs of the body tissues.
- Exerts a therapeutic influence on the electrical activities of the heart.
    - Decreases sympathetic stimulation, and returns normal vagal activity to the sinoatrial (SA) and atrioventricular (AV) nodes.
        - These actions reduce impulse formation in the sinoatrial (SA) node, and decrease the conduction of electrical activity between the atria and the ventricles.
        - In higher doses, atrioventricular (AV) conduction is depressed, which benefits the client with atrial flutter or fibrillation.

Digitoxin (Crystodigin)

- This agent is quickly absorbed from the gastrointestinal tract.
- It has the most extended duration of action, ranging from 1-3 weeks.

Digoxin Immune Fab (fragment antigen binding) (Digibind)

- This agent is given to treat life-threatening digitalis toxicity.
- It is administered by IV, and is excreted by the kidneys within 15-20 hours.

Therapeutic Nursing Interventions

- Obtain a complete health and medication history.
    - Inquire if the client has taken digitalis glycosides in the past, and if so, determine the client's reaction to the medication.
- Monitor the client for signs and symptoms of heart failure.
- Administer a "loading dose" of cardiac glycosides if ordered.
    - Check the client's apical pulse rate before the administration of the drug.
- Administer digitalis glycosides at the same time every day.
- Monitor the client's apical heart rate for one full minute prior to administering the drug, and record the heart rate and rhythm.
    - You will need to know the specific pulse limitations for your client.
    - Usually you will need to withhold the drug, and contact the primary care provider for orders if the apical pulse rate is < 60 bpm in an adult, < 70 bpm in a child, or < 90 bpm in an infant, or if you have noted a dysrhythmia.
    - A lower pulse rate than usual may indicate an increase in the serum level of digitalis. The primary care provider may need to order a lower dose of the medication.
    - A faster pulse rate than usual may signal the need for a higher dose of digitalis glycoside.
- Administer digitalis glycosides orally if possible, because the administration of IM or IV digitalis may irritate the client's subcutaneous and muscular tissues.
    - Use the gluteus maximus or ventrogluteal sites when administering an IM injection.
    - Avoid using the deltoid muscle for IM injections.

- Slowly administer intravenous cardiac glycosides.
  - An IV infusion of cardiac glycosides should take between 10-30 minutes.
  - Rapid IV administration is dangerous because it can cause severe arteriolar vasoconstriction resulting in hypertension.
- Assess the client for signs and symptoms of digitalis toxicity.
- Assess serum digitalis levels (therapeutic digoxin level, 0.8-2 ng/mL). Immediately report high serum levels to the primary care provider (e.g., > 2.5 mg/mL for digoxin).
- Monitor:
  - Serum levels of:
    - Potassium
    - Calcium
    - Magnesium
  - Acid-base balance
  - Kidney function studies
  - Liver function studies
  - Vital signs
- Take and record daily weight.
- Treat digitalis toxicity as ordered. Standard treatment includes:
  - Withdrawal of the digitalis glycoside
  - IV fluids, if indicated
  - Administration of:
    - Potassium, if potassium levels are low
    - Lidocaine or phenytoin to correct ventricular dysrhythmias
    - Atropine to treat:
      - Bradydysrhythmias
      - Sinoatrial (SA) arrest
      - Atrioventricular (AV) block
    - Digoxin Immune Fab (fragment antigen binding) (Digibind), a digoxin-binding antidote, for severe digitalis toxicity
- Assess the client for hypersensitivity reactions to the medication.
  - These reactions may not develop for 5-7 days after the start of therapy.
- Schedule regular appointments with the primary care provider for evaluation of the client's heart failure and reaction to the digitalis glycosides.
- Teach client how to check pulse and blood pressure, and tell them to report significant findings to the health care provider.

Client Education

- Take the medication exactly as ordered, and at the same time every day.
- Take the daily dosage when fully awake, so pulse can be checked accurately prior to taking the medication. Being awake and active is especially important for older clients because they usually have a low heart rate upon rising. Thus, it may be best for older clients to take their medication around noon.

- Take pulse for one full minute before taking digitalis glycosides.
- Contact the primary care provider if the pulse rate is irregular, or the pulse rate is outside of the limitations set by the primary care provider, which is usually <60 or >100.
- Immediately report signs of digitalis toxicity to the health care provider.
- Avoid taking antacids or antidiarrheals or eating bran within two hours of taking digitalis glycosides.
    - Digitalis glucosides absorb aluminum-containing antacids and bran.
- Consult with the health care provider before taking any OTC drugs because of the risk of adverse drug interactions.
- Carry an identification card at all times that outlines the medication regimen and states the primary care provider's name and telephone number.
- Schedule regular follow-up appointments with the health care provider.

Other Cardiotonic Inotropic Drugs

Amrinone (Inocor)

- This cardiotonic-inotropic agent is a bipyridine derivative.
    - It differs from the digitalis glycosides because it also acts as a vasodilator.
- Amrinone relaxes the arteries, thereby increasing cardiac output, stroke volume, and myocardial contractility.
    - This agent does not significantly affect heart rate or blood pressure.
- Amrinone is a short-term intravenous drug that is prescribed for clients with heart failure, who have not improved despite the use of digitalis glycosides, diuretics, and other vasodilators.
- Before starting therapy with amrinone, the client's fluid and electrolyte status must be in balance to fully benefit from the drug.
    - Clients who have been vigorously treated with diuretics are at risk of fluid and electrolyte imbalance.
    - Amrinone should not be infused with furosemide (Lasix) because a precipitate forms.
- Common adverse effects include:
    - Supraventricular and ventricular dysrhythmias
    - Thrombocytopenia
    - Hypotension
    - Nausea
    - Vomiting
    - Anorexia
- Platelet count should be monitored weekly.
- Hypersensitivity reactions can occur up to two weeks after starting this drug.
- Dosage should be reduced if the client experiences severe gastrointestinal symptoms.
- Amrinone should not be added to intravenous glucose mixtures because an adverse chemical reaction may occur.

Milrinone (Primacor)

- This agent is also a bipyridine derivative, and is similar in structure, action, and adverse effects to amrinone.
- Milrinone can be administered in an intravenous solution for short-term care.
- Long-term use of milrinone can cause headaches and aggravate the symptoms of angina.

Nesiritide (Natrecor)

- Nesiritide treats clients with decompensated heart failure.
- This agent is not an inotropic drug, but a brain natriuretic peptide (BNP).
- Nesiritide promotes diuresis and vasodilation.
- It may cause hypotension.

Drugs That Treat Angina

Overview

Angina is a syndrome of paroxysmal left-sided chest pain, which is produced when the oxygen demands of the heart exceed the oxygen supply.

There are four major types of angina:

- Stable angina is precipitated by stress and relieved by rest or nitroglycerin (NTG).
- Unstable angina is characterized by more severe symptoms, and it is less responsive to treatment. It is the intermediate syndrome between stable angina and myocardial infarction.
- Variant (Prinzmetal's) angina is not caused by atherosclerotic narrowing, but results from a coronary artery spasm. This angina does not necessarily occur with exertion.
- Refractory (intractable) angina is characterized by incapacitating pain that does not respond to standard therapy.

Angina is treated with coronary vasodilators (antianginal drugs), rest, oxygen, and control of precipitating factors such as stress and smoking. Antianginal drugs act to reduce the oxygen requirements of the myocardium and increase the blood flow to the ischemic heart muscle. Acute anginal attacks are treated with short-acting NTG products. Long-term stable angina is treated with oral or topical nitrates, beta-adrenergic blockers, and calcium channel blockers. These medications are also used to prevent anginal attacks.

Organic Nitrates

Overview

Organic nitrates are the first line of defense in the prevention and treatment of angina. These agents relax smooth muscle in the blood vessel walls, and thus, help to stop the pain of anginal attacks.

Organic nitrates:

- Redistribute blood flow to ischemic areas of the myocardium, improving the perfusion of the heart

- Dilate the veins, reducing venous pressure and venous return
- Decrease blood volume and pressure within the heart, thereby reducing preload. Preload is the distending force that stretches the ventricular muscle prior to electrical excitation and contraction of the heart muscle.
- Dilate coronary blood arteries and increase blood flow to ischemic areas by dilating collateral vessels
- Dilate arterioles, which lowers peripheral vascular resistance
- Reduce afterload. Afterload is the load the heart muscle must move during contraction.

Tolerance to organic nitrates may develop with sustained, long-term use.

Uses

- Acute anginal attacks
- Unstable angina
- Chronic angina
- Acute and chronic heart failure

Adverse Effects

- Pounding or pulsating headache (the most frequent side effect)
- Hypotension
- Dizziness and weakness
- Syncope
- Nausea and vomiting
- Facial flushing

Precautions

- Organic nitrates are contraindicated for clients who are hypersensitive to nitrates, clients with severe anemias, and clients with head trauma because nitrates increase intracranial pressure.
- Nitrates should not be given IV to clients with severe hypotension or hypovolemia because they can cause shock due to vasodilation.
- Nitrates should be administered cautiously to clients with:
    - Ventricular outflow obstruction disease
    - Severe hypertension
    - Carotid disease
    - Renal or hepatic dysfunction
    - Fluid depletion due to diuretic therapy
    - Low blood pressure (< 90 mmHg systolic)
    - Constrictive pericarditis
    - Cardiac tamponade
- Clients taking nitrates should avoid alcohol and other vasodilators unless they've obtained permission from their primary care provider.

Important Drugs

Nitroglycerin (NTG) (Nitro-Bid, Nitrostat, Nitrodisc, Nitrogard, Nitro-Dur)

- NTG is the prototype for the organic nitrates. Nitroglycerin decreases both preload and afterload.
  - NTG tablets (Nitrostat) are taken sublingually to relieve an anginal attack. Nitrostat has a rapid onset (1-3 minutes), and a short duration (1-2 hours).
  - The client usually takes one tablet every 5-10 minutes, 3 times.
  - If the pain is not relieved, the client should call an ambulance immediately because of the risk of developing a myocardial infarction.
  - NTG tablets may be also be taken to prevent anginal attacks.
  - The client should place a tablet under the tongue prior to mild or moderate activity or sexual activity.
  - NTG is available as an ointment or patch. These are worn for 12 hours and then removed for 12 hours to avoid tolerance.
  - Nitroglycerin sustained-release tablets are administered every 8-12 hours.
- Nitroglycerin translingual (Nitrolingual) is a metered aerosol spray.
  - The client can use the spray to relieve an acute anginal attack or to prevent an attack.
- NTG IV (Nitro-Bid IV, Tridil) is used to treat acute unstable angina, acute heart failure, and hypertension.
  - NTG IV is usually mixed with D5W or 0.9% sodium chloride solution.

Isosorbide dinitrate (Isordil) is a nitrate taken sublingually or orally. It is prescribed for long-term prophylaxis.

Therapeutic Nursing Interventions

- Assess the client for signs of coronary artery disease, and ask the client to describe the anginal attacks.
  - Inquire about:
    - Pain:
      - Onset
      - Type
      - Location
      - Frequency
      - Intensity
      - Pattern of radiation of anginal pain
    - What activities appear to precipitate attacks
    - The client's current use of medications to relieve the pain, including NTG or other coronary vasodilators
- Advise the client to summon a health care professional when an anginal attack occurs.
- Assess the client's ability to apply and remove NTG (nitroglycerin) patches or ointment.
  - For example, clients with arthritis may find it difficult to work with a patch.

- Monitor the client's apical pulse rate and quality, and the blood pressure for hypertension or hypotension.
    - Withhold the drug and notify the primary care provider if the client's systolic blood pressure is below 90 mmHg.
- Teach the client how to accurately take his or her own blood pressure and pulse.
- Check the client for skin irritation if NTG patches are used.
- Access the client for facial flushing and other side effects of NTG.
- Use care when mixing NTG with D5W or normal saline solution for an intravenous infusion.
    - Use glass IV bottles and non-polyvinyl chloride tubing because plastic bottles and PVC tubing adsorb NTG.
- Assess the client's blood pressure and pulse every 5 minutes after starting the IV.
- Use an IV pump and titrate the dose every 3-5 minutes, using the client's level of pain, blood pressure, and pulse as your guide.
- Wean the client gradually from IV NTG as ordered.
- Notify the primary care provider immediately if the pain returns or the blood pressure rises during the weaning period.
- The therapeutic effects of NTG should continue for 30-60 minutes following weaning.

Client Education

- When taking organic nitrates:
    - Take one tablet every 5 minutes, 3 times upon the start of an acute anginal attack.
    - Dissolve tablets slowly under the tongue.
    - Do not swallow tablets whole or chew them.
    - Lie or sit down to prevent falling due to dizziness.
    - If the pain is completely relieved, expel any remaining tablet from the mouth.
    - If the pain is not relieved, call the primary care provider and an ambulance.
        - It is best to go immediately to the emergency department because of the risk of myocardial infarction.
- Store NTG tablets away from light, heat, and moisture to prevent a loss of potency.
    - Keep tablets in the original glass container or in specially designed metal containers.
    - Do not keep medications in the glove compartment of an automobile.
    - Replace tablets that are 3-6 months old or tablets that do not "tingle" under the tongue.
- Rise from a lying position and change positions slowly to prevent orthostatic hypotension.
- Dangle legs for a couple of minutes when getting out of bed.

- Notify the primary care provider if NTG produces a severe headache that lasts more then 15-20 minutes. The primary care provider may need to change the drug dosage. A short-term headache is a normal side effect.
- Do not drink alcohol after taking NTG because alcohol acts as a vasodilator, and can cause an acute drop in blood pressure and extreme dizziness.
- Spray NTG lingual aerosol onto or under the tongue.
    - Do not inhale the aerosol and try not to swallow it.
    - Do not spray more than 3 metered doses during a 15-minute period.
- Use the special application paper supplied by the manufacturer when applying NTG paste to the skin.
    - Always apply the paste to clean, dry skin.
    - Do not rub the paste into the skin.
    - Rotate application sites.
    - Remove the application paper for 12 hours each day according to the primary care provider's directions.
    - Keep the paste tightly closed and store it in a dry place.
    - Wash hands immediately after application and/or use of gloves.
- Prevent anginal attacks by taking NTG around 5-10 minutes prior to moderate physical or sexual activity.
- Avoid strenuous physical exercise, emotional stress, and cold. For example, do not shovel snow.
- Stop smoking because nicotine acts as a vasoconstrictor.
- Carry an identification card at all times that outlines the medication regimen and states your primary care provider's name and telephone number.
- Notify dentists and other health care professionals of the NTG medication regimen.
- Schedule regular follow-up appointments with the primary care provider.

Beta-Adrenergic Blockers

Overview

Beta-adrenergic blocking agents act to interrupt adrenergic stimulation to beta$_1$- or beta$_2$-receptors by competing with norepinephrine for available beta-adrenergic receptor sites.

Beta blockers that block beta$_1$-receptors act to decrease blood pressure, the contraction of the heart muscle, and cardiac output.

- These agents are used to control angina pectoris.
- Beta blockers that inhibit beta$_2$-receptors cause vasodilatation in skeletal muscle arterioles. They are used to control angina pectoris and lower blood pressure.

Beta-blocking agents are used for prophylaxis only in the treatment of coronary artery disease. They do not act quickly enough to alleviate an ongoing anginal attack. Beta blockers are the mainstay of prophylactic treatment for chronic stable angina. Clients usually report that they have an increased tolerance to activity and fewer anginal attacks. Beta-adrenergic blockers are often combined with isosorbide dinitrate (Isordil) because the combined effects are more therapeutic.

Uses

- Chronic stable angina: Given to decrease oxygen demand, myocardial contractility, heart rate, and blood pressure
- Dysrhythmias: Given to slow sinus node conduction and prolong conduction through the atrioventricular (AV) node, thereby slowing ventricular response
- Hypertension: Given to lower blood pressure. The mechanism of action is unclear.
- Myocardial infarction: Given to decrease the incidence of catecholamine-induced dysrhythmias following attack

Adverse Effects

- Bradycardia
- Orthostatic hypotension
- Shortness of breath
- Edema
- Reduced tolerance to exercise
- Congestive heart failure (CHF)
- Hypoglycemia n
- Fatigue
- Nausea, vomiting, and diarrhea
- Bronchospasm
- Impotence
- Depression
- Sleep disorders

Precautions

- Beta-adrenergic blocking agents should be administered cautiously to clients with:
    - A history of asthma, emphysema, heart failure, cerebral vascular accident, hypotension, sinus bradycardia, heart block, and peptic ulcer.
    - Diabetics who are taking insulin or oral hypoglycemic agents because they may mask the symptoms of hypoglycemia.
    - Peripheral vascular insufficiency because they reduce blood flow to the extremities.
    - Kidney or liver disease because they accumulate in the serum of clients with these diseases, and cause toxic effects.
- Beta-adrenergic blocking agents should not be stopped abruptly, particularly in clients with ischemic heart disease.
    - These agents are titrated down slowly, usually over a week or two.
    - The client with angina who abruptly discontinues beta blockers is at four times greater risk of developing an anginal attack, or a mild myocardial infarction within 30 days of discontinuation.
- Beta-adrenergic blocking agents should not be taken with alcohol, CNS depressants, or OTC decongestants.

- Beta-adrenergic blocking agents are not always effective for African-American clients, and thus are usually combined with a diuretic.
  - The reason why this combination is therapeutic is not clearly understood.
- These agents should be administered with caution to elderly clients because they are more at risk of adverse effects.

Important Drugs

Propranolol hydrochloride (Inderal)

- Propranolol is the prototype for beta-adrenergic blocking agents.
- It is used to treat angina, dysrhythmias, and myocardial infarction.
- Propranolol is available in a wide dosage range. Clients vary greatly in the amount of oral drug that survives hepatic metabolism to reach the systemic circulation.

Atenolol (Tenormin) is used to treat angina pectoris, hypertension, and myocardial infarction.

Pindolol (Visken) is used to treat angina pectoris and hypertension.

Therapeutic Nursing Interventions

- Assess the client for signs of coronary artery disease, and ask the client to describe his or her anginal attacks. Inquire about the onset, type, location, frequency, intensity, and pattern of radiation of anginal pain, and what activities appear to precipitate episodes.
- Inquire about the client's current use of beta blockers or other medications to relieve the pain, including nitroglycerin (NTG) or calcium channel blockers.
- Obtain a baseline weight before starting the administration of beta blockers.
- Check the client's pulse rate before administration, because beta blockers slow the sinus rate and may produce bradycardia.
- Monitor the client's blood pressure for hypotension.
- Teach the client how to accurately measure own blood pressure and pulse.
- Monitor for hypoglycemia, which is indicated by a blood glucose level of less than 60 mg/dl.
- Carefully evaluate therapeutic effect of the medication. Because the first dose of a beta blocker is almost completely metabolized by the liver, the dosage may need to be increased for a therapeutic effect.

Client Education

- Learn to take own pulse and blood pressure, and identify low values.
- Learn to monitor blood sugar level for low blood sugar. Beta blockers may mask the symptoms of hypoglycemia in clients who are diabetic and are taking insulin or oral hypoglycemic agents.
- Change positions slowly to prevent orthostatic hypotension.
- Never stop medication abruptly because of the risk of an anginal attack or myocardial infarction.
- Take beta blockers at the same time each day.

- Avoid taking beta blockers with antacids without the primary care provider's permission because of the risk of a drug interaction.
- Avoid taking beta blockers and OTC drugs at the same time without the primary care provider's permission.
- Avoid prolonged exposure to the sun, taking hot showers, sitting in hot tubs, or visiting locations with very hot climates.
- Use caution when driving a vehicle or operating heavy machinery because beta blockers can cause dizziness.
- Avoid drinking alcoholic beverages because the interaction of alcohol and beta blockers may cause adverse effects.
- Store beta blockers in dry, moisture-proof, childproof bottles.
- Schedule regular follow-up appointments with primary care provider.

Calcium Channel Blockers

Overview

Calcium channel blockers act to:

- Prevent the flow of calcium ions into the cells
- Relax arterial smooth muscle and decrease contraction of the heart muscle
- Slow atrioventricular (AV) conduction
- Reduce the heart rate
- Dilate coronary and peripheral arteries
- Decrease coronary vascular resistance
- Increase coronary blood flow
- Reduce myocardial oxygen demand

Calcium channel blockers appear to work as effectively as the organic nitrates and beta-adrenergic blockers in the treatment of unstable angina.

Uses

- Prevent and control supraventricular tachyarrhythmias
- Prevent post-myocardial infarction complications
- Treat hypertension
- Treat chronic stable angina
- Treat and prevent unstable angina
- Treat and prevent vasospastic angina

Adverse Effects

- Constipation
- Nausea
- Headache
- Hypotension
- Dizziness

- Bradycardia
- Heart block
- Dyspnea and wheezing
- Peripheral edema

Precautions

- Calcium channel blockers are contraindicated for clients with these conditions:
    - Hepatic or renal disease
    - Heart block
    - Hypotension
    - Severe bradycardia
    - Aortic stenosis
    - Severe left ventricular dysfunction
    - Women who are pregnant or lactating
- These agents should be administered with caution to clients with serious respiratory disorders, and to clients with heart failure because calcium channel blockers can worsen heart failure.
- Calcium channel blockers should be administered with caution to elderly clients because they experience a more pronounced hypotensive effect than younger clients.
- The effects of calcium channel blockers may be augmented when administered with beta blockers.
- The administration of calcium channel blockers with digoxin can cause a significant increase in the blood digoxin concentration.
- Discontinuation of calcium channel blockers should be gradual and under the primary care provider's supervision to prevent untoward effects.

Important Drugs

Verapamil hydrochloride (Calan, Covera-HS, Isoptin, Verelan)

- Verapamil reduces arterial pressure, increases coronary perfusion, reduces heart rate, and decreases atrioventricular conduction.
- It is used for angina pectoris, essential hypertension and cardiac dysrhythmias.

Nifedipine (Adalat, Nifedical, Procardia)

- Nifedipine is classified as a dihydropyridine, which blocks calcium channels in vascular smooth muscles (VSM) and promotes vasodilation.
- It is used for vasospastic angina, angina of effort, and hypertension.

Diltiazem hydrochloride (Cardizem) is used to treat spastic (Prinzmetal's) angina, chronic stable angina, and hypertension.

Amlodipine (Norvasc) is used to treat vasospastic (Prinzmetal's) angina, chronic stable angina, and hypertension.

Nicardipine hydrochloride (Cardene SR) is used to treat chronic stable angina, and is frequently given in combination with beta blockers.

Therapeutic Nursing Interventions

- Assess the client for signs of coronary artery disease, and ask the client to describe his/her anginal attacks.
- Inquire about:
  - Pain:
    - Onset
    - Type
    - Location
    - Frequency
    - Intensity
    - Pattern of radiation of anginal pain
  - What activities appear to precipitate attacks
  - The client's current use of calcium channel blockers to relieve the pain, or other medications including NTG or beta blockers.
- Monitor the client's blood pressure, and apical pulse rate and quality before, during, and after the administration of calcium channel blockers.
- Do not give the medication if the client has signs of a heart block.
- Call the primary care provider immediately.
- Teach the client how to accurately measure own blood pressure and pulse.
- Give calcium channel blockers with food or milk to prevent gastric discomfort.
- Measure intake and output (I & O).
- Report oliguria to the primary care provider.
- Monitor laboratory studies for increased serum creatinine.
- Monitor the client with heart failure for worsening symptoms (e.g., increased peripheral edema, increased fatigue, rales in the lungs, more severe dyspnea and orthopnea, and weight gain).
- Have emergency equipment nearby when administering calcium channel blockers IV.
- Monitor the client's vital signs continually during administration.

Client Education

- Take sustained-release forms of calcium channel blockers with food or milk to prevent gastric discomfort.
- Get up from a lying position and change positions slowly to prevent orthostatic hypotension. Dangle the legs for a couple of minutes when getting out of bed. If hypotension develops, notify the primary care provider, and remain lying down for one hour after taking the medication.
- Do not drink alcohol with calcium channel blockers because alcohol acts as a vasodilator and can cause an acute drop in blood pressure and extreme dizziness.
- Report dizziness, irregular pulse, shortness of breath, edema of the feet, and constipation to the health care provider.
- Avoid discontinuing medication abruptly without consulting the primary care provider.

- Carry an identification card at all times that outlines the medication regimen and states the primary care provider's name and telephone number.
- Notify dentists and other health care professionals of medication regimen.
- Schedule regular follow-up appointments with the health care provider.

Lipid-lowering Drugs

Overview

Hyperlipidemias are disorders characterized by abnormally elevated serum levels of cholesterol or triglycerides. Cholesterol is a waxy sterol that is produced in the liver and is found in egg yolks, some fats and oils, brain and spinal cord nerve tissue, the liver, the kidneys, the adrenal glands, and in bile. Triglycerides, also called neutral fats, are composed of 3 molecules of fatty acid combined with one molecule of glycerol. They are the fats most frequently found in humans. Cholesterol and triglycerides are carried in lipoproteins. Lipoproteins are conjugated compounds that contain:

- **Chylomicrons**, which are the largest lipoproteins.
- **Very low-density lipoproteins** (VLDL), which transport triglycerides.
- **Low-density lipoproteins** (LDL), which convey cholesterol in the circulation and are the most injurious form of lipoprotein. LDL is sometimes called "bad cholesterol." The major goal of antihyperlipidemic therapy is to lower LDL.
- **High-density lipoproteins** (HDL), which are the smallest and most dense lipoprotein, also transport cholesterol. HDL is sometimes called "good cholesterol."

A high cholesterol level in adults (depending on their age) is >200 mg/dl, and a high triglyceride level is >140-160 mg/dl. Elevated levels of cholesterol and triglycerides may stimulate the development of atherosclerosis and the complications of coronary artery disease (e.g., thrombosis or myocardial infarction). A low-cholesterol diet is the first line of therapy against hyperlipidemias. Drug therapy is prescribed only if diet therapy and an exercise program fail to lower serum lipid levels to normal values. In addition to medication, it is important to identify and control modifiable risk factors such as smoking, obesity, excessive alcohol ingestion, hypertension, and diabetes mellitus. Lipid-lowering medications that are used to treat hyperlipidemias include bile acid sequestrants, HMG-CoA reductase inhibitors, and fibric acid derivatives.

Bile Acid Sequestrants

Overview

Bile acid sequestrants reduce the concentration of cholesterol by binding bile acids in the gastrointestinal tract, and increasing the excretion of bile acids in the feces. These agents are prescribed when diet has failed to control hyperlipidemia. Bile acid sequestrants may be administered concurrently with HMG-CoA reductase inhibitors to control severe hyperlipidemia.

Uses

- Bile acid sequestrants are the first-line drugs used to treat hypercholesterolemia in adults.

Adverse Effects

- Constipation
- Bloating and flatulence
- Nausea
- Headache
- Pruritus
- Less common effects include:
    - Fecal impaction
    - Intestinal obstruction
    - Exacerbation of hemorrhoids
    - Decreased absorption of the fat-soluble vitamins A, D, E, and K
    - Prolonged prothrombin time (PT)

Precautions

- Bile acid sequestrants are contraindicated for clients who are hypersensitive to these products or who have complete biliary obstruction.
- Bile acid sequestrants should be administered with caution to clients with a history of constipation or bowel obstruction.
- These agents should be given with great caution to children who are at risk of intestinal obstruction.

Important Drugs

Colestipol (Colestid) should be used in combination with diet and exercise to control hyperlipidemia.

Cholestyramine (Questran, Prevalite Powder) should be used in combination with diet and exercise to control hyperlipidemia. The powder should be thoroughly mixed into liquids or moist foods.

Therapeutic Nursing Interventions

- Obtain a complete health and medication history.
- Assess for signs and symptoms of coronary artery disease.
- Obtain a diet history, and ask the client about his or her daily dietary intake of fats.
    - Ask if the client includes high-fiber foods in the daily diet.
- Ask the client about daily activities and exercise.
- Inquire if the client has been taking any lipid-lowering medications, and if so, if there have been any adverse effects.
- Weigh the client and continue to monitor weight throughout the treatment program.
- Examine the client for xanthomas, which are lipid deposits in the skin due to hyperlipidemia.

- Monitor:
  - Serum cholesterol and triglyceride levels before starting lipid-lowering therapy. Monitor laboratory results frequently during the first months of therapy, and then on a periodic basis.
  - Prothrombin time (PT) and observe client for bruising and petechiae
  - The client for gastrointestinal symptoms and constipation
- Provide the client with a written plan for dietary limitations, and an exercise plan. Help the client set realistic goals for lowering lipids.

Client Education

- Take the medication exactly as directed, before meals.
- Follow a low-fat, low-cholesterol diet, which will augment the therapeutic effects of the medication. Control sugar intake and avoid "empty calories" in food items such as cakes, candies, and doughnuts.
- Eat foods that are high in fiber (whole grain cereals, vegetables, and fruits), and drink at least 6-8 glasses of fluid a day to prevent constipation.
- Follow a program of exercise, which will help to lower low-density lipoprotein (LDL) cholesterol and reduce weight.
- Restrict alcohol and stop smoking to reduce the risk of coronary artery disease.
- Mix fiber powder into moist foods such as cereals or pulpy fruits, or into 4-6 ounces of water, fruit juice, milk, or carbonated beverages. Mix or shake liquids thoroughly. Mix the product ahead and refrigerate it to improve the flavor. Suck the fluid through a straw to decrease a gritty, sandy taste.
- Increase fluids and take a stool softener if constipation develops. Notify the primary care provider if constipation, nausea, or flatulence persist.
- Report unusual bleeding, tarry stools, or bruising to the primary care provider who may need to prescribe vitamin K.
- If surgery is planned, inform the surgeon of medication regimen.
- Schedule regular appointments with health care professionals for re-evaluation and ongoing laboratory studies.

HMG-CoA Reductase Inhibitors

Overview

HMG-CoA reductase inhibitors (also called "statins") inhibit the enzyme HMG-CoA (3- hydroxy-3-methylglutaryl coenzyme A) reductase that is involved in the synthesis of cholesterol. These agents decrease the concentration of total and LDL cholesterol and triglycerides, and increase the concentration of high-density level (HDL) cholesterol. HMG-CoA reductase inhibitors are powerful and effective in controlling lipid levels.

Uses

- HMG-CoA reductase inhibitors are used to treat primary hypercholesterolemia, and appear to slow the progress of atherosclerosis.

Adverse Effects

- HMG-CoA reductase inhibitors may produce the following adverse effects, which usually decrease or disappear after a period of time:
    - Constipation
    - Diarrhea
    - Abdominal distention
    - Belching
    - Hemorrhoid irritation
    - Nausea and vomiting
    - Increased creatine phosphokinase (CPK)
    - Headache
    - Fatigue
    - Unexplained elevated liver function tests

Precautions

- HMG-CoA reductase inhibitors are contraindicated for pregnant clients because they may harm the fetus.
- These agents are also contraindicated for clients with acute liver disease.
- HMG-CoA reductase inhibitors should be administered cautiously to clients with suspected liver dysfunction and/or alcoholism.

Important Drugs

Atorvastatin (Lipitor) is a lipid-lowering agent that is able to cross the blood-brain barrier, and has a long half-life.

Simvastatin (Zocor) is a lipid-lowering agent that is able to cross the blood-brain barrier, and has a long half-life.

Fluvastatin (Lescol) is a lipid-lowering agent that is not able to cross the blood-brain barrier, and has a short plasma half-life.

Pravastatin (Pravachol) is a lipid-lowering agent that is not able to cross the blood-brain barrier, and has a short plasma half-life.

Lovastatin (Mevacor) is a lipid-lowering agent that is not able to cross the blood-brain barrier, and has a short plasma half-life.

Therapeutic Nursing Interventions

- Record the client's complete health, diet, family, medication, and exercise history.
- Weigh the client and examine the skin for xanthomas.
- Monitor:
    - Serum cholesterol
        - Triglyceride levels
    - Liver function tests:
        - Aspartate aminotransferase (AST); also called SGOT: serum glutamic oxaloacetic transminase)– an enzyme found in the liver, and elsewhere in the body

      - Alanine aminotransferase (ALT); also called SGPT: serum glutamic pyruvic transaminase)–an enzyme found primarily in liver cells, before starting lipid-lowering therapy.
- Monitor laboratory results frequently during the first months of therapy, and then on a periodic basis.
- Monitor the client for gastrointestinal symptoms and constipation.
- Assess client for muscle tenderness.
  - If tenderness develops, monitor CPK levels.
  - If CPK levels are elevated, medication should be discontinued.
- Provide the client with a written plan for dietary limitations, and an exercise plan. Help the client set realistic goals for lowering lipids.

Client Education

- Take the medication exactly as directed, and do not skip doses. Take daily dose in the evening to maximize the drug effects. (Lipitor is an exception).
- Follow a low-fat, low-cholesterol diet and control sugar intake.
- Eat foods that are high in fiber, and drink at least 6-8 glasses of fluid a day to prevent constipation.
- Follow an exercise program.
- Restrict alcohol and stop smoking to reduce the risk of coronary artery disease.
- Report muscle pain and serious gastrointestinal side effects to the primary care provider.
- If pregnant or pregnancy is planned or suspected, notify health care professional.
  - HMG-CoA reductase inhibitors can harm the fetus.
- If surgery is planned, inform the surgeon of medication regimen.
- Schedule regular appointments with health care professionals for reevaluation and ongoing laboratory studies.

Fibric Acid Derivatives

Overview

Fibric acid derivatives reduce plasma triglycerides by increasing the enzyme lipoprotein lipase, which helps to break down cholesterol. These agents increase high-density lipoprotein (HDL) cholesterol 10-15% and decrease triglycerides 20-50%. Fibric acid derivatives are prescribed for short-term therapy only.

Uses

- Fibric acid derivatives are used to treat clients with hyperlipidemia who fail to respond to diet therapy or who are at risk of pancreatitis.

Adverse Effects

- Abdominal pain and diarrhea
- Fatigue
- Headache

- Eczema
- Cholelithiasis, especially in clients with a history of gallstones
- Liver tumors

Precautions

- Fibric acid derivatives are contraindicated for clients with a history of renal or liver disease, primary biliary cirrhosis, gallstones, or hypersensitivity to these agents.
- These agents should not be administered to women who are pregnant or lactating.
- Fibric acid derivatives should be administered with caution to clients with a history of jaundice, peptic ulcer, or gout.

Important Drugs

Gemfibrozil (Lopid) is a lipid-lowering agent that is used to manage hyperlipidemia in clients who do not have symptoms of coronary artery disease, and who have had poor results with diet therapy.

Fenofibrate (Lipidil) is a lipid-lowering agent that is used to manage hyperlipidemia in conjunction with diet therapy. It is prescribed for clients who are at risk of pancreatitis.

Therapeutic Nursing Interventions

- Record the client's complete health, diet, family, medication, and exercise history.
- Weigh the client and examine the skin for xanthomas.
- Monitor:
    - Serum cholesterol
        - Triglyceride levels
    - Liver function tests:
        - Aspartate aminotransferase (AST); also called SGOT: serum glutamic oxaloacetic transminase)– an enzyme found in the liver, and elsewhere in the body
        - Alanine aminotransferase (ALT); also called SGPT: serum glutamic pyruvic transaminase)– an enzyme found primarily in liver cells
        - Prothrombin time (PT) before starting lipid-lowering therapy
- Monitor these laboratory studies frequently during the first months of therapy, and then on a periodic basis.
- Monitor the client for gastrointestinal symptoms, and report severe symptoms to the primary care provider.
- Monitor the client for signs of cholelithiasis.
    - Manifestations of gallstones include intolerance to fatty foods, nausea sometimes accompanied by vomiting, upper right quadrant abdominal pain, clay-colored stools, and low-grade fever.
    - Report these signs to the health care provider who will likely discontinue the drug.
- Provide the client with a written plan for dietary limitations, and an exercise plan. Help the client set realistic goals for lowering lipids.

Client Education

- Take the medication exactly as directed, and do not skip doses.
- Follow a low-fat, low-cholesterol, high-fiber diet and follow an exercise program.
- Drink adequate fluids to prevent constipation.
- Restrict alcohol and stop smoking to reduce the risk of coronary artery disease.
- Report serious gastrointestinal side effects and other adverse effects to the health care provider.
- Report signs and symptoms of gallstones immediately to the health care provider.
- Schedule regular appointments with a health care professional for reevaluation and ongoing laboratory studies.

Drugs That Treat Dysrhythmias

Overview

Automaticity is defined as the ability of the heart to generate an electrical impulse, and conductivity is the ability of the heart to conduct an electrical impulse. Dysrhythmias are disturbances in the electrical conduction system of the heart. Dysrhythmias may be produced by drugs, cardiac diseases, congenital anomalies, stress, electrolyte imbalances, hypoxia, ischemia, shock, imbalances of the autonomic nervous system, and substance abuse of alcohol, caffeine, nicotine, or "recreational" drugs. Dysrhythmias are classified by their site of origin as follows:

- Sinus dysrhythmias (e.g., sinus bradycardia and sinus tachycardia)
- Atrial dysrhythmias (e.g., atrial flutter, atrial fibrillation, premature atrial contraction)
- Junctional nodal dysrhythmias (e.g., junctional escape rhythm, junctional tachycardia)
- Conduction dysrhythmias (e.g., first degree, second degree, and complete heart block)
- Ventricular dysrhythmias (e.g., premature ventricular contraction, ventricular fibrillation)
- Ectopic beats (e.g., beats that originate outside of the sinoatrial (SA) node)

Dysrhythmias may be benign or life-threatening and may or may not require drug therapy. Many dysrhythmias are more effectively treated with cardioversion, countershock, or pacemakers. Antidysrhythmic agents are used to treat, suppress, or prevent dysrhythmias and relieve symptoms. Unfortunately, antidysrhythmic drugs can cause dysrhythmias. For example, antidysrhythmics that prolong the QT interval predispose the client to torsades de pointes (a form of ventricular tachycardia where the morphology of the QRS complexes varies from beat to beat); it can cause death.

Antidysrhythmic agents are grouped or classified according to their mechanism of action and their electrophysiologic effects on the heart. Major groups of antidysrhythmic drugs include:

- Group I: Sodium channel blockers
    - IA
    - IB
    - IC
- Group II: Beta-adrenergic blockers
- Group III: Potassium channel blockers
- Group IV: Calcium channel blockers

Group I—Sodium Channel Blockers

Group IA

Overview

Group IA antidysrhythmic drugs alter the myocardial cell membrane, and interfere with the autonomic nervous system control of pacemaker cells. This group of drugs blocks the fast channel in the myocardial cell membrane, reducing the influx of sodium. This action results in:

- A reduction in the rate of automaticity of the ectopic foci
- An increase in the refractory period
- A reduction in the speed of conductivity

Group IA drugs also block parasympathetic discharges to the sinoatrial (SA) and atrioventricular (AV) nodes, and they prolong the QRS interval.

Uses

- Atrial fibrillation (AF)
- Premature ventricular contractions (PVCs)
- Ventricular tachycardia (VT)

Adverse Effects

- Diarrhea, nausea, and vomiting (especially quinidine)
- Hypotension (especially procainamide)
- Dizziness and confusion in elderly clients
- Tinnitus and visual disturbances (quinidine)
- Delirium, confusion, psychosis
- Drug-induced systemic lupus erythematosus (especially procainamide)
- Fever and chills
- Thrombocytopenia
- Dysrhythmias

Precautions

- All class IA drugs are contraindicated for clients who are hypersensitive to them.
- These agents are also contraindicated for clients with:
  - Complete atrioventricular (AV) block
  - Conduction defects
  - Myasthenia gravis
- Class IA drugs are given cautiously to clients with kidney or liver disorders because these drugs may not be adequately biotransformed and eliminated by diseased organs.
- All class 1A drugs can produce serious dysrhythmias.
  - They prolong the QT interval, thereby predisposing the client to torsades de pointes (a form of ventricular tachycardia where the morphology of the QRS complexes varies from beat to beat).
  - These drugs can also precipitate heart failure. Early signs include hypotension, edema, and irregular heartbeat.

Important Drugs

Quinidine sulfate (Cin-Quin, Quinora) is used to convert atrial fibrillation and atrial flutter, and to suppress ventricular premature contractions and recurrent ventricular tachycardia.

- It should be administered with extreme caution to clients with incomplete atrioventricular (AV) block, digitalis toxicity, and congestive heart failure.
- Cardiac adverse effects are most likely to occur when quinidine is administered IV at high concentrations.
- Gastrointestinal symptoms are signs of quinidine toxicity.

Procainamide hydrochloride (Pronestyl) is used to prevent, but not to convert, recurrences of atrial fibrillation and other atrial dysrhythmias.

- This agent slows cardiac conduction and decreases cardiac conductivity.
- It should be used with caution for clients with acute myocardial infarction and renal failure.
- Procainamide (Pronestyl) has a higher margin of safety than quinidine.

Disopyramide phosphate (Norpace) is used to treat atrial and ventricular dysrhythmias.

- This agent is used when clients are unable to tolerate quinidine because of severe gastrointestinal side effects.
- This drug can cause torsades de pointes.

Therapeutic Nursing Interventions

- Obtain a complete nursing, drug, and family medical history. Ask the client about problems with heart disease and irregular heart rate or rhythm. Inquire if the client is taking or has ever taken medications to correct dysrhythmias.
- Monitor electrocardiogram (ECG), including QRS and widening of the QT interval), apical pulse rate and rhythm, and blood pressure before giving medication, after administration, and on a regular basis thereafter.
- Monitor serum magnesium and potassium levels.

- Monitor client for dysrhythmias possibly due to the medication, and report symptoms to the primary care provider.
- Monitor client for signs of heart failure, kidney disease, or liver disease.
- Monitor for gastrointestinal symptoms because they are early signs of drug toxicity. Notify the primary care provider if the client has diarrhea or other gastrointestinal problems.
- Monitor for tinnitus and visual disturbances in clients who are taking quinidine.
- Give medication around the clock to maintain steady therapeutic blood levels, unless a sustained-release form of the drug has been ordered.
- Crush tablets and open capsules if necessary, and mix medication with food for clients who have difficulty swallowing.
  - Do not crush sustained-release tablets.
- Use an infusion pump to accurately administer quinidine in an intravenous infusion.
- Teach client or family members how to accurately take client's pulse and blood pressure and report important findings.
- Provide ice chips for dry mouth.
- Provide adequate fluids.
- Decrease roughage to control diarrhea.
- Expect to adjust drug dosages for clients with liver or kidney disease because these agents are metabolized in the liver and excreted by the kidney.
- Schedule regular appointments for reevaluation following discharge.

Client Education

- Take the medication around the clock, exactly as directed, and do not skip doses.
- Take pulse prior to and after taking medication.
  - Report alterations in rate or rhythm to the primary care provider.
- Crush tablets and mix with food if you have difficulty swallowing. Do not crush sustained- release tablets.
- Drink adequate fluids and decrease roughage to prevent diarrhea.
- Report gastrointestinal side effects and other adverse effects to the primary care provider.
- Avoid driving and other activities that require alertness until effects of drug are known.
  - Group IA drugs may cause dizziness and confusion.
- Consult with the primary care provider before taking any OTC drugs because of the risk of drug interactions.
- Carry an identification card at all times that outlines the medication regimen and states the name and telephone number of your primary care provider.
- Schedule regular appointments with a health care professional for reevaluation and ongoing laboratory studies.

Group IB

Overview

The major action of Group IB antidysrhythmic drugs is to decrease the action potential duration, and decrease automaticity in the ventricles. It also slows conduction velocity in the Purkinje system. (The Purkinje system is a network of fibers which branch out and deliver the electrical impulse in uniform fashion to the right and left ventricular myocardium). The action potential is the change in the intracellular charge as sodium and calcium flow into the cell and potassium flows out of the cell. Group IB agents do not slow the speed of AV (atrioventricular) conduction, and therefore do not cause heart blocks as can Group IA agents.

Uses

- Group IB antidysrhythmic drugs are used to treat acute and chronic ventricular dysrhythmias, including:
    - Premature ventricular contractions
    - Ventricular tachycardia

Adverse Effects

- A high incidence of brief, dose-related CNS effects:
    - Drowsiness
    - Confusion (initial sign of toxicity)
    - Paresthesias
    - Slurred speech
    - Visual and hearing disturbances
    - Seizures
    - Hallucinations
- Respiratory arrest
- Hypotension
- Bradycardia
- Heart block (with very high serum concentrations)
- Upper gastrointestinal distress (with tocainide)

Precautions

- Group IB antidysrhythmic drugs are contraindicated for clients who are hypersensitive to the drug, women who are pregnant or lactating, and clients with a second- or third-degree heart block.
- These drugs should be administered with caution to elderly clients and to clients with renal or hepatic disorders or acute myocardial infarction. Drug dosage may need to be adjusted.

Important Drugs

Lidocaine hydrochloride (Xylocaine)

- Lidocaine is the drug of choice for premature ventricular contractions.
- This agent acts as a local heart anesthetic.

- Lidocaine is the most widely used drug for the emergency management of ventricular dysrhythmias.
    - Suppresses premature ventricular contractions (PVCs), converts ventricular tachycardia, and reduces the frequency of ventricular tachycardia
- This agent is usually administered IV for treatment of ventricular dysrhythmias, but may also be administered via the endotracheal route.
- Lidocaine may produce serious central nervous system side effects, and it has a low margin of safety.

Mexiletine hydrochloride (Mexitil) suppresses ventricular ectopy. It can be administered orally to prophylactically treat the same ventricular dysrhythmias that are treated with lidocaine.

Tocainide hydrochloride (Tonocard) is considered to be the oral equivalent of lidocaine. Like mexiletine, tocainide is given orally for prophylactic treatment of the same ventricular arrhythmias that would be treated with lidocaine.

Therapeutic Nursing Interventions

- Obtain a complete nursing, drug, and family medical history, and obtain information about the dysrhythmia(s) the client is experiencing.
- Inquire about medications the client has taken for problems of heart rate and rhythm.
- Ask the client if he or she has experienced adverse reactions to local anesthetics because lidocaine is also used as a local/topical anesthetic.
- When administering lidocaine IV, use a rate-controlling pump, and have an emergency cart readily available.
- Monitor electrocardiogram (ECG), apical pulse rate and rhythm, and blood pressure before giving medication, during administration, and on a regular basis thereafter. Report deviations from target rates and rhythm.
- Monitor serum potassium frequently because hypokalemia exacerbates dysrhythmias.
- Monitor client for dysrhythmias, and report occurrence to the primary care provider.
- Monitor client for signs of heart failure, kidney disease, or liver disease.
- Administer mexiletine and tocainide with food to decrease gastrointestinal distress. Report gastrointestinal symptoms. The dose may need to be adjusted.
- Monitor for confusion, drowsiness, tinnitus, and visual disturbances, which are side effects of these agents. Report adverse effects to the primary care provider.
- Teach client or family member how to accurately take the client's pulse and blood pressure, and when to report findings to the primary care provider.
- Expect to adjust drug dosages for clients with liver or kidney disease because these agents are metabolized in the liver and excreted by the kidneys.
- Schedule regular appointments for re-evaluation following discharge.

Client Education

- Take the medication exactly as directed, and do not skip doses.

- Take pulse prior to and after taking the medication. Report alterations in rate or rhythm.
- Report gastrointestinal side effects and other adverse effects to the primary care provider.
- Avoid driving and other activities that require alertness until effects of the drug are known. Class 1B drugs may cause dizziness and confusion.
- Consult with the primary care provider before taking any OTC drugs because of the risk of adverse drug interactions.
- Carry an identification card at all times that outlines the medication regimen and states the name and telephone number of your primary care provider.
- Schedule regular appointments with a health care professional for reevaluation and ongoing laboratory studies.

Group IC

Overview

Group IC antidysrhythmic drugs primarily block the influx of sodium into the cell membrane, thereby stabilizing the cell membrane and decreasing depolarization. These agents depress automaticity of the sinus node, and they slow impulse conduction in the atria, atrioventricular (AV) node, ventricle, and Purkinje muscle fibers. Group IC drugs are administered to clients with life-threatening ventricular dysrhythmias that have not been controlled with other less toxic agents.

Uses

- Life-threatening ventricular arrhythmias
- Atrial fibrillation
- Atrial flutter

Adverse Effects

- Dysrhythmias
- Dizziness
- Headache
- Fatigue
- Tremor
- Exacerbation of symptoms of heart failure
- Visual disturbances

Precautions

- Group IC drugs are contraindicated for clients who are hypersensitive to these drugs or who have heart block.
- These drugs should not be administered to women who are pregnant or lactating, or to children, because safety of use has not been established.
- These agents should be administered cautiously to clients with heart failure, liver impairment, sick sinus syndrome, hyperkalemia, or hypokalemia.

Important Drugs

Propafenone hydrochloride (Rythmol) is administered for life-threatening ventricular dysrhythmias, paroxysmal supraventricular tachycardia (PSVT), and atrial fibrillation that has not been controlled by other agents.

Flecainide acetate (Tambocor) is administered for life-threatening ventricular dysrhythmias and disabling supraventricular tachycardias.

Therapeutic Nursing Interventions

- Obtain a complete nursing, drug, and family medical history, and obtain information about the dysrhythmia(s) the client is experiencing.
- Monitor ECG, apical pulse rate and rhythm, and blood pressure before giving medication, during administration, and on a regular basis thereafter. Report deviations from target rates and rhythm to the primary care provider. These drugs may worsen existing dysrhythmias or cause new dysrhythmias.
- Monitor serum potassium frequently because hypokalemia exacerbates dysrhythmias.
- Monitor client for dysrhythmias, and for signs and symptoms of heart failure. Report any adverse manifestations to the primary care provider.
- Schedule client for eye examinations on a regular basis while taking these medications.
- Administer flecainide acetate and propafenone hydrochloride with food to decrease gastrointestinal distress. Report gastrointestinal symptoms. The dose may need to be adjusted.
- Teach client or family member how to accurately take client's pulse and blood pressure, and when to report findings to the primary care provider.

Client Education

- Take the medication exactly as directed, and do not skip doses.
- Take pulse prior to and after taking medication, and report alterations in rate or rhythm.
- Report gastrointestinal side effects and other adverse effects to the primary care provider.
- Avoid driving and other activities that require alertness until effects of drug are known. Group 1C drugs may cause dizziness and confusion. Report CNS adverse effects to health care provider.
- Consult with the primary care provider before taking any OTC drugs because of the risk of adverse drug interactions.
- Carry an identification card at all times that outlines the medication regimen and states the name and telephone number of your primary care provider.
- Schedule an appointment for an eye examination. Report any visual changes to the primary care provider.
- Schedule regular appointments for reevaluation of the dysrhythmia, an ECG, and ongoing laboratory studies.

Group II Beta-Adrenergic Blockers

Overview

Group II beta blockers play an important role in the treatment of dysrhythmias. They block adrenergic stimulation to $beta_1$- or $beta_2$-receptors by competing with norepinephrine for available beta-adrenergic receptor sites. Group II agents are given to slow sinus node conduction and prolong conduction through the atrioventricular (AV) node, thereby slowing ventricular response. These agents block excessive sympathetic stimulation at the sinus node, which substantially reduces tachycardia induced by exercise or increased activity.

Uses

Group II beta-adrenergic blocking agents are used to treat the following dysrhythmias:

- Atrial fibrillation
- Atrial flutter
- Tachydysrhythmias
- Wolf-Parkinson-White syndrome (also called atrioventricular nodal reentrant tachycardia). The electrical impulse may return to the upper chamber over an abnormal extra connection that typically has been present since birth. The returning electrical impulse may once again go down the "normal" conduction system, creating an additional heartbeat. Each time this cycle repeats itself, the heart beats. Rapid heart beating is simply the repeating of this kind of cycle many times. This process is the most common mechanism of an arrhythmia in clients with extra connections.
- Ventricular dysrhythmias

Adverse Effects

- Bradycardia
- Orthostatic hypotension
- Edema
- Reduced tolerance to exercise
- Exacerbation or precipitation of heart failure (these agents reduce the force of myocardial contraction and increase preload)
- Bronchoconstriction and bronchospasm
- Shortness of breath
- Hypoglycemia
- Fatigue
- Nausea, vomiting, and diarrhea
- Impotence
- Depression
- Sleep disorders

Precautions

- Group II beta-adrenergic blockers should be administered cautiously to clients with:
  - A history of asthma, emphysema, heart failure, cerebral vascular accident (CVA), hypotension, sinus bradycardia, or heart block
  - Diabetics who are taking insulin or oral hypoglycemic agents because these drugs may mask the symptoms of hypoglycemia
  - Peripheral vascular insufficiency because they constrict peripheral blood vessels and thus reduce blood flow to the extremities
  - Kidney or liver disease because they accumulate in the serum of clients with these diseases, and cause toxic effects
- These agents should not be stopped abruptly, particularly in clients with ischemic heart disease.
- Beta blockers should not be taken with alcohol, central nervous system depressants, or OTC decongestants.
- These agents should be administered with caution to elderly clients because they are more at risk of adverse effects.

Important Drugs

Propranolol hydrochloride (Inderal)

- This agent is the prototype for beta-adrenergic blocking agents.
- It is most effective for clients with dysrhythmias associated with excess catecholamines.
- Propranolol is available in a wide dosage range. Clients vary greatly in the amount of oral drug that survives hepatic metabolism to reach the systemic circulation.

Esmolol hydrochloride (Brevibloc) is used to treat sinus tachycardia and supraventricular dysrhythmias.

Sotalol (Betapace) is given to control the ventricular rate in life-threatening ventricular tachycardia.

Metoprolol (Lopressor) is used to treat ventricular dysrhythmias.

Acebutolol (Monitan) is used to treat ventricular tachydysrhythmia.

Therapeutic Nursing Interventions

- Obtain a complete nursing, drug, and family medical history and obtain information about the dysrhythmia(s) the client is experiencing.
- Inquire about the client's current use of beta blockers or other medications to relieve dysrhythmias.
- Check the client's apical pulse rate before administration because beta blockers slow the sinus rate and may produce bradycardia. If the pulse rate is < 50 bpm, withhold the drug and notify the primary care provider.
- Monitor the client's blood pressure for hypotension.
- Teach the client how to accurately measure own blood pressure and pulse.
- Monitor for hypoglycemia, which is indicated by a blood glucose level of < 60 mg/dl.

- Assess breath sounds and listen for wheezing because beta blockers may cause bronchoconstriction.
- Carefully evaluate the therapeutic effects of the medication. Because the first dose of a beta-blocker is almost completely metabolized by the liver, the dosage may need to be increased for a therapeutic effect.

Client Education

- Learn to take own pulse and blood pressure.
- Do not take the medication and call the primary care provider if pulse rate is < 50 bpm.
- Take beta blockers at the same time each day.
- Learn to monitor blood sugar level for low blood sugar.
- Change positions slowly to prevent orthostatic hypotension.
- Never stop medication abruptly because of the risk of an anginal attack or myocardial infarction.
- Avoid taking beta blockers with antacids without the primary care provider's permission because of the risk of a drug interaction.
- Avoid taking beta-blockers and OTC drugs at the same time without the primary care provider's permission.
- Avoid prolonged exposure to the sun, taking hot showers, sitting in hot tubs, or visiting locations with very hot climates.
- Use caution when driving a vehicle or operating heavy machinery because beta blockers can cause dizziness.
- Avoid drinking alcoholic beverages because the interaction of alcohol and beta blockers may cause adverse effects.
- Store beta blockers in dry, moisture-proof, childproof bottles.
- Schedule regular follow-up appointments.

Group III—Potassium Channel Blockers

Overview

Group III antidysrhythmic drugs each have pharmacokinetic and electrophysiologic properties very different from each other. All of the Group III drugs interfere with norepinephrine. These agents also increase action potential duration (APD) and the effective refractory period (ERP).

Uses

Group III antidysrhythmic drugs are used to treat:

- Ventricular dysrhythmias
- Some atrial dysrhythmias

Adverse Effects

Group III antidysrhythmic drugs may produce the following adverse effects, depending on the specific drug:

- Nausea and vomiting

- Orthostatic hypotension
- Dizziness
- Acute respiratory distress syndrome (ARDS)
- Skin photosensitivity (blue-gray skin discoloration)
- Hypothyroidism
- Hyperthyroidism
- Torsades de pointes
- Visual disturbances (photophobia, halos around lights, decreased visual acuity that may be permanent)

Precautions

- Bretylium should be administered with caution to clients with renal failure, aortic stenosis, pulmonary hypertension, and postural hypotension.
- Amiodarone is contraindicated for clients with bradycardia and severe sinus node dysfunction.
- Amiodarone should be administered with caution to clients with liver disease or pulmonary disease.

Important Drugs

Bretylium tosylate (Bretylol)

- This agent is given intravenously and is used for short-term therapy for life-threatening dysrhythmias. Monitor vital signs carefully.
- Over the first 30 minutes of intravenous therapy, the client may experience hypertension, vomiting, and dysrhythmias. This is because of the release of norepinephrine. Unless the situation is urgent, such toxic effects can be avoided by infusing the drug more slowly.
- A large percentage of clients may experience hypotension that is sufficiently severe to warrant discontinuation of the drug.

Amiodarone (Cordarone)

- This highly toxic, potent antidysrhythmic drug may be administered orally or IV.
- Amiodarone reduces the frequency and duration of life-threatening ventricular dysrhythmias that have not responded to other antidysrhythmic agents.
- Nausea and vomiting are fairly common side effects.
- Almost all clients who receive this agent develop a bluish-gray skin discoloration.
- Because amiodarone is a potentially dangerous drug, the client must be closely monitored for toxic effects such as central nervous system disturbances, acute respiratory distress syndrome (ARDS), and severe hypotension.
- Amiodarone significantly increases digoxin level. For clients taking digoxin, the digoxin dose should be decreased by 50%.

Ibutilide (Covert) is given to treat atrial fibrillation and atrial flutter. Because it can produce life-threatening dysrhythmias the client must be closely monitored.

Therapeutic Nursing Interventions

- Obtain a complete nursing, drug, and family medical history, and obtain information about the dysrhythmia(s) the client is experiencing.
- Monitor the client's electrocardiogram (ECG), blood pressure, and apical pulse continually during intravenous administration of these potent and dangerous antidysrhythmic drugs. Rotate IV sites.
- Observe client closely for the development of new dysrhythmias during IV infusion.
- Notify the primary care provider if the systolic blood pressure drops below 80 mmHg, because the client may require dopamine or norepinephrine and/or blood products for volume correction.
- Monitor liver, kidney, and thyroid function tests for clients receiving amiodarone. Findings may not be available for 1-3 weeks.
- Observe for signs of acute respiratory distress syndrome (ARDS) throughout treatment. Report dyspnea, tachypnea, cough, pleuritic pain, and crackles immediately to the primary care provider. The client will require a chest x-ray and possibly bronchoscopy.
- Observe the client receiving amiodarone for a blue-gray skin discoloration, which is a very common side effect of the drug.
- Schedule ophthalmic examinations before, during, and after therapy with amiodarone because there is a risk of permanent loss of vision.
- Assess client for signs of thyroid dysfunction.
  - Hypothyroidism is manifested by weight gain, lethargy, cool pale skin, and edema of the hands and feet. If these symptoms appear, drug dosage may need to be reduced.
  - Hyperthyroidism is manifested by weight loss, nervousness, tachycardia, insomnia, and skin that is warm and flushed. If these symptoms appear, the drug may need to be discontinued and antithyroid agents administered.
  - Provide emotional support to the client and family while client is taking these potentially toxic Group III drugs.

Client Education

- Take the medication exactly as directed, and do not skip doses.
- Take pulse prior to and after taking medication, and report alterations in rate or rhythm to the primary care provider.
- Report gastrointestinal side effects, signs of thyroid dysfunction, and respiratory distress immediately.
- Avoid driving and other activities that require alertness until effects of the drug are known.
- Change positions slowly to prevent orthostatic hypotension.
- Use sunscreen and stay out of direct sunlight to lessen skin photosensitivity.

- Consult with the primary care provider before taking any OTC drugs because of the risk of adverse drug interactions.
- Carry an identification card at all times that outlines the medication regimen and states the name and telephone number of your primary care provider.
- Schedule an appointment for an eye examination. Report any visual changes to the primary care provider.
- Schedule regular appointments for reevaluation of the dysrhythmia, an ECG, thyroid function tests, and ongoing laboratory studies.

Group IV—Calcium Channel Blockers

Overview

Group IV antidysrhythmics (calcium channel blockers) are used to treat supraventricular arrhythmias with rapid ventricular response rates. Calcium channel blockers act as antidysrhythmics to:

- Prevent the flow of calcium (Ca^+) ions into the cells
- Relax arterial smooth muscle and decrease contraction of the heart muscle
- Slow atrioventricular (AV) conduction
- Reduce the heart rate
- Dilate coronary and peripheral arteries
- Decrease coronary vascular resistance
- Increase coronary blood flow
- Reduce myocardial oxygen demand

Uses

- Calcium channel blockers are used to prevent and control supraventricular tachyarrhythmias.

Adverse Effects

- Constipation (most common side effect)
- Nausea
- Headache
- Leg and muscle cramps
- Orthostatic hypotension (especially when given intravenously)
- Dizziness
- Bradycardia
- Heart block
- Precipitation or worsening of heart failure
- Precipitation of myocardial infarction
- Dyspnea and wheezing
- Hepatic toxicity

Precautions

- Group IV antidysrhythmic agents are contraindicated for clients with these conditions:
  - Hepatic or renal disease
  - Heart block
  - Hypotension
  - Severe bradycardia
  - Aortic stenosis
  - Severe left ventricular dysfunction
- Calcium channel blockers are also contraindicated for women who are pregnant or lactating.
- These agents should be administered with caution to clients with serious respiratory disorders or heart failure because calcium channel blockers can worsen heart failure.
- Calcium channel blockers should be administered with caution to elderly clients because they experience a more pronounced hypotensive effect than do younger clients.
- Discontinuation of these agents should be gradual and under the primary care provider's supervision to prevent untoward effects.

Important Drugs

Verapamil hydrochloride (Calan, Isoptin)

- Verapamil depresses the myocardium and prolongs AV conduction time.
- It is the drug of choice for clients with supraventricular tachycardias who may or may not have angina.

Diltiazem hydrochloride (Cardizem) is used to treat:

- Paroxysmal supraventricular tachycardia (PSVT)
- Atrioventricular node re-entry tachycardia
- Wolf-Parkinson-White syndrome (also called atrioventricular nodal reentrant tachycardia). The electrical impulse may return to the upper chamber over an abnormal extra connection that typically has been present since birth. The returning electrical impulse may once again go down the "normal" conduction system, creating an additional heartbeat. Each time this cycle repeats itself, the heart beats. Rapid heart beating is simply the repeating of this kind of cycle many times. This process is the most common mechanism of an arrhythmia in clients with extra connections.
- Atrial flutter or fibrillation

Therapeutic Nursing Interventions

- Obtain a complete nursing, drug, and family medical history, and obtain information about the dysrhythmia(s) the client is experiencing.
- Inquire about the client's current use of antidysrhythmic agents, including Group IV agents. Ask about the client's response to the drug and any adverse effects.

- Monitor the client's blood pressure and the apical pulse rate and quality before and after the administration of the drug.
  - Do not give the medication if the client has signs of a heart block.
  - Call the primary care provider immediately.
- Teach the client how to accurately measure own blood pressure and pulse.
- Give these agents with food or milk to prevent gastric discomfort.
- Monitor the client for signs of respiratory distress. Observe the client for dyspnea and wheezing. Report respiratory symptoms to the primary care provider.
- Monitor the client with heart failure for worsening symptoms (e.g., increased peripheral edema, increased fatigue, rales in the lungs, more severe dyspnea and orthopnea, and weight gain).
  - Report these findings immediately to the primary care provider.
- Have emergency equipment nearby during IV administration of calcium channel blockers.
- Monitor the client's vital signs continually during administration. Administer IV slowly and monitor ECG findings for abnormalities.

Client Education

- Take medication with food or milk to prevent gastric discomfort.
- Get up from a lying position and change positions slowly to prevent orthostatic hypotension.
- Do not drink alcohol with calcium channel blockers because alcohol acts as a vasodilator and can cause an acute drop in blood pressure and extreme dizziness.
- Report all adverse effects to the health care provider. The drug dosage may need to be adjusted or the drug discontinued.
- Avoid discontinuing medication abruptly without consulting with the primary care provider.
- Carry an identification card at all times that outlines the medication regimen and states the name and telephone number of your primary care provider.
- Notify dentists and other health care professionals of medication regimen.
- Schedule regular follow-up appointments.

Drugs That Treat Hypertension

Overview

Hypertension is usually defined as a systolic blood pressure > 140 mmHg or a diastolic blood pressure > 90 mmHg. Primary or essential hypertension (no cause can be found) comprises 90% of the cases of hypertension. Secondary hypertension results from a specific cause such as renal, endocrine, or CNS disorder. For example, pheochromocytoma is a tumor of the sympathoadrenal system that produces severe hypertension.

The two major determinants of arterial blood pressure are cardiac output (systolic blood pressure) and peripheral resistance (diastolic blood pressure). Cardiac output = heart rate x stroke volume, which is the amount of blood ejected during ventricular contraction. Drugs that lower blood pressure reduce either cardiac output and/or peripheral resistance.

Antihypertensive drugs act at the following sites:

- Kidneys: To increase sodium and water loss and lower blood volume
- Arterioles: To decrease peripheral resistance
- Veins: To decrease venous return and lower cardiac output
- Heart: To reduce cardiac output
- Sympathetic centers in the brain: To lower sympathetic stimulation

The major goals of antihypertensive therapy are to:

- Lower blood pressure to the lowest reading that can be tolerated by the client (usually less than 90 mmHg diastolic)
- Prevent complications of hypertension, including kidney damage, heart failure, myocardial infarction, retinal hemorrhage, cerebral vascular accident (stroke), acute pulmonary edema, transient ischemic attacks (TIA), and hypertensive encephalopathy

There are many different types of antihypertensive agents. The major groups include:

- Angiotensin-converting enzyme (ACE) inhibitors
- Angiotensin-II receptor antagonists
- Antiadrenergics/sympatholytics
- Beta-adrenergic blockers
- Calcium channel blockers
- Direct-acting vasodilators

The drug regimen needs to be individualized for each client for optimum compliance. Usually a stepped-care approach is prescribed to minimize side effects:

- Step 1: The client should stop smoking, lose weight, exercise, restrict alcohol, restrict sodium intake, and reduce stress.
- Step 2: The client should continue to observe Step 1 restrictions. In addition, the primary care provider will prescribe a low dosage of one or two antihypertensive agents.
- Step 3: If the client's blood pressure is not under control, the primary care provider will change drugs or add another antihypertensive agent.
- Step 4: The primary care provider reevaluates the client and prescribes another medication for better blood pressure control.

Special considerations for clients receiving antihypertension therapy include:

- Perioperative period: Give the drug until surgery, and then restart the medication as soon as possible following surgery.
- During pregnancy: Beta blockers are safe, but angiotensin-converting enzyme (ACE) inhibitors are contraindicated.
- Pediatrics: Blood pressure is more labile in children, so it is important to take multiple blood pressure readings. Also, as a general rule, administer the smallest number of drugs and the lowest dosages.
- Geriatrics: Administer a lower dosage of antihypertensives. It is essential to reduce blood pressure slowly to facilitate adequate flow through arteriosclerotic blood vessels.
- Genetic/ethnic considerations: Asians generally need smaller doses of beta blockers. ACE inhibitors and beta blockers are less effective as monotherapy for African-American clients.

Angiotensin-Converting Enzyme (ACE) Inhibitors

Overview

Angiotensin-converting enzyme (ACE) inhibitors inhibit the conversion of angiotensin I to angiotensin II, which is a powerful vasoconstrictor. This action reduces peripheral vascular resistance, and thus lowers blood pressure. These agents reduce aldosterone secretion, which then increases renal sodium and water excretion. ACE inhibitors also reduce metabolic inactivation of bradykinin, a hormone with vasodilator activity. Clients need to have normal renal function to use these drugs as starting antihypertensive agents.

Uses

- Mild to moderate hypertension
- Heart failure, given in conjunction with cardiac glycosides

Adverse Effects

- Renal tubular damage
- Hyperkalemia
- Orthostatic hypotension
- Rash
- Urticaria
- Dysgeusia (an altered sense of taste)
- Cough (affects one-third of clients)
- Renal dysfunction
- Angioedema

Precautions

- ACE inhibitors are contraindicated for clients who previously developed angioedema after taking these agents.
- ACE inhibitors should be administered with caution to clients with renal disorders, sodium depletion, hypovolemia, or coronary insufficiency.
- These agents should be given cautiously to clients who are on dialysis or who are taking diuretics.

Important Drugs

Captopril (Capoten) is given to treat hypertension and heart failure. It is often administered concurrently with a loop diuretic.

Lisinopril (Prinivil) is given to treat hypertension. It is administered alone or in combination with a thiazide diuretic.

Enalapril maleate (Vasotec) is given to treat hypertension and heart failure. It is also available in an intravenous formulation (Enalaprilat).

Quinapril hydrochloride (Accupril) is given to treat hypertension and heart failure.

Moexipril hydrochloride (Univasc) is given alone to treat hypertension, or in combination with a low dose of a thiazide diuretic.

Ramipril (Altace) is given to treat hypertension and hypertensive/renal crisis in clients with scleroderma.

Fosinopril (Monopril) is given to treat hypertension. It is administered alone or in combination with a thiazide diuretic.

Therapeutic Nursing Interventions

- Obtain a complete nursing, drug, and family medical history. Inquire if the client has had a history of high blood pressure.
- Assess the client's lifestyle. Inquire about exercise level, diet, amount of salt and fat intake, daily stress level, smoking habits, and the amount of daily alcohol intake.
- Inquire if the client is taking any cardiovascular drugs, especially any medications to control hypertension. If so, have there been any adverse effects?
- Take the client's blood pressure standing, sitting, and in the supine position prior to beginning antihypertensive drug therapy and then throughout the course of therapy.
    - Also take the apical pulse rate, and note heart rate and any irregularities.
- Instruct the client how to take the blood pressure and pulse at home, and record it properly.
    - Discuss the various types of equipment that can be purchased for taking home blood- pressure readings.
- Take and record the client's weight. If overweight, provide dietary guidelines for weight reduction.
- Monitor the client's intake and output, and monitor renal function tests. ACE inhibitors can cause renal tubular damage.
- Monitor serum electrolytes, in particular potassium and magnesium levels.
- Monitor blood count for signs of neutropenia and agranulocytosis (a significant decrease in the number of neutrophils).
- Assess for angioedema, which is characterized by edema and facial swelling.
    - Report signs to the primary care provider.

Client Education

- Take the medication exactly as ordered, at the same time every day.
- Take and record blood pressure and pulse daily.
    - Contact primary care provider if blood pressure is outside the parameters set by the primary care provider (e.g., usually a blood pressure higher than 140/90 mmHg and a pulse rate that is higher than 100 bpm).
- Stop smoking, restrict intake of alcohol, exercise, avoid stressful situations, learn to control responses to stress, eat a healthy, low-calorie, low-fat diet, and reduce sodium intake.
    - These additional non-pharmacologic therapies will help to lower blood pressure and maintain normal blood pressure readings.
- Change positions slowly to prevent orthostatic hypotension.
- Never stop the medication abruptly because of the risk of rebound hypertension.

- Report side effects such as coughing, itching, or a rash to the primary care provider, who may need to adjust the dosage or change drugs.
- Consult with the primary care provider before taking any OTC drugs because of the risk of adverse drug interactions.
- Carry an identification card at all times that outlines the medication regimen and states the name and telephone number of your primary care provider.
- Schedule regular follow-up appointments for ongoing laboratory studies, and to have blood pressure and pulse rechecked.
    - The primary care provider will need to adjust the antihypertensive drugs if blood pressure remains high.

Angiotensin-II Receptor Antagonists

Overview

Instead of decreasing production of angiotensin like the ACE inhibitors, angiotensin-II receptor antagonists compete with angiotensin II for tissue binding sites. These agents block the vasoconstriction and aldosterone secretion produced by angiotensin, thus lowering blood pressure.

Uses

- Angiotensin-II receptor antagonists are used to treat hypertension.

Adverse Effects

- Diarrhea
- Dyspepsia
- Dizziness
- Orthostatic hypotension
- Cough (less common than with ACE inhibitors)
- Renal dysfunction
- Angioedema

Precautions

- Use cautiously in clients with volume depletion or hyponatremia.
- Clients with liver dysfunction may not be candidates for treatment with angiotensin-II receptor antagonists.
- The efficacy is reduced in African-Americans treated with losartan (Cozaar) monotherapy.

Important Drugs

Losartan potassium (Cozaar) is a new antihypertensive drug that may be used alone or in combination with other drugs.

- Appears to lower blood pressure more substantially in Caucasian clients than in African-American clients

Therapeutic Nursing Interventions

- Obtain a complete health history, including baseline blood pressure prior to treatment with angiotensin-II receptor antagonist.

- Inquire about the lifestyle of the client with hypertension.
  - Assess areas associated with risk for hypertension, including sedentary activity, diet high in fat and cholesterol, consumption of alcohol and nicotine, high salt intake, low dietary fiber, and perceived stress level in daily living.
- Obtain medication history, including antihypertensives and the effect on blood pressure.
  - Information about the side effects the client experiences with various medications is important.
- Monitor blood pressure in standing, sitting, and recumbent positions periodically during course of treatment.
- Monitor serum electrolytes, including sodium, potassium, and magnesium.
  - Report abnormalities to primary care provider.
- Monitor client's weight.
  - Rapid change in weight is a sensitive indicator of fluid balance, which can directly affect the blood pressure.
- Assess for peripheral, periorbital, facial, and generalized edema.
- Monitor the intake and output.
- Monitor serum kidney function tests (BUN and creatinine) and report abnormal findings.
  - Angiotensin-II receptor antagonists can cause kidney impairment.

Client Education

- Emphasize the need to take medication as prescribed even when feeling well.
- If a dose is missed, do not skip it. It is advisable to take the dose as soon as it is remembered.
- Take the medication at the same time daily.
- Notify health care provider if pregnancy is suspected.
  - The treatment regime may need to be altered.
- Notify health care provider prior to surgery or major dental procedures.
- Orthostatic hypotension commonly occurs in persons treated with antihypertensive medications, particularly in hot weather.
- Educate the client regarding the proper method to monitor own blood pressure at home. Provide parameters for the client to report deviations to the health care provider.

Beta-Adrenergic Blockers

Overview

Beta-adrenergic blockers are a group of medications used for the treatment of hypertension, dysrhythmias, and angina pectoris. Beta-adrenergic blockers play an important role in the treatment of hypertension. Beta blockers reduce cardiac contractility, thereby reducing arterial pressure.

- Beta blockers also block sympathetic stimulation at the sinus node, which decreases the heart rate and cardiac output, thereby lowering blood pressure.

The advantages of using beta blockers to treat hypertension are:

- Relief from symptoms of anxiety
- Less fluid volume retention
- Protection from anginal attacks, dysrhythmias, and some complications that follow myocardial infarction

The disadvantages of using beta blockers are the side effects. Beta blockers increase serum lipid levels, cause hypoglycemia, and aggravate heart failure, asthma, or emphysema. From 50% to 70% of clients respond to the blood-pressure-lowering effects of beta blockers.

Uses

- Beta-adrenergic blocking agents are used to treat hypertension, often in combination with a diuretic or other antihypertensive agents.

Adverse Effects

- Bradycardia
- Orthostatic hypotension
- Exacerbation or precipitation of heart failure
- Edema
- Reduced tolerance to exercise
- Bronchoconstriction and bronchospasm
- Shortness of breath
- Hypoglycemia
- Fatigue
- Nausea, vomiting, and diarrhea
- Impotence
- Depression
- Sleep disorders

Precautions

- Beta-adrenergic blocking agents should be administered cautiously to clients with:
  - A history of asthma, emphysema, heart failure, cerebral vascular accident, hypotension, sinus bradycardia, heart block, and peptic ulcer
  - Diabetics who are taking insulin or oral hypoglycemic agents because they may mask the symptoms of hypoglycemia
  - Peripheral vascular insufficiency because they constrict peripheral blood vessels and thus reduce blood flow to the extremities
  - Kidney or liver disease because they accumulate in the serum of clients with these diseases, and cause toxic effects
- These agents should not be stopped abruptly, because abrupt discontinuation may cause rebound hypertension (acute increases in blood pressure that may exceed pre-drug levels).

- Beta blockers should not be taken with alcohol, CNS depressants, or OTC decongestants.
- These agents should be administered with caution to elderly clients because they are more at risk of adverse effects.

Important Drugs

Propranolol hydrochloride (Inderal)

- This agent is the prototype for beta-adrenergic blocking agents.
- It is used to manage hypertension and other cardiovascular conditions.
- Propranolol is available in a wide dosage range.
  - Clients vary greatly in the amount of oral drug that survives hepatic metabolism to reach the systemic circulation.

Atenolol (Tenormin) is prescribed to manage hypertension and reduce heart rate.

Acebutolol (Monitan) is used to treat hypertension and other cardiovascular conditions.

Metoprolol tartrate (Lopressor) is used to treat hypertension and other cardiovascular disorders.

- If metoprolol is given IV, it is essential to monitor vital signs and ECG (electrocardiogram) every 5-15 minutes during administration, and then for several hours following IV infusion.

Labetalol (Normodyne, Trandate) is used to manage hypertension.

Therapeutic Nursing Interventions

- Obtain a complete nursing, drug, and family medical history.
  - Inquire if the client has had a history of high blood pressure.
- Assess the client's lifestyle.
  - Inquire about exercise level, diet, amount of salt and fat intake, daily stress level, smoking habits, and amount of daily alcohol intake.
- Inquire if the client is taking or has ever taken beta blockers for a cardiovascular disorder.
  - If so, ask if the drug helped to control hypertension and if any adverse effects were experienced.
- Take the client's pulse and blood pressure prior to beginning antihypertensive drug therapy and throughout the course of therapy.
- Instruct the client in how to take own blood pressure and pulse at home, and record it properly.
- Take and record the client's weight.
  - If overweight, provide dietary guidelines for weight reduction.
- Monitor for hypoglycemia, which is indicted by a blood glucose level of < 60 mg/dl.
- Carefully evaluate the therapeutic effect of the medication.
  - The first dose of a beta blocker is almost completely metabolized by the liver, therefore the dosage may need to be increased for a therapeutic effect.

Client Education

- Take and record blood pressure and pulse daily.
    - Contact the primary care provider if blood pressure is outside of the parameters set by the primary care provider (e.g., usually a blood pressure higher than 140/90 and a pulse rate that is higher than 100 bpm).
- Take beta blockers at the same time each day.
- Learn to monitor blood sugar level for low blood sugar.
- Make lifestyle changes (lower stress, reduce dietary sodium and fat, exercise) to augment the effects of the medication.
- Change positions slowly to prevent orthostatic hypotension.
- Report side effects to the primary care provider, who may need to adjust the dosage or change drugs.
- Never stop beta blockers abruptly because of the risk of rebound hypertension, anginal attack, or myocardial infarction.
- Avoid taking beta blockers with antacids without the primary care provider's permission because of the risk of a drug interaction.
- Avoid taking beta blockers and OTC drugs at the same time without the primary care provider's permission.
- Avoid prolonged exposure to the sun, taking hot showers, sitting in hot tubs, or visiting locations with very hot climates.
- Schedule regular follow-up appointments.

Calcium Channel Blockers—Calcium Antagonists

Overview

Calcium channel blockers (calcium antagonists) are used to treat hypertension, dysrhythmias, and angina pectoris. Calcium channel blockers lower blood pressure by inhibiting the influx of calcium into muscle cells, which reduces vasoconstriction and dilates coronary and peripheral arteries. These agents also relax arterial smooth muscle and decrease contraction of the heart muscle, thereby lowering blood pressure. Calcium channel blockers are frequently prescribed during the early stages of hypertension.

Uses

- Calcium channel blockers are used to treat and control hypertension.

Adverse Effects

- Constipation (most common side effect)
- Nausea (a sign of overdose)
- Headache
- Leg and muscle cramps
- Orthostatic hypotension (especially when give intravenously)
- Dizziness
- Bradycardia

- Heart block
- Precipitation or worsening of heart failure
- Precipitation of myocardial infarction
- Dyspnea and wheezing
- Hepatic toxicity

Precautions

- Calcium channel blockers are contraindicated for clients with:
  - Hepatic or renal disease
  - Heart block
  - Hypotension
  - Severe bradycardia
  - Aortic stenosis
  - Severe left ventricular dysfunction
- Calcium channel blockers are also contraindicated for women who are pregnant or lactating.
- These agents should be administered with caution to clients with serious respiratory disorders, and to clients with heart failure because calcium channel blockers can worsen heart failure.
- Calcium channel blockers should be administered with caution to elderly clients because they experience a more pronounced hypotensive effect than younger clients.
- Discontinuation of these agents should be gradual and under the primary care provider's supervision to prevent untoward effects.

Important Drugs

Nifedipine (Procardia) is used to treat hypertension and other cardiovascular disorders. It should be administered cautiously to clients with serious cardiac disease because it may precipitate heart failure or myocardial infarction.

Amlodipine besylate (Norvasc) is used to treat hypertension.

- Reduces blood pressure by causing systemic vasodilation
- May be used alone or with other agents

Diltiazem hydrochloride (Cardizem) is used to treat hypertension and other cardiovascular disorders. It reduces blood pressure by causing systemic vasodilation.

Verapamil hydrochloride (Isoptin) is used to treat hypertension and other cardiovascular disorders.

Felodipine (Plendil) is used to treat hypertension and other cardiovascular disorders.

Therapeutic Nursing Interventions

- Obtain a complete nursing, drug, and family medical history.
  - Inquire if the client has had a history of high blood pressure.
- Assess client's lifestyle for controllable risk factors that may contribute to high blood pressure.

- Ask if the client is taking any drugs to control hypertension, including calcium channel blockers.
- Take the client's apical pulse and blood pressure prior to beginning antihypertensive drug therapy and throughout the course of therapy.
- Instruct the client how to take own blood pressure and pulse at home, and record it properly.
- Give calcium channel blockers with food or milk to prevent gastric discomfort.
- Assess the client for dyspnea and wheezing.
  - Report respiratory symptoms to the primary care provider.
- Monitor the client with heart failure for worsening symptoms due to the action of calcium channel blockers.
- Have emergency equipment nearby when administering calcium channel blockers by IV:
  - Monitor the client's vital signs continually during administration.
  - Administer intravenous infusions slowly.
  - Closely monitor ECG findings for abnormalities.

Client Education

- Take calcium channel blockers at the same time each day.
- Take these agents with food or milk to prevent gastric discomfort.
- Take and record blood pressure and pulse rate daily.
  - Contact the primary care provider if blood pressure is outside of the parameters set by the primary care provider.
- Make lifestyle changes (lower stress, reduce dietary sodium and fat, exercise) to augment the effects of the medication.
- Do not drink alcohol with calcium channel blockers because alcohol acts as a vasodilator and can cause an acute drop in blood pressure and extreme dizziness.
- Report all adverse effects to the health care provider.
  - The drug dosage may need to be adjusted or the drug discontinued.
- Avoid discontinuing medication abruptly without consulting with the primary care provider.
- Carry an identification card at all times that outlines the medication regimen and states the name and telephone number of your primary care provider.
- Notify other health care professionals of medication regimen.
- Schedule regular follow-up appointments.

Other Antihypertensive Agents

Prazosin hydrochloride (Minipress) is a peripherally acting alpha-adrenergic blocking agent.

- Dilates both arteries and veins by blocking alpha1-adrenergic receptors. This agent is used to treat mild to moderate hypertension

Reserpine (Serpasil, Sandril) is a peripherally acting alpha-adrenergic blocking agent.

- The most powerful of the rauwolfia compounds
- Used to treat mild to moderate hypertension, and is often combined with diuretic therapy.

Clonidine hydrochloride (Catapres) is a centrally acting sympathetic nervous system inhibitor.

- These alpha$_2$-agonists are used to treat mild to moderate hypertension.
- Major side effects involve the central nervous system and include drowsiness, poor concentration, forgetfulness, and vivid dreams.

Hydralazine (Apresoline) is a direct-acting vasodilator.

- This agent directly dilates arterioles, resulting in decreased peripheral resistance and lowered blood pressure.
- Common adverse effects include tachycardia, palpitations, nausea, and anorexia.

Minoxidil (Loniten) is a powerful, oral, direct-acting vasodilator that is similar to hydralazine.

- It is given once daily and is used for severe hypertension.
- It is also prescribed for clients with hypertension who have not responded to other antihypertensive medications.

Diazoxide (Hyperstat) is a direct-acting vasodilator.

- Used to treat clients with severe hypertension, or those who are in hypertensive crisis
    - Hypertensive crisis is any condition that demands an immediate reduction in blood pressure (e.g., toxemia of pregnancy, pheochromocytoma crisis, hypertensive encephalopathy).

Sodium nitroprusside (Nipride) is a mixed arterial and venous vasodilator.

- This agent is given to rapidly reduce blood pressure in clients who have developed hypertensive crisis.
- Cyanide is a metabolite of this drug.
- Cyanide poisoning may result from prolonged use.
    - Overdose causes profound hypotension and reflex tachycardia.

Drugs That Treat Hypotension and Shock

Overview

The major factor regulating blood flow through the coronary and cerebral vessels is the mean diastolic blood pressure. Hypotension is below normal systolic and diastolic blood pressure, which results in a decreased blood flow through the coronary and cerebral vessels, and decreased profusion of vital organs. Hypotension develops as a result of shock, hemorrhage, severe infections, fevers, cancer, anemia, and debilitating or wasting diseases. It is also a sign of approaching death. Shock is a condition caused by acute peripheral circulatory failure. It is characterized by severe hypotension.

- **Anaphylactic shock** results from extensive vasodilation and decreased peripheral resistance.

- **Cardiogenic shock** is characterized by decreased cardiac output.
- **Hypovolemic shock** results from a decreased volume of circulating blood.
- **Septic shock** results from profound vasodilation and decreased peripheral resistance. It is usually caused by gram-negative bacteria.
- **Traumatic shock** is due to injury or surgery.

Adrenergic Drugs

Overview

The goal of therapy for all forms of shock is to increase blood flow through the coronary and cerebral vessels, and to correct the hypoperfusion of vital organs. The adrenergics are the major drugs used to treat shock. Adrenergic (sympathomimetic) drugs mimic the actions of the sympathetic nervous system. The sympathetic nervous system prepares the body to meet stress with either a fight or flight reaction. Major therapeutic uses and adverse effects of adrenergic drugs stem from drug actions on the heart, lungs, and blood vessels. Some adrenergic drugs act on both the heart and lung receptors. Stimulation of the sympathetic nervous system by adrenergic drugs increases the heart rate, dilates the bronchioles, and takes blood from the gastrointestinal tract and sends it to the skeletal muscles.

Adrenergic agents mimic functions of the sympathetic nervous system by stimulating alpha-adrenergic, beta-adrenergic, and dopaminergic receptors. Alpha receptors are primarily found in blood vessels. Activation results in vasoconstriction, which then raises blood pressure and helps reverse shock. $Beta_1$-receptors are found primarily in the heart. Activation results in increased heart rate, increased force of heart contraction, and increased automaticity and conduction velocity. $Beta_2$-receptors are found primarily in the lungs and peripheral blood vessels. Activation in the lungs results in bronchodilation. Activation in the blood vessels results in vasodilation, with increased blood flow to skeletal muscles, the heart, and the brain. The body needs this increased blood flow to recover from the effects of hypotension and shock.

Uses

Primarily emergency drugs, which are given to treat:

- Cardiac arrest: Given to stimulate the heart
- Hypotension: Given to increase blood pressure
- Shock: Given to increase profusion of blood to the vital organs
- Allergic reactions: Given for vasoconstriction and decongestant effects that relieve edema
- Bleeding: given to constrict blood vessels and stop the bleeding

Adverse Effects

- Nervousness and restlessness
- Sweating

- Hypertension
- Tachycardia and palpitations
- Hyperglycemia
- Nausea and vomiting

Precautions

- Adrenergics are contraindicated for clients with cardiac dysrhythmias, angina, hypertension, and narrow-angle glaucoma.
- Use adrenergics cautiously with children.
- Adrenergics are contraindicated for pregnant women.

Important Drugs

Catecholamine

Epinephrine hydrochloride (Adrenalin)

- The prototype of the adrenergics
- The drug of choice for anaphylaxis
- The active ingredient in OTC asthma preparations
- Effects:
  - Stimulates both alpha and beta receptors
  - Increases blood pressure
  - Increases heart rate
  - Increases blood flow to brain, heart, and skeletal muscles
  - Constricts peripheral vessels
  - Relaxes gastrointestinal smooth muscle
- Administered by:
  - Intravenous injection
  - Subcutaneous injection
  - Intraosseous (in children)
  - Inhalation
  - Injection directly into the heart (intracardially)
  - Cannot be given orally because gastrointestinal enzymes destroy it

Norepinephrine (Levophed)

- Potent vasoconstrictor
- Used to treat:
  - Hypotension
  - Cardiac arrest

Dopamine hydrochloride (Intropin)

- The immediate precursor of norepinephrine
- Dosage effects:
  - Low doses (1-3 mcg/kg/min) cause increased renal perfusion.
  - Intermediate doses (3-10 mcg/kg/min) cause increased cardiac output.
  - Higher doses (>10 mcg/kg/min) cause vasoconstriction and increase blood pressure.

Dobutamine hydrochloride (Dobutrex)

- A synthetic catecholamine
- Acts directly on the heart muscle to increase the force of contraction

Isoproterenol hydrochloride (Isuprel)

- A synthetic catecholamine
- A bronchodilator
- Stimulates both $beta_1$ and $beta_2$ receptors
- Used to control shock and some dysrhythmias
- Absorption effect
  - Good by injection or aerosol
  - Poor by oral or sublingual

Therapeutic Nursing Interventions

- Obtain a short history of the client in shock, and conduct a quick but thorough physical assessment of the client.
- Monitor vital signs and ECG for increased heart rate, decreased blood pressure, and dysrhythmias.
- It is important to check the client's records and obtain a baseline blood pressure if possible.
  - A person who has hypertension, but who suddenly has a "normal" blood pressure reading, may actually be going into shock.
- Monitor respirations and lung sounds for bronchial congestion and difficult breathing.
- Monitor blood glucose levels for elevated blood sugar.
- Monitor I & O for signs of renal failure due to shock.
- Administer plasma expanders or blood transfusions as ordered.
  - Observe for and immediately report any adverse effects.
- Administer emergency drugs such as epinephrine as ordered.
  - Observe for and immediately report any adverse effects.
- Avoid infiltration of IV infusion into the tissues, especially when infusing norepinephrine bitartrate (Levophed) or dopamine (Intropin).
  - Never leave the client unattended while receiving norepinephrine IV.
  - Inspect the intravenous site every 15 minutes for edema and coolness.
  - Compare the injection site with the opposite extremity.
  - Observe for a decreased or stopped drip rate.
  - If infiltration is suspected, discontinue the infusion immediately and notify the primary care provider. Phentolamine (Regitine) may be prescribed to treat the extravasation.
  - Once shock has been reversed, the client will need to be gradually weaned off of the norepinephrine drip.
- This drug can cause tissue necrosis, which may result in the amputation of the involved extremity.
- Continually monitor the client's blood pressure, pulse, respirations, ECG tracings, and laboratory reports until shock is reversed.

Client Education

- Following treatment for hypotension and shock, schedule follow-up visits to evaluate progress.

Critical Thinking Exercise: Drugs Affecting the Cardiovascular System

Note: *It is recommended that the following exercises be reviewed with a partner or in a small group to achieve maximum student interaction and to enhance critical thinking skills.*

1. Heart failure develops when the following occurs:

   a. The cardiac and pulmonary vessels become occluded with plaque.

   b. When the pulse pressure drops too rapidly.

   c. When the heart muscle fails to pump effectively and sufficient blood does not circulate to the lungs and body tissue.

   d. When the ventricles become hypertrophied due to viral or bacterial infection.

2. List four types of angina.

3. Hypertension is usually defined as:

   a. Systolic blood pressure <90 mm Hg and diastolic blood pressure >60 mm Hg

   b. Diastolic blood pressure >90 mm Hg and systolic blood pressure >140 mm Hg

   c. Diastolic blood pressure <60 mm Hg and systolic blood pressure >80 mm Hg

   d. Systolic blood pressure >120 mm Hg and diastolic blood pressure <80 mm Hg

4. Digoxin has the following action:

    a. Increases the ability of the heart to respond to adrenal hormones

    b. Strengthens atrial contractility and decreases pulmonary artery resistance

    c. Decreases atrial irritability and restores normal conduction

    d. Increases cardiac contracility without elevating the oxygen requirement of the myocardium

5. The primary goal of andrenergic therapy for all forms of shock is to:

    a. Decrease the likelihood of myocardial infarction

    b. Increase blood flow to maintain adequate kidney function

    c. Increase blood flow through the coronary and cerebral vessels

    d. Stimulate the release of stress hormones to reduce peripheral perfusion

6. Drugs that affect the cardiovascular system are often given to counteract the effects of shock. In the table below, draw a line from the description of the shock (left) to the correct type of shock (right).

Table 1

Description	Type of shock
Characterized by decreased cardiac output	Traumatic
Results from profound vasodilation and decreased peripheral resistance often resulting from gram-negative bacteria	Anaphylactic
Results from a decreased volume of circulating blood	Septic
Generally due to injury	Cardiogenic
Extensive vasodilation and decreased peripheral resistance often resulting from systemic allergic responses	Hypovolemic

---

Situation: S.M is a 64-year-old with heart failure who has been maintained on digoxin 0.125 mg, PO daily for a number of years without problems. He is now admitted to the hospital with bilateral ankle edema, weight gain of 12 pounds, dyspnea on exertion and fatigue. His admission ECG (electrocardiogram) showed atrial fibrillation. His digoxin level was 0.9 ng/ml. He was placed on the following medications:

- Digoxin 0.125 mg, PO daily
- Lasix 80 mg IVP now, then Lasix 40 mg, PO BID
- K-Dur 20 mEq, PO BID
- Amiodarone (Cordarone) 200 mg, PO daily
- Heparin 1000 units/hour, IV (after a loading dose of 5,000 units)

---

7. What is the primary nursing concern when digoxin and Lasix are given simultaneously?

8. What are the signs of digitalis toxicity?

9. Based on the above clinical scenario, what do you think are the clinical indications for administering heparin to this client?

10. What must the nurse consider about the dosage of either digoxin or amiodarone when they are being administered together?

CHAPTER 7

Drugs Affecting the Blood

Key Points

- Anticoagulants, antiplatelets, and thrombolytic agents are used in the prevention and treatment of thrombotic and thromboembolic disorders.
- Anticoagulant therapy:
  - Anticoagulant drugs are given to prevent formation of new clots and extension of existing clots.
  - They are also given to prevent or treat thrombosis or alter some aspect of the blood coagulation process.
  - Parenteral heparin and oral warfarin (Coumadin) are the two most commonly used anticoagulants.
  - Low-molecular-weight (LMW) heparins are a new type of antithrombin drug. LMW heparins, also called heparinoids, have a longer half-life and requires less laboratory monitoring than heparin sodium.
  - Venipunctures and injection sites of clients on anticoagulant therapy require application of pressure to prevent bleeding or hematoma formation.
  - Intramuscular injections of other medications should be avoided to prevent the development of hematomas.
  - A heparin dose should be checked by second licensed personnel, prior to administration.
  - Clotting status is monitored by the activated partial thromboplastin time (APTT) and partial thromboplastin time (PTT) at 1.5-2.5 times the normal.
  - Mild thrombocytopenia is expected to appear on the 4th day of heparin therapy; it resolves itself despite continued therapy.
  - Protamine sulfate can be given as a slow IV push over 10 minutes to neutralize heparin activity.
  - In clients requiring long-term anticoagulation, oral anticoagulant therapy should be instituted 3-5 days prior to discontinuing heparin therapy.
  - Coumadin dosage is adjusted by the prothrombin time (PT) at 1.3-1.5 times the normal or the International Normalized Ratio (INR) at 2-3 times the control value.
  - Vitamin K is the antidote to reverse anticoagulation effects of Coumadin.
  - Missed doses should be taken as soon as possible, unless it is almost time for the next dose. Clients taking Coumadin should not double-dose to catch up.
- Antianemic therapy:
  - Erythropoietin (Epogen) is a hormone used to treat anemia primarily associated with chronic renal failure. It stimulates the bone marrow to increase the production of red blood cells.

    - Erythropoietin can be administered either intravenously for hemodialysis clients or subcutaneously for those clients not on dialysis three times per week.
- Thrombolytic therapy:
    - Thrombolytic therapy is used for the treatment of an acute myocardial infarction.
    - Thrombolytic agents are given to dissolve thrombi and reperfuse the myocardium before cellular death occurs.
    - The choice of a thrombolytic agent depends mainly on the risks of adverse effects and costs.
    - All thrombolytics may cause either internal or external bleeding and should be administered by experienced personnel in the intensive care unit setting.
    - Commonly used thrombolytics include alteplase (Activase), anistreplase (Eminase), streptokinase (Streptase), and urokinase (Abbokinase).
- Antiplatelet therapy:
    - Antiplatelet drugs prevent platelet aggregation, interfering with initial phase of blood coagulation.
    - Commonly known antiplatelet drugs are aspirin, dipyridamole (Persantine), ticlopidine (Ticlid), and abciximab (ReoPro).
    - Do not crush or chew enteric-coated tablets, and do not take antacids within 1-2 hours of consuming enteric-coated aspirin tablets.
    - Chewable aspirin tablets may be chewed, dissolved in liquid, or swallowed whole.
    - Drink a full glass of water and sit up for 15-30 minutes following dosage.
- Blood replacement therapy:
    - Reactions to blood transfusions are more likely to occur within the first 15 minutes of administration.
    - Blood transfusion has broadened to include the administration of specific blood components, such as packed red blood cells (RBCs), platelets, fresh-frozen plasma, albumin, and cryoprecipitate.
    - Infuse blood products through a 19-gauge or larger needle into a free-flowing IV line with a Y-connector and filter.
    - No other additives should be given via the same tubing as the blood.
        - Insert another peripheral IV for infusion of medications and other fluids.

Blood Coagulation

Overview

Platelets are essential for blood coagulation. Blood coagulation is a normal body defense mechanism to prevent blood loss. Normal blood coagulation is a complex process caused by injury to a blood vessel. When injury occurs to a blood vessel wall, platelets respond within seconds to form a platelet plug and stop bleeding. Simultaneously, the fragile cell membrane disintegrates, allowing platelet contents to leak, causing vasoconstriction and activation of prothrombin. After 24 hours, fibrin replaces platelets at the blood clot. Blood coagulation causes hemostasis 1-2 minutes following platelet aggregation. The blood coagulation process involves the:

- Release of thromboplastin by disintegrating platelets and damaged tissue
- Conversion of prothrombin to thrombin requiring thromboplastin and calcium ions
- Conversion of fibrinogen to fibrin by thrombin

There is a sequential activation of clotting factors normally present in the blood and tissues. The blood coagulation factors and functions are outlined below:

- **Fibrinogen** forms fibrin, the insoluble protein strands that compose the supporting framework of a blood clot.
- **Prothrombin** forms thrombin, which catalyzes the conversion of fibrinogen to fibrin; thrombin and calcium are required for the conversion.
- Tissue thromboplastin (**tissue factor**) converts prothrombin to thrombin.
- **Calcium** catalyzes the conversion of prothrombin to thrombin.
- **Labile factor** is required for the formation of active thromboplastin.
- **Platelet coagulant activities** (PF_3 and PF_4)
- Proconvertin, or **stable factor**, accelerates action of tissue thromboplastin.
- **Antihemophilic factor** promotes breakdown of platelets and formation of active platelet thromboplastin.
- **Christmas factor** acts similar to Factor VIII.
- **Stuart-Prower factor** promotes action of thromboplastin.
- **Plasma thromboplastin antecedent** promotes platelet aggregation and breakdown, with subsequent release of platelet thromboplastin.
- **Hageman factor** is similar to Factor XI.
- **Fibrin-stabilizing factor** converts fibrin meshwork to the dense, tight mass of the completely formed clot.

Anticoagulants

Overview

Anticoagulation therapy is widely used in thrombotic disorders. Thrombus formation is the development of a blood clot in the vascular system. An embolus occurs when part of a thrombus breaks off and travels to another part of the body. Thrombi and emboli that lodge in vital organs are major causes of morbidity and mortality. Thrombosis may occur in both arteries and veins. Arterial thrombosis is usually associated with atherosclerotic plaque, hypertension, and turbulent blood flow, causing partial or complete obstruction. Venous thrombosis is usually associated with venous stasis, and is less cohesive than an arterial thrombus, and more likely to become an embolus. Anticoagulant therapy is more effective in preventing venous, rather than arterial, thrombosis. Anticoagulants do not dissolve clots, improve blood flow in the surrounding tissue of a clot, nor prevent ischemic damage to tissues beyond the clot. Anticoagulant drugs are given to prevent clot extension and formation. The two types of anticoagulants most commonly used are parenteral heparins and oral warfarin. These drugs act by different mechanisms to interfere with certain coagulation factors.

Heparin

Overview

Heparin is a pharmaceutical preparation of the natural anticoagulant produced primarily by mast cells in connective tissue. Standard heparin is a mixture of high and low molecular weights with most anticoagulant activity attributed to low molecular weights.

Heparin:

- Acts directly on the intrinsic and common pathways of blood coagulation.
- Inhibits thrombin-mediated conversion of fibrinogen to fibrin.
- Prevents thrombus formation effectively when antithrombin deficiency (also called: antithrombin III) is present in the blood.
- Potentiates the actions of antithrombin III, inhibits the activation of factor IX, and neutralizes activated factor X by activating factor X inhibitor.
- Is metabolized in the liver and excreted in the urine.
- Possesses a half-life of 1-2 hours; increases with increasing dosage.
- Does not cross the placental barrier and is not secreted in breast milk.
- In low doses, prevents the conversion of prothrombin to thrombin.
- In high doses, neutralizes thrombin and prevents the conversion of fibrinogen to fibrin.

A new type of antithrombin drug, the low-molecular-weight (LMW) heparin, may be more effective than heparin sodium for the prevention and management of clotting disorders. This type of drug requires less laboratory monitoring.

Uses for Heparin Sodium

- Prophylaxis and treatment of various thromboembolic disorders, including:
  - Venous thromboembolism (e.g., deep venous thrombosis [DVT] and thrombophlebitis)
  - Pulmonary emboli
  - Atrial fibrillation with embolization
  - Acute and chronic consumptive coagulopathies
  - Peripheral arterial thromboembolism
- Maintains patency of IV catheters as a heparin flush in very low doses of 10-100 units
- Acts immediately after intravenous (IV) administration and within 20-30 minutes after subcutaneous injection
- Prevents clotting during cardiac and vascular surgery, extracorporeal circulation, hemodialysis, blood transfusions, and in blood samples used for laboratory testing
- Effective in preventing embolization from prosthetic heart valves
- Used in disseminated intravascular coagulation (DIC)—a life-threatening condition characterized by widespread clotting, which depletes the blood coagulation factors

    - Goal of heparin therapy in DIC is to prevent blood coagulation long enough for clotting factors to be replenished and thus be able to control hemorrhage.

Uses for Low-Molecular-Weight (LMW) Heparins

- Prevention of thromboembolic phenomena including DVT
- Pulmonary emboli after surgical procedures known to increase the risk of such complications (e.g., knee/hip replacement, abdominal surgery)

Adverse Effects

- Life-threatening adverse reaction is bleeding.
- Most commonly encountered problems include anemia and thrombocytopenia.
- Local pain or discomfort may be experienced at injection site.
- Gastrointestinal effect includes drug-induced hepatitis.
- Increased risk of bleeding can occur when used concurrently with:
    - Antiplatelet drugs, such as aspirin, nonsteroidal anti-inflammatory drugs (NSAIDs), clopidogrel (Plavix), dipyridamole (Persantine)
    - Drugs that cause hypoprothrombinemia, including quinidine and cephalosporins
    - Thrombolytic agents
- Anticoagulant effect of heparin may be increased by:
    - Digitalis glycosides
    - Tetracyclines
    - Nicotine
    - Antihistamines
- Long-term use causes:
    - Alopecia
    - Osteoporosis

Precautions

- Contraindicated for the client with:
    - Active hemorrhage
    - Gastrointestinal ulcerations (e.g., peptic ulcer disease, ulcerative colitis)
    - Blood dyscrasias, such as hemophilia, thrombocytopenia, or polycythemia vera
    - Severe liver or kidney disease
    - Severe uncontrolled or untreated hypertension
    - Recent CNS surgery, spinal cord injury, brain injury, or hemorrhagic stroke
    - Recent ophthalmologic surgery or retinopathy associated with hypertension or diabetes mellitus
- Use cautiously for clients with:
    - Mild hypertension
    - Severe diabetes
    - Bacterial endocarditis
    - Renal or hepatic disease

- Alcoholism
- History of gastrointestinal ulcerations
- Presence of drainage tubes (e.g., nasogastric tubes, indwelling urinary catheters)
- History of congenital or acquired bleeding disorder
- Malignancy
- Women >60 years old who have an increased risk of bleeding
- Last trimester of pregnancy and the immediate postpartum period
- Any occupations with high risk of traumatic injury

- Thrombocytopenia not resolved by the 8th day of therapy necessitates discontinuing medication.
- Low-dose heparin prophylaxis is either ineffective or contraindicated in abdominal prostatectomy, and brain surgery.
- aPTT (activated partial thromboplastin time) or PTT (partial thromboplastin time) monitoring is not necessary with low-dose conventional heparin given subcutaneously for prophylaxis of thromboembolism, or with enoxaparin or dalteparin (LMW heparins).
- Heparin has not been proven effective in preventing further thromboembolic problems, despite its use in arterial occlusive disease, myocardial infarction (MI), and stroke.
- Protamine sulfate acts as an antidote or antagonist for heparin by neutralizing heparin activity.

Important Drugs

Heparin sodium

- Low-molecular-weight heparins/heparinoids:

  Enoxaparin (Lovenox)
  - Treats DVT
  - Prevents ischemic complications in clients with unstable angina and non-Q-wave MI when combined with aspirin

  Dalteparin (Fragmin)
  - Prevents ischemic complications in clients with unstable angina and non-Q-wave MI when combined with aspirin

  Danaparoid (Orgaran)

  Ardeparin (Normiflo)

Therapeutic Nursing Interventions

- Obtain a health history, specifically pertaining to bleeding disorders and preexisting conditions that may increase the risk for bleeding complications.
- Check PTT each day before administering the drug. The therapeutic level for PTT is 1.5 to 2.5 times the "normal" (control) value. Standards vary by institution and range from a low of 20 seconds to generally not more than 35 seconds duration.
- Assess client for bleeding gums, nosebleeds, unusual bruising, decreased hematocrit or blood pressure, hematuria, guaiac-positive stools, and prolonged bleeding from puncture sites or minor wounds.

- Assess client for evidence of additional or increased thrombosis.
- Monitor client for hypersensitivity reactions, such as chills, fever, and urticaria.
- Observe injection sites for hematomas, ecchymosis, or inflammation.
- Reduce the risk for hematomas and bleeding at injection sites by using 25- or 26-gauge needles or tuberculin syringes for the subcutaneous route, rotating and not massaging sites.
    - Apply steady pressure for 1-2 minutes or longer if needed.
    - Do not aspirate prior to injection.
- Avoid injection near scarred tissue.
- Administer heparin using the "bunching" technique into the fatty tissue in the abdomen and area above the iliac crest.
- Document the sites for injection using a graphic record.
- Careful attention to dosage is critical because of the different concentration supplied to pharmacies.
    - The most common medication error is the confusion between the 1,000 USP units/mL and the 10,000 USP units/mL vials.
- For heparin therapy administered intravenously, diligently check the equipment, tube connections, and IV patency for appropriate delivery of medication.
- Monitor activated partial thromboplastin time (aPTT) or partial thromboplastin time (PTT) and hematocrit prior to and regularly throughout therapy.
- Observe for therapeutic levels of the aPTT and the PTT.
- For intermittent IV therapy, draw aPTT or PTT levels 30 minutes before each dose during initial therapy and then regularly every 6 hours.
- During continuous administration, monitor aPTT or PTT levels every six hours during early therapy.
- For subcutaneous therapy, draw blood 4-6 hours after injection.
- Avoid use of heparin containing the preservative benzyl alcohol in premature infants.
- Monitor platelet count every 2-3 days throughout therapy for the development of thrombocytopenia.
- Expect mild thrombocytopenia to appear on the 4th day of therapy; this effect is transient.
- Dose adjustment is needed for weight <45 kg with low-molecular-weight heparins/ heparinoids.

Client Education

- Wear Medic Alert identification indicating what type of anticoagulant is being taken.
- Make appointments for regular follow-up with blood tests to assess blood clotting and whether a change in drug dosage is required.
- Avoid vigorous activities leading to injury that might cause bleeding.

- Contact primary care provider immediately for:
  - Any bleeding that does not stop after a reasonable amount of time
  - Blood in urine or stool, or black, tarry stools
  - Unusual bleeding from gums, throat, skin, or nose
  - Severe headaches or stomach pains
  - Weakness and dizziness
- Avoid alcohol or consume less than one alcoholic beverage per day because of the potential for liver impairment, which can lead to increased sensitivity to anticoagulation therapy.
- Avoid aspirin-containing drugs and NSAIDs due to a compounding anticoagulation effect.
- Alopecia may occur with long-term therapy but hair growth will return to normal after discontinuation of the drug.
- Diet can alter the effectiveness of anticoagulant therapy.
  - Foods high in vitamin K (green vegetables, foods in the cabbage family, and spinach) or the consumption of supplemental vitamin containing high vitamin K can interfere with warfarin (Coumadin).
- Persons with malabsorption disease, chronic diarrhea, or vitamin C deficiency may experience an increased anticoagulant effect.
- Clients should be instructed to use an electric shaver when shaving, a soft toothbrush, and protective gear as necessary.
- Inform primary care providers, dentists, and other health care providers of anticoagulant therapy before invasive procedures.

Warfarin

Overview

Warfarin (Coumadin) is the most commonly used coumarin anticoagulant.

Coumadin:

- Inhibits hepatic synthesis of vitamin K-dependent clotting Factors (II, VII, IX, and X)
  - Vitamin K is normally required for the synthesis of these factors.
- Acts as a competitive antagonist to hepatic use of vitamin K because Coumadin is structurally similar to vitamin K
- Has no effect on circulating clotting factors or on platelet function
- Is absorbed well in the gastrointestinal tract following oral administration
- Is metabolized by the liver and excreted by the kidneys
- Is highly bound to plasma proteins, mainly albumin
- Has a half-life of 0.5 to 3 days
- Crosses the placenta, but does not enter breast milk

Uses

Long-term prevention or treatment of venous thromboembolic disorders:

- Deep vein thrombosis (DVT)
- Pulmonary embolism
- Atrial fibrillation with embolization

Management of myocardial infarction (MI):

- Decreases risk of:
  - Death
  - Subsequent MI
  - Future thromboembolic events

Prevention of thrombus formation and embolization after prosthetic valve placement.

Adverse Effects

Contraindications include:

- Gastrointestinal ulcerations (e.g., peptic ulcer disease, ulcerative colitis)
- Blood dyscrasias (e.g., hemophilia, thrombocytopenia)
- Severe kidney or liver disease
- Severe hypertension
- Recent surgery of the eye, spinal cord, or brain
- Pregnancy

Use cautiously in:

- Hypertension
- Renal or hepatic disease
- Alcoholism
- History of gastrointestinal ulcerations
- Drainage tubes (e.g., nasogastric [NG] tubes, indwelling urinary catheters)
- Occupations with high risk of traumatic injury

Increased risk of bleeding can occur when used concurrently with:

- Antiplatelet drugs, such as salicylates, clopidogrel, NSAIDs
- Cephalosporins
- Thrombolytic agents

Anticoagulant effect of warfarin (Coumadin) may be decreased by:

- Estrogens or oral contraceptives
- Phenytoin
- Nutritional supplements containing vitamin K

Adverse effects include:

- Cramps and nausea on initial therapy
- Possible dermal necrosis
- Rare, severe reactions can occur following IV infusion. The client may exhibit dizziness, flushing, confusion, thready pulse, chest pain, and shortness of breath.

Precautions

- Anticoagulant effects do not occur for about 3-5 days after warfarin (Coumadin) is started because clotting factors already in the blood follow their normal pathway of elimination.
- Oral anticoagulants are begun while heparin is still being administered, overlapping 3-5 days to maintain therapeutic control of clotting.
- Initiate therapy with lower doses in geriatric or debilitated clients.
- There is no advantage in therapeutic effect, if warfarin is given parenterally.
- Coumadin is not indicated in arterial thrombosis because arterial thrombi are composed primarily of platelets.
- Withholding one or more doses of medications is usually sufficient if prothrombin time (PT) is excessively prolonged or if minor bleeding occurs.
- If overdose occurs or anticoagulation needs to be immediately reversed, the antidote is vitamin K.
- Administration of whole blood plasma also may be required in severe bleeding because of delayed onset of vitamin K.

Important Drugs

Warfarin (Coumadin) is the prototype.

Therapeutic Nursing Interventions

- Assess client for signs of bleeding and hemorrhage from gums, skin, nose, urine, and stools.
- Warfarin (Coumadin) is usually given orally.
- Monitor PT or INR (International Normalized Ratio) regularly during therapy.
- Check for a therapeutic PT level of 1.3-1.5 times the control or an INR of 2-3 times the control value.
- Adjust oral dosage of 2.5-10 mg tablets per day by lab results.
- Monitor stool and urine periodically for blood.

Client Education

- Take medication at the same time each day.
- If dose is missed, take it as soon as possible.
- Do not double-dose to catch up and inform a health care professional of current dosage at time of lab tests.
- Diet can alter the effectiveness of anticoagulant therapy.
    - Keep diet consistent. Avoid foods or vitamins high in vitamin K, including turnip greens, asparagus, broccoli, watercress, cabbage, beef liver, lettuce, and green tea because they decrease anticoagulant action or warfarin. If your diet changes, alert your primary care provider.
- Wear Medic Alert identification indicating what type of anticoagulant is being taken.
- Avoid alcohol or consume less than one alcoholic beverage per day because of the potential for liver impairments, which can lead to increased sensitivity to anticoagulation therapy.

- Contact primary care provider immediately if any of the following occurs:
  - Any bleeding that does not stop after a reasonable amount of time
  - Blood in urine or stool, or black, tarry stools
  - Unusual bleeding from gums, throat, skin, or nose
  - Severe headaches or stomach pains
  - Weakness and dizziness
- Avoid aspirin-containing drugs and NSAIDs.
- Inform the client receiving heparin that alopecia may occur with long-term therapy but hair growth will return to normal after discontinuation of the drug.

Anti-Anemics

Erythropoietin

Overview

Erythropoietin is a hormone produced by the kidneys to stimulate the bone marrow to produce red blood cells (RBCs). Erythropoiesis is:

- The production of erythrocytes, or RBCs
- Largely regulated by cellular oxygen requirements and general metabolic activity
- A process stimulated by hypoxia and controlled hormonally by erythropoietin
- Influenced by the availability of nutrients. The essential nutrients are iron, vitamin B_{12}, and folic acid
- Influenced by the number of reticulocytes as this number predicts the adequacy of erythrocyte production

Uses

- Treatment of anemia associated with chronic renal failure
- Management of anemia secondary to azidothymidine (AZT or zidovudine) (Retrovir) therapy in HIV-infected clients
- Management of anemia from chemotherapy in clients with nonmyeloid malignancies
- Reduction of need for transfusions after surgery

Adverse Effects

- Risk of seizures is greatest during the first 90 days of therapy
- May cause transient rashes and petechiae

Precautions

- Institute seizure precautions in clients who experience greater than a 4 percentage point increase in hematocrit in a 2-week period or exhibit any change in neurologic status.
- Contraindicated in uncontrolled hypertension and clients with erythropoietin levels >200 mU/mL

- Clients receiving zidovudine with endogenous serum erythropoietin levels > 500 mU/mL may not respond to therapy.
- Use cautiously in clients with:
    - History of seizures
    - History of porphyria
    - Pregnancy or who are lactating

Important Drugs

Epoetin alfa (Epogen, EPO, Procrit)

Therapeutic Nursing Interventions

- Monitor for manifestations of anemia:
- Dyspnea
- Fatigue
- Tachycardia, palpitations
- Pallor of nail beds and mucous membranes
- Low hemoglobin and hematocrit levels
- Easy bruising
- Assess level of consciousness for changes in neurological response:
    - Speech disturbances
    - Sudden headache
    - Numbness, tingling
- Monitor lab values, including complete blood count (CBC) with reticulocyte count.
- Monitor blood pressure before and throughout therapy. Note any increases in blood pressure before and throughout therapy.
- Administer intravenously and undiluted.
    - Do not shake vial.
    - Discard immediately upon withdrawing single dose.
    - Refrigerate multi-dose vial.
    - Stable for 21 days after opening.
- Use subcutaneous route for clients not requiring dialysis.
- Monitor serum ferritin, transferring, and iron levels during iron supplementation therapy.
- Transfuse blood for severe symptomatic anemia as ordered.
- For anemia of chronic renal failure:
    - Assess dialysis shunt for the presence of thrill and auscultate the bruit to determine the capacity for hemodialysis.
    - Check hematocrit before and twice weekly during initial therapy, for 2-6 weeks after a change in dose, and regularly after target range of 30-36% has been reached and maintenance dose is determined.
    - Monitor renal function studies and electrolytes closely; for clients with chronic renal failure expect abnormal values in blood urea nitrogen (BUN), creatinine, phosphorus, and potassium.

    - Initially administer 50-100 units/kg either subcutaneously or intravenously 3 times weekly, and then adjust dosage based on hematocrit.
- For anemia secondary to zidovudine therapy:
    - Determine serum erythropoietin level before therapy.
    - Monitor hematocrit weekly during dosage adjustment.
    - Administer 100 units/kg either subcutaneously or intravenously 3 times weekly for 8 weeks; if response adequate, may increase by 50-100 units/kg every 4-8 weeks, up to 300 units/kg 3 times weekly.
- For anemia from chemotherapy:
    - Monitor hematocrit weekly until stable.
    - Administer 150 units/kg subcutaneously 3 times weekly.
        - May increase after 8 weeks up to 300 units/kg for 3 times weekly.
- For anemia from surgery:
    - Determine hematocrit at >10 to <13 g/dL before therapy.
    - Administer 300 units/kg/day for 10 days before surgery, the day of surgery, and 4 days after; or 600 units/kg at 21, 14, and 7 days before surgery and on day of surgery.

Client Education

- Understand the rationale for concurrent iron therapy because it is required to increase RBC production.
- Monitor activities, such as driving, when there is an increased risk of seizures.
- Comply with dietary and fluid restrictions.
- Take medications as prescribed.

Thrombolytics

Overview

Thrombolytic therapy is used in the treatment of acute myocardial infarction (MI). The overall goal of thrombolytic therapy is to re-establish blood flow and prevent or limit tissue damage. Thrombolytic agents:

- Dissolve thrombi
- Stimulate conversion of plasminogen to plasmin (also called fibrinolysins)
- Degrade fibrin present in clots because plasmin is a proteolytic enzyme that breaks down fibrin, the framework of a thrombus

Uses

- Acute management of coronary thrombosis, or the treatment of an acute MI
- Lysis of thrombi in coronary arteries, with preservation of ventricular function
- Lysis of pulmonary emboli or deep vein thrombosis
- Decreased neurologic sequelae with stroke
- Dissolving of clots in intravascular catheters
- Iliofemoral thrombosis

Adverse Effects

- Bleeding is the most common adverse effect.
  - Internal (e.g., intracranial, gastrointestinal, genitourinary)
  - External (e.g., venous or arterial puncture sites, surgical incisions)
- Exercise extreme caution in using thrombolytic agents in:
  - Clients receiving warfarin therapy
  - Clients within 10 days of childbirth (early postpartum period)
- Alteplase and anistreplase may act more specifically on the fibrin in a clot and cause less systemic depletion of fibrinogen, but they are very expensive.
- Streptokinase is the least expensive agent, but may cause an allergic reaction because it is a foreign protein.

Precautions

- Although these drugs have different mechanisms of action and different pharmacokinetics, they all produce an open artery by lysis of the thrombus in the coronary artery.
- It is important to decrease the risks of bleeding by carefully selecting recipients, avoiding invasive procedures when possible, and omitting anticoagulant or antiplatelet drugs while thrombolytics are being given.
- If bleeding cannot be controlled with local pressure, the thrombolytic drug should be stopped and fibrinogen replaced with whole blood plasma or cryoprecipitate.
- Before initiating thrombolytic therapy, determine blood coagulation by checking baseline values of lab tests for:
  - Prothrombin time (PT) or International Normalized Ratio (INR)
  - Activated partial thromboplastin time (aPTT) and partial thromboplastin time (PTT)
  - Platelet count
  - Fibrinogen
- Contraindicated in clients with:
  - Active internal bleeding
  - History of cerebrovascular accident, recent CNS trauma or surgery, neoplasm, or arteriovenous malformation
  - Severe uncontrolled hypertension
  - Known bleeding tendencies
- Use with caution in clients with:
  - Recent major surgery (within 10 days), trauma, gastrointestinal, or genitourinary bleeding
  - Left heart thrombus
  - Severe hepatic or renal disease
  - Hemorrhagic ophthalmic conditions
  - Septic phlebitis
  - Previous puncture of a noncompressible vessel
  - Subacute bacterial endocarditis or acute pericarditis

- Recent streptokinase infection or previous therapy within the previous 6 months
- Clients >75 years old
- Pregnancy, lactation, or in children

Important Drugs

Alteplase (Activase)

- Produced by recombinant deoxyribonucleic acid (DNA) technology
- Referred to as t-PA (tissue plasminogen activator)
- Used in acute MI to dissolve clots obstructing coronary arteries and reestablish tissue perfusion beyond the thrombotic area
- Binds to fibrin in clot and acts locally to dissolve the clot with minimal systemic effects
- Administered as an IV infusion, 100 mg over 3 hours with a standard regimen of:
  - 60 mg with a bolus of 6-10 mg over 1-2 minutes in first hour
  - 20 mg in the second hour
  - 20 mg in the third hour
- Administered as an IV infusion in an accelerated or front-loading regimen of:
  - 15 mg initially
  - Then 0.75 mg/kg (up to 50 mg) over 30 minutes
  - Then 0.5 mg/kg (up to 35 mg) over next 60 minutes
  - Usually accompanied by heparin therapy

Anistreplase (Eminase)

- Combination of human plasminogen and streptokinase
- Breaks down fibrin similar to t-PA
- Used to lyse coronary artery clots in acute MI
- Administer as a single IV injection of 30 units over 2-5 minutes

Streptokinase (Streptase)

- Protein derived from streptococci
- Interacts with a plasminogen proactivator
- Catalyzes conversion of plasminogen to plasmin
- Used for treatment of acute pulmonary emboli or iliofemoral thrombophlebitis
- Administer intravenously for pulmonary emboli, or into arterial or venous cannula for catheter occlusion
- Use direct intracoronary administration to dissolve a thrombus if done within 6 hours from the onset of symptoms

Urokinase (Abbokinase)

- Proteolytic enzyme that catalyzes conversion of plasminogen to plasmin
- Recommended for use in clients allergic to streptokinase
- Contraindicated in children, pregnancy, open wounds, malignancies, and recent strokes

- Heparin and warfarin are started after urokinase therapy is completed
- Administered intravenously for pulmonary embolus
- Administer intracoronary for coronary thrombosis
- Used for treatment of catheter occlusion

Therapeutic Nursing Interventions

- Begin therapy immediately following the onset of symptoms.
- Assess client for bleeding every 15 minutes during the first hour of therapy, every 30 minutes for the next hour, every hour for the next 4 hours, then every 4 hours for the duration of therapy.
- Assess client for hypersensitivity reaction; notify health care provider immediately.
- Monitor vital signs with oral temperature, at least every 4 hours.
- Do not use lower extremities to monitor blood pressure because of the risk of dislodging a deep vein thrombosis.
- Apply pressure to site and reinforce original dressing, if local bleeding occurs.
- Discontinue therapy and notify the primary care provider, if uncontrolled bleeding occurs.
- Assess for changes in neurologic status, indicating possible intracranial bleeding.
- Monitor ECG continuously for dysrhythmias.
- Check cardiac enzymes.
- Assess intensity, character, location, and radiation of chest pain. Note presence of associated symptoms.
- Administer medications for chest pain and discomfort.
- Monitor heart and lung sounds every 4 hours for gallops and adventitious sounds.
- Observe extremities and palpate pulses of affected extremities every hour.
- Monitor ability to aspirate blood as indicator of catheter patency.
- Evaluate lab tests and expect changes:
  - Hematocrit (Hct)
  - Hemoglobin (Hgb)
  - Platelet count
  - Fibrin/fibrin degradation product titer
  - Fibrinogen concentration
  - Prothrombin time (PT)
  - Thrombin time
  - Activated partial thromboplastin time (aPTT)
- Type and crossmatch for possible blood transfusion at all times in case of hemorrhage.
- Test stool for occult blood loss and urine for hematuria.
- Mix constituted drug gently to prevent foaming.
  - The bubbles will disappear; allow the solution to settle for a few minutes.

- Do not add any other medication to the bag because of the drug incompatibility.
- Avoid unnecessary handling or repositioning of the client to avoid bruising.

Client Education

- Understand purpose of medication administration.
- Maintain bedrest during therapy.
- Avoid trauma to lower extremities.
- Perform passive range-of-motion (ROM) leg exercises.
- Wear antiembolic hose; remove every 8 hours.
- Maintain fluid intake at 1500-3000 mL/dL to avoid dehydration and hemoconcentration.

Antiplatelets

Overview

Increased platelet aggregation is associated with atherosclerosis and thromboembolic disorders. Arterial thrombi are mainly composed of platelets that can embolize from abnormal heart valves, mural thrombi, or atherosclerotic plaque. Antiplatelet agents:

- Prevent platelet aggregation
- Interfere with the initial phase of blood coagulation

Uses

- Abciximab (ReoPro), tirafiban (Aggrastat), eptifibatide (Integrilin) are used with aspirin and heparin to prevent reclosure of treated coronary arteries after percutaneous transluminal angioplasty or atherectomy, or to prevent acute cardiac ischemic complications.
- Other drugs, such as dipyridamole (Persantine), clopidogrel (Plavix) and ticlopidine (Ticlid), are used to prevent:
  - MI
  - Stroke in clients with transient ischemic attack (TIA)
  - Thromboembolism in clients with prosthetic heart valves

Adverse Effects

- Use of antiplatelet agents may cause an increased risk of bleeding.
- Routine use of aspirin may cause gastrointestinal bleeding, dyspepsia, epigastric distress, heartburn, and nausea, but the small doses of aspirin for antiplatelet effects will most likely not cause adverse effects.

Precautions

- Contraindicated in bleeding disorders and thrombocytopenia, or a cross-sensitivity with NSAIDs
- Use cautiously with:
  - History of gastrointestinal bleeding or ulcer disease
  - Chronic alcohol use/abuse

    - Severe renal or hepatic disease
    - Geriatric clients
    - Pregnancy and lactating mothers
- Thiazide diuretics, alcohol, estrogen, and chemotherapeutic agents can suppress platelet production.
- Abnormal platelet aggregation is caused by:
    - NSAIDs, such as ibuprofen, indomethacin, and naproxen
    - Antibiotics, such as penicillins and cephalosporins
    - Analgesics, such as aspirin and aspirin-containing drugs
    - Spices, such as ginger, cumin, turmeric, cloves, and garlic
    - Vitamins C and E
- Aspirin is a commonly used analgesic-antipyretic-anti-inflammatory drug with potent antiplatelet effects and minimal adverse effects.
- If platelet count is <80,000, discontinue ticlopidine. Platelet transfusions can reverse the effects of antiplatelet agents.

Important Drugs

Aspirin

- Produces analgesia and reduces inflammation and fever
- Decreases platelet aggregation by inhibiting the production of prostaglandins
- Reduces the incidence of transient ischemic attacks (TIAs) and MI
- Exerts antiplatelet effects with small dosages

Dipyridamole (Persantine)

- Decreases platelet aggregation by inhibiting the enzyme phosphodiesterase
- Produces coronary vasodilation by inhibiting adenosine uptake
- Recommended for prevention of thromboembolism after cardiac valve replacement when given in combination with warfarin
- Dilates normal coronary arteries, reducing flow to vessels that are narrowed and causing abnormal thallium distribution during diagnostic thallium imaging

Ticlopidine (Ticlid)

- Inhibits platelet aggregation by altering the function of platelet membranes
- Prolongs bleeding time
- Indicated for prevention of thrombosis in coronary artery or cerebral vascular disease
- Prevents stroke in clients who have had a completed thrombotic stroke, experienced TIAs, and are unable to tolerate aspirin

Abciximab (ReoPro)

- A monoclonal antibody that binds with platelets and inhibits platelet aggregation
- Abciximab is used with percutaneous transluminal coronary angioplasty to prevent rethrombosis of treated arteries, and prevention of acute cardiac ischemic complications.

- Contraindicated in clients who have recently received an oral anticoagulant or IV dextran
- Monitor femoral site access for bleeding.

Clopidogrel (Plavix)

- Inhibits platelet aggregation by altering the platelet membrane
- Prevents heart attack and stroke
- Prolongs bleeding time

Eptifibatide (Integrillin)

- Used in the treatment of clients with acute coronary syndrome
- Used for the treatment of clients undergoing percutaneous coronary intervention (PCI)

Tirofiban (Aggrastat)

- Used in the treatment of clients with acute coronary syndrome
- Used for the treatment of clients undergoing PCI

Therapeutic Nursing Interventions

- Monitor blood pressure and pulse before instituting therapy.
- Monitor vital signs routinely.
- Obtain an ECG.
- Assess for symptoms of stroke.
- Monitor lab tests for bleeding time, CBC with differential, and platelet count every two weeks for three months.
- Administer medications after meals or with food or an antacid to minimize gastric irritation.

Client Education

- Drink salicylates with a full glass of water and sit up for 15-30 minutes.
- Take only prescribed dosage; increasing the dosage will not provide additional benefits.
- Take missed doses as soon as possible unless it is almost time for the next dose; do not double-dose to catch up.
- Do not change brands; notify the primary care provider for any changes in medication.
- Report tinnitus, unusual bleeding of gums, bruising, black, tarry stools, or fever lasting longer than three days.
- Avoid concurrent use of alcohol to minimize gastric irritation.
- Avoid taking concurrently with OTC drugs (e.g., NSAIDs).
- Change positions slowly to minimize orthostatic hypotension.
- Follow up with routine visits and lab work, especially during the first three months of therapy to monitor for side effects.

Blood Products

Overview

Hematologic System: Blood nourishes and oxygenates all body cells, protects the body from invading microorganisms, and initiates hemostasis by carrying platelets to injured areas. Plasma comprises about 55% of the total blood volume, and is more than 90% water. Erythrocytes, or red blood cells (RBCs), have a lifespan of 120 days, and function to transport oxygen. Leukocytes, or white blood cells (WBCs), have a lifespan of a few hours, produce antibodies, and function as a defense mechanism against microorganisms through phagocytosis. Platelets, or thrombocytes, are fragments of large cells called megakaryocytes that circulate in the bloodstream for 7-10 days before the spleen removes them. Serum albumin helps maintain blood volume by exerting colloidal osmotic pressure, moving water from extravascular space into intravascular space.

Blood component therapy is used to manage and treat many hematologic disorders. However, it is only temporary support for the client because ultimately the underlying problem must be resolved for true control. Blood transfusion traditionally has meant the administration of whole blood only. However, plasma is rich in clotting factors, but does not contain platelets. Therefore, blood transfusion has broadened to include the administration of specific blood components, such as:

Packed RBCs are prepared from whole blood by sedimentation or centrifugation; one unit contains 250-350 mL.

Platelets are prepared from fresh whole blood within 4 hours after collection; one unit contains 30-60 mL of platelet concentrate.

Fresh-frozen plasma is the liquid portion of whole blood separated from cells and frozen; one unit contains 200-250 mL and must be used within 2 hours after thawing. Plasma is rich in clotting factors, but does not contain platelets.

Albumin is prepared from plasma and is available in 5%-25% solution.

Cryoprecipitate is prepared from fresh-frozen plasma, with 10-20 mL per bag; it must be used once it is thawed.

Uses

- Transfusion of packed RBCs is indicated for:
  - Severe or symptomatic anemia
  - Acute blood loss
- Autotransfusion of frozen RBCs is done for clients with previous febrile reactions to transfusions. It is infrequently used because filters remove most of the WBCs.
- Transfusion of platelets is indicated for bleeding caused by thrombocytopenia and platelets levels 10,000/µL to 20,000/µL; expect an increase of 10,000 µL/unit.
- Infusion of fresh-frozen plasma is used for bleeding caused by a deficiency in clotting factor (e.g., DIC [disseminated intravascular coagulation], hemorrhage, massive transfusion).
  - Also used for blood volume expansion in clients with extensive burn injury, shock, or protein deficiency

- Albumin is given for hypovolemic shock, hypoalbuminemia, and treatment of cerebral edema.
- Cryoprecipitate replaces clotting factors, especially Factor VIII and fibrinogen.
- Blood transfusion has broadened to include the administration of specific blood components, such as packed RBCs, fresh-frozen plasma, albumin, and cryoprecipitate.

Adverse Effects

- Blood transfusion reactions are more likely to occur within the first 15 minutes of administration.
- Rapid infusion of cold blood may cause the client to become chilled. If rapid replacement is necessary, a blood-warming device should be used.
- Acute blood transfusion reactions include: acute hemolytic reactions, febrile reactions, mild allergic reactions, circulatory overload, sepsis, and massive blood transfusion reaction. They will usually occur within the first 15 minutes of blood transfusion.
- Delayed blood transfusion reactions include: delayed hemolytic reactions, iron overload, and Graft-versus-Host-Disease (GVHD).
    - They will occur 2-4 days after the administration of blood/blood products.
- The most common cause of hemolytic reactions is transfusion of incompatible blood when antibodies in the recipient's serum react with antigens on the donor's RBCs.

Precautions

- Larger than 19-gauge needles may be preferred to prevent hemolysis of RBCs if rapid transfusion is needed.
- Smaller size needles can be used for platelets, albumin, and cryoprecipitates.
- Dextrose solutions or lactated Ringer's solutions should not be used because they induce RBC hemolysis.
- Blood administration tubing should have a filter and a Y-connector with an isotonic saline solution; may connect a stopcock to control flow and maintain a closed system.
- Other additives, especially medications, should not be given via the same tubing as the blood, unless the tubing is cleared completely with saline solution.
- Do not refrigerate blood on the nursing unit; it should be administered immediately upon collecting from the blood bank.
- Blood should be infused within 4 hours. Any blood remaining after 4 hours should not be infused.
- Infuse blood products between 2-4 hours safely through a 19-gauge or larger needle into a free-flowing IV line with a Y-connector and filter.
- No other additives should be given via the same tubing as the blood. Insert another peripheral IV for infusion of medications and other fluids.

Important Blood Components

- Packed RBCs
- Frozen RBCs

- Platelets
- Fresh-frozen plasma
- Albumin
- Cryoprecipitate and commercial concentrates

Therapeutic Nursing Interventions

- Verify consent for blood administration and treatment.
- Position the person in a comfortable, reclining position.
- Check with a second licensed personnel to make a positive identification of donor blood and recipient. Errors in transfusions given to the wrong client can result in transfusion reaction and adverse effects.
- Use universal precautions for handling blood products and intravenous insertion equipment because of the risk of blood-borne pathogens (e.g., hepatitis, acquired immune deficiency syndrome [AIDs]).
- Administer blood components safely with a 19-gauge or larger needle into a free-flowing IV line.
- Connect filter and prime tubing with saline solutions.
    - Do not use dextrose or other solutions with blood products because it may cause cell lysis.
- Do not administer other drugs with blood products.
- To achieve transfusion infusion rate, the nurse may raise the level of the bed, utilizing the force of gravity.
    - A pressure bag may be inflated to 300 mmHg to increase the rate, however, excessive pressure may cause the blood bag to burst.
- Document the client's baseline vital signs, time the transfusion started and was completed, total volume, and client's response to transfusion.
    - Medical record must contain the signatures of the nurse responsible for the transfusion and the person double-checking the correct product with the client.
- Avoid overly rapid transfusion, particularly for persons with congestive heart failure. Assess for signs of circulatory overload (edema, enlarged liver, distended neck veins, tachypnea, oxygen need).
- Complete the infusion of blood products over a 2-4 hour period.
- To avoid blood incompatibility:
    - Do not give the client with type A blood either B or AB blood.
    - Do not give the client with type B blood either A or AB blood.
    - Persons with type O blood (universal donor) can only receive type O transfusions.
- Monitor for clinical manifestations of an acute hemolytic reaction:
    - Chills
    - Fever
    - Low back pain
    - Flushing

  - Tachycardia
  - Tachypnea
  - Hypotension
  - Vascular collapse
  - Hemoglobinuria
  - Acute jaundice
  - Dark urine
  - Bleeding
  - Acute renal failure
  - Shock
  - Cardiac arrest
  - Death
- If a blood transfusion reaction occurs, then:
  - Stop the infusion.
  - Maintain a patent IV line with saline solution.
  - Notify the blood bank and the primary care provider immediately.
  - Recheck identifying tags and numbers.
  - Monitor vital signs and urine output.
  - Treat symptoms per primary care provider orders.
  - Save the blood bag and tubing and send them to the blood bank for examination.
  - Complete transfusion reaction reports.
  - Collect required blood and urine specimens at intervals stipulated by hospital policy to evaluate for hemolysis.
  - Document on transfusion reaction form and client chart.

Client Education

- Understand treatment and give consent.
- Understand the cause or reason for treatment.
- Maintain bedrest during blood administration.
- Report any pain or discomfort, flushed skin, chills, headache, or burning sensation.

Blood Chelation Therapy

Uses

- Chelating agents attract calcium within the bloodstream and calcium stores within the bones to form a water-soluble compound to reduce lead levels in the body. The excess lead is then excreted through the urinary system.

Adverse Effects

- Nausea
- Vomiting
- Anorexia
- Fatigue
- Headache
- Glycosuria
- Anemia
- Arrhythmias (prolonged QT and inverted T)

Precautions

- Use only when severe blood lead levels (BLL) exist: 45 micrograms/deciliter or higher
- Monitor VS and ECG before and during therapy
- Monitor serum electrolytes carefully (especially calcium)
- IV extravasation may cause peripheral tissue necrosis

Important Drugs

Ethylenediaminetetraacetic acid (commonly called calcium disodium edetate [EDTA]) is the most common chelating agent.

- Administered IV or IM
- Used most commonly when BLL is 45 micrograms/deciliter or higher.
- Adult/pediatric dose: 40 mg/kg every 24 hours in divided doses (Q 6-12 hour intervals)
- Monitor BLL, serum electrolytes, urine and serum renal studies, renal function, CBC, and liver function tests.

Succimer (Chemet) is another common chelating agent

- Administered orally
- Pediatric dose: 10 mg/kg TID times 5 days, then follow with same dosage BID for two weeks.
- Comes in capsules that can be broken and placed in food or liquid to facilitate administration

Therapeutic Nursing Interventions

Monitor:

- Neurologic deficit (decreased LOC)
- Alterations in behaviors

- Loss of appetite; nausea
- ECG changes (inverted T waves)
- Seizures

Client Education

- Educate client about lead hazards, including environmental testing in the home and removal of causative agent
- Review medication administration (dosing and scheduling)
- Observe client carefully for any physical changes in health
- Instruct client to avoid folk remedies; instead seek professional medical assistance
- Dietary considerations:
    - Encourage drinking from cold water tap (hot water tap may contain more lead
    - Eat foods with adequate iron and calcium

Critical Thinking Exercise: Drugs Affecting the Blood

Note: *It is recommended that the following exercises be reviewed with a partner or in a small group to achieve maximum student interaction and to enhance critical thinking skills.*

Situation: M.S. is a 54-year-old man who began having chest pain during lunch while at work. On admission to the emergency department via ambulance one hour later, M.S. was pale, diaphoretic, and complained of shortness of breath. He was diagnosed with unstable angina to rule out myocardial infarction (MI). The client reported no previous episodes of chest pain or pressure. He has smoked two packs of cigarettes daily for 25 years. There is no family history of heart disease.

After evaluation of initial lab results, presenting symptoms, and ECG, the diagnosis of an extensive anterolateral MI was made. The client was considered a candidate for thrombolytic therapy; tissue plasminogen activator (t-PA) was started immediately, using front-loaded dosing technique. A nitroglycerin (NTG) drip (50 mg/250 mL D5W) was started at 1.5 mL/h (5 mcg/min). A heparin bolus of 8000 units given IVP, and a drip was hung at 1000 units/hour. Metoprolol tartrate 25 mg and an aspirin were given orally. The client was transferred to ICU.

After 1.5 hours of t-PA, his chest pain returned and blood pressure was 96/60. NTG was given sublingually with no relief, and no ECG changes were noted. M.S. was sent to the cardiac catheterization lab for an emergency cardiac catheterization and possible percutaneous transluminal coronary angioplasty (PTCA). Results showed 90% blockage of left anterior descending coronary artery, and a successful PTCA was performed. A total of 23,000 units of heparin was given IVP, and 500,00 units of urokinase was given intracoronary.

1. What are the pharmacologic actions of heparin?

2. What are the indicators for use of heparin in the client after a myocardial infarction (MI)?

3. What is the effect of a thrombolytic agent on the MI client?

4. What made the client eligible to receive thrombolytics?

CHAPTER 8

Drugs Affecting the Respiratory System

Key Points

- Antihistamines are used to:
  - Treat various allergic reactions
  - Induce sleep
  - Relieve nausea
  - Prevent motion sickness
- Antihistamines are classified as first or second generation. The primary difference is that first-generation drugs cause more drowsiness and have more anticholinergic side effects.
- Antihistamines are generally contraindicated with:
  - Narrow-angle glaucoma
  - Prostatic hypertrophy
  - Pregnancy
  - Bladder neck obstruction
  - Peptic ulcer disease
- Antitussives suppress the cough center in the medulla.
- The two types of antitussives are opioids and non-opioids.
- Antitussives should be used to suppress a cough that is nonproductive, painful, or preventing sleep.
  - Contraindicated for clients with severe chronic respiratory disorders and with productive cough
- Codeine is often added to cough medicines to suppress a cough.
  - The most serious adverse effect of opioids is respiratory depression.
- Bronchodilators are used to relax the smooth muscle in the bronchi and bronchioles in conditions such as asthma, bronchitis, and emphysema.
- Adrenergic bronchodilators that affect both beta1- and beta2-receptors can cause tachycardia and cardiac arrhythmias.
- Selective beta2-adrenergic agonists produce bronchodilation with minimal symptoms of cardiac stimulation.
- Excessive use of adrenergic bronchodilators can cause paradoxical bronchoconstriction.
- Anticholinergic bronchodilators do not relieve acute bronchoconstriction, but enhance the bronchodilating effects of adrenergics.
- When taking more than one medication by inhalation:

  - Wait at least one minute between puffs of a single drug.
  - Wait at least five minutes between inhaling different drugs.
- When taking multiple inhaled drugs, take the bronchodilator first and the corticosteroid last.
- Clients on xanthines such as theophylline (Theo-Dur) must have serum drug levels monitored regularly because the drugs have a narrow margin of safety and toxicity can cause fatal arrhythmias. Therapeutic serum theophylline levels are 10-20 mcg/mL.
- Children and cigarette smokers generally need higher doses of theophylline (Theo-Dur) preparations because they metabolize theophylline rapidly.
- Topical adrenergics relieve nasal congestion, but can cause rebound congestion if used for more than 3 days.
- Although some experts dispute their effectiveness, expectorants may be ordered to stimulate respiratory secretions and thin mucus for easier expectoration.
- Inhaled corticosteroids reduce airway inflammation and increase the number and sensitivity of beta2-receptors to adrenergic bronchodilators.
- Inhaled corticosteroids are unlikely to have systemic effects, and therefore are much safer than oral corticosteroids.
- Rinsing the mouth with water after using a corticosteroid inhaler helps to prevent oral irritation and fungal infection.
- Leukotriene modifiers prevent symptoms of asthma by suppressing synthesis of leukotrienes or blocking their receptors.
- Periodic liver function tests should be done for clients taking zileuton (Zyflo) or zafirlukast (Accolate).
- Cromolyn and the leukotriene inhibitors are used for prevention, NOT for acute attacks.
- Mast cell stabilizers reduce symptoms of inflammation in the respiratory tract by preventing the release of histamine from mast cells.
- Mucolytics react directly with mucus to make it thinner and more easily expectorated.
- Mucomyst is the antidote for acetaminophen overdose.

Antihistamines

Overview

Histamine is an important chemical mediator that is stored in mast cells located in almost all body tissues. Histamine is released in response to antigens for which a person has developed antibodies. The effects of histamine include:

- Contraction of smooth muscle in the bronchi, gastrointestinal tract, and uterus
- Vasodilation and increased capillary permeability (edema)
- Increased secretion of gastric juicealso increases bronchial, intestinal, and salivary secretions.
- Pain and itching caused by sensory nerve stimulation

Antihistamines prevent the effects of histamine by occupying the histamine receptors. The two types of histamine receptors are H_1- and H_2-receptors; antihistamines are H_1- antagonists. Antihistamines are classified as first or second generation. The primary difference is that first-generation drugs cause more drowsiness and anticholinergic side effects. Antihistamines are used to treat symptoms caused by histamine in a variety of allergic disorders. Because there are other substances that produce allergic reactions besides histamine, antihistamines may provide only partial relief of the symptoms.

Uses

Allergic reactions, such as:

- Rhinitis
- Common cold
- Contact dermatitis
- Drug reactions
- Anaphylaxis
- Insomnia
- Urticaria
- Pruritus
- Nausea and vomiting

Antihistamines are used to prevent:

- Motion sickness
- Allergic reactions to transfusions of blood or blood products

Adverse Effects

- The elderly are at higher risk for dizziness, confusion, hypotension, unsteady gait, and CNS stimulation. Antihistamine dosage should be lower for them.
- Most antihistamines have anticholinergic side effects, including dry mouth and blurred vision.
- Central nervous system (CNS) effects
  - CNS effects of first-generation antihistamines vary with the dosage.
    - Usual doses: drowsiness, blurred vision
    - High doses: CNS stimulation
    - Phenothiazines: convulsive seizures
  - Second-generation antihistamines can cause:
    - Fatigue
    - Headache
    - Drowsiness (usually less than first generation)
    - Hypertension
- Gastrointestinal effects
  - First-generation antihistamines can cause:
    - Dry mouth

- Constipation
- Anorexia
- Nausea
- Vomiting
- Second-generation antihistamines may cause dry mouth and gastrointestinal distress.
- Genitourinary effects
    - First-generation antihistamines can cause urinary retention, especially in older males with prostatic enlargement.
- Drug allergy
    - Anaphylaxis may occur in clients who are allergic to antihistamines.

Precautions

- First-generation antihistamines taken with other CNS depressants can cause excessive sedation.
- Some antibiotics enhance the effects of loratadine (Claritin).
- Antihistamines are generally contraindicated with narrow-angle glaucoma, prostatic hypertrophy, pregnancy, bladder neck obstruction, and peptic ulcer disease.
- Antihistamines are not recommended with bronchitis or pneumonia because they dry secretions, making them more difficult to remove.
- Monoamine oxidase inhibitors (MAO) inhibitors inhibit metabolism of antihistamines and enhance their effects.
- The anticholinergic adverse effects of antihistamines are enhanced by the henbane leaf herb.
- Children may experience drowsiness with first few administrations and CNS excitation with repeated use.

Important Drugs

Fexofenadine (Allegra) is the prototype second-generation antihistamine used for rhinitis.

Loratadine (Claritin) is an effective antihistamine for seasonal allergies given in the tablet or syrup form.

Cetirizine (Zyrtec) is an H1-receptor antagonist used for allergic rhinitis and urticaria.

Dimenhydrinate (Dramamine) and meclizine (Antivert) are used to prevent and treat motion sickness.

Promethazine (Phenergan) and hydroxyzine (Vistaril) are used to treat nausea and vomiting, and increase CNS depression.

Diphenhydramine hydrochloride (Benadryl) is used to treat allergic responses and to promote sleep.

Therapeutic Nursing Interventions

- Monitor for therapeutic and adverse effects.
- Administer intravenous antihistamines slowly to prevent severe hypotension.

- Give oral antihistamines with food to decrease gastrointestinal distress.
- Caution the client about drowsiness and institute safety precautions.
- Offer fluids often and assist with oral hygiene as needed for dry mouth.
- Assess for urinary retention, especially in older male clients.
- Document stools and encourage extra fluids and fiber to prevent constipation.
- Notify primary care provider of constipation and discuss possibility of using stool softeners or bulk laxatives.

Client Education

- Do not drive when you are drowsy.
- Taking antihistamines (except loratadine) with food usually controls gastrointestinal distress.
- Antihistamines will manage allergies more effectively if they are taken regularly rather than only after symptoms develop.
- To prevent constipation, increase your physical activity and your intake of fluids and fiber.
- To prevent motion sickness, take antihistamines 30-60 minutes before travel.
- If you have prostate enlargement, ask your primary care provider to recommend the most appropriate antihistamine.

Antitussives

Overview

Antitussives are drugs used to relieve cough by suppressing the cough center in the medulla. Coughing is usually caused by irritation of the bronchial mucosa. Coughing is a protective mechanism in that it helps to remove foreign matter and excess secretions from the airway.

The two types of antitussives are opioids and non-opioids. Codeine is an opioid used as an antitussive. Antitussive mixtures that contain codeine are classified under Schedule V of the Controlled Substances Act. Dextromethorphan is a non-opioid antitussive that is as effective as codeine, but lacks the potential for abuse.

Uses

- Suppresses a cough that is nonproductive, painful, or prevents sleep

Adverse Effects

- Central nervous system effects
  - Opioids can cause:
    - Drowsiness
    - Sedation
    - Dizziness
    - Respiratory depression
  - Less commonly, opioids cause:
    - Restlessness

        - Agitation
        - Euphoria
        - Seizures
    - Dizziness and sedation (Dextromethorphan)
- Gastrointestinal effects
    - Opioid effects on the gastrointestinal tract include:
        - Nausea
        - Vomiting
        - Anorexia
        - Constipation
    - Nausea (Dextromethorphan)
- Respiratory effects
    - Respiratory depression is the most serious adverse effect of opioids.
    - The antidote for opioid toxicity is naloxone (Narcan).
- Cardiovascular effects
    - Opioids can cause:
        - Circulatory collapse
        - Hypotension
        - Tachycardia or bradycardia
- Genitourinary effects
    - Clients on codeine may have urinary retention, especially if they have prostate enlargement.
- Integumentary effects
    - Codeine can cause:
        - Rash
        - Itching
        - Flushing
        - Urticaria (hives)
- Drug allergy
    - Opioids may cause anaphylaxis in the client who is allergic to it.

Precautions

- The sedative effects of antitussives are enhanced by other CNS depressants and by the herb kava.
- Older adults should be given lower doses of antitussives to avoid excessive sedation and dizziness.
- Both codeine and dextromethorphan are contraindicated with severe respiratory disorders (e.g., asthma, chronic obstructive pulmonary disease [COPD]), hypersensitivity, and productive cough.
- Codeine is contraindicated with increased intracranial pressure.
- Opioids must be used cautiously in older adults and in clients with cardiac dysrhythmias.
- In clients taking MAO inhibitors, codeine must be used cautiously; dextromethorphan should not be used at all.

- A productive cough in a client with chronic respiratory disease should not be suppressed.

Important Drugs

Codeine is an opioid most often used as an analgesic.

- A low dose of codeine is often combined with other drugs in cough suppressant preparations.

Dextromethorphan is the most prominent non-opioid antitussive.

- It is an ingredient in numerous cough and cold remedies.

Therapeutic Nursing Interventions

- Assess cough and sputum characteristics.
- Unless contraindicated, encourage high fluid intake to thin secretions.
- Monitor urinary and bowel elimination.
- Monitor respirations.
    - Report rate < 10 breaths/minute to primary care provider.
- Promote safety with opioid use: Put side rails up; place call button in client's reach; turn night-light on.
- Monitor mental status and vital signs.

Client Education

- See your primary care provider if cough persists more than 2-3 days.
- Avoid smoke, dust, and other respiratory irritants.
- Do not drink alcohol while taking opioids.
- Caution outpatients that drowsiness may make driving unsafe.
- Advise clients to call for assistance getting up if dizzy or sedated.
- Change positions and rise slowly to prevent dizziness.

Bronchodilators

Overview

Constriction of the bronchi and bronchioles occurs in response to various stimuli. Severe bronchoconstriction is life-threatening, so prompt relief is vital to client survival. Bronchodilators are drugs that relax the smooth muscles in bronchi and bronchioles.

Bronchodilators are often used with drugs that reduce inflammation in the airways. Three types of drugs used as bronchodilators are:

Adrenergics:

- Act on beta$_2$-adrenergic receptors in the smooth muscles of the bronchi and bronchioles. They stimulate increased production of cyclic adenosine monophosphate (cAMP), which induces relaxation of the smooth muscle and allows the airways to dilate.
- Some adrenergics act on beta1-adrenergic receptors as well, which results in cardiac stimulation.
- Adrenergics that affect primarily beta$_2$-adrenergic receptors are said to be selective adrenergics.

Xanthines:

- Increase cAMP, but by a different mechanism. Xanthines inhibit the enzyme that normally breaks down cAMP.
- Cause mild diuresis by increasing blood flow to the kidneys.

Anticholinergics:

- Given by inhalation reduce intracellular cyclic guanosine monophosphate (cGMP), a substance that blocks the action of acetylcholine in bronchial smooth muscle.

Uses

- Bronchodilators are used to prevent or to treat bronchial constriction in conditions such as asthma, bronchitis, and emphysema.

Adverse Effects

- CNS effects
  - Both adrenergics and xanthines stimulate the central nervous system, which can result in restlessness, agitation, and insomnia.
  - Xanthines may cause convulsions.
  - Anticholinergic bronchodilators can cause nervousness, headache, and dizziness.
- Cardiovascular effects
  - Adrenergics that affect beta1-adrenergic receptors as well as beta2-adrenergic receptors can cause tachycardia, hypertension, and cardiac arrhythmias.
    - Xanthines also stimulate the heart, possibly causing tachycardia and cardiac arrhythmias.
  - The anticholinergic bronchodilator ipratropium (Atrovent) can cause hypotension, cough, and gastrointestinal distress.
- Gastrointestinal effects
  - Gastrointestinal adverse effects of xanthines include:
    - Irritation of the gastric mucosa
    - Increased mucosal blood flow
    - Pain
    - Nausea
    - Anorexia
    - Vomiting
  - The anticholinergic bronchodilator ipratropium (Atrovent) can cause gastrointestinal distress.
- Respiratory effects
  - Anticholinergic bronchodilators can cause coughing.
- Drug allergy
  - People who are allergic to atropine or belladonna alkaloids may also be allergic to ipratropium.

Precautions

- Adrenergics and xanthines must be used cautiously in clients with congestive heart failure, hypertension, liver disease, and in people over age 60.
- Adrenergics must also be used cautiously with diabetes and glaucoma because they can increase blood glucose and intraocular pressure.
- Toxicity onset may be sudden, with arrhythmias and seizures as the first signs.
- Adrenergics and xanthines are contraindicated with hyperthyroidism and uncontrolled arrhythmias.
- The margin of safety for xanthines is narrow, especially in the young, elderly, and debilitated.
- Tremors occur with high serum levels of theophylline; the nurse should report this symptom to the prescribing practitioner for serum monitoring and possible dosing changes.
- Ipratropium (Atrovent) must be used cautiously with narrow-angle glaucoma and prostatic hypertrophy.
- Ipratropium (Atrovent) is not the first choice for acute bronchoconstriction because the onset of action is too long.

Important Drugs

- Examples of adrenergic bronchodilators are **albuterol** (Proventil), salmeterol (Serevent Diskus), and **terbutaline** (Brethine).
    - All of these are inhaled drugs that can be used for treatment of bronchoconstriction.
    - All but salmeterol are also useful for prevention of exercise-induced asthma symptoms.
- **Salmeterol** (Serevent Diskus) is a long-acting drug with a slow onset of action that is useful only for prevention of bronchoconstriction.
- Bronchodilators, such as **levalbuterol** (Xopenex), that have less beta1-adrenergic action cause fewer cardiac side and adverse effects.
- The adrenergic agonist epinephrine can be administered subcutaneously to treat acute bronchoconstriction.
- The xanthine bronchodilator is theophylline (Theo-Dur and other brands) for oral use, and aminophylline (Phyllocontin) for IV use.
- **Ipratropium** (Atrovent) is an anticholinergic bronchodilator.
    - Often used in combination with an adrenergic bronchodilator because it enhances the bronchodilating effects
    - Does not relieve acute bronchoconstriction

Therapeutic Nursing Interventions

- With adrenergic and xanthine bronchodilators, monitor pulse, blood pressure, respiratory status, and mental status.
- Review reports of serum theophylline levels; notify prescriber if higher than 20mcg/mL. Draw blood for peak levels 15-30 minutes after IV loading dose, 1-2 hours after rapid-acting forms, and 4-12 hours after extended-release forms.

- When ipratropium (Atrovent) is given with other inhalation medications, give other medications first and wait 5 minutes before giving ipratropium (Atrovent). If a corticosteroid is also prescribed, it should be used last.
- Children and cigarette smokers usually need higher dosages to maintain therapeutic blood levels because they metabolize theophylline (Respbid, Theo-Dur) rapidly.
- Because there is no antidote for xanthine, standard first-aid measures (charcoal, emesis, gastric lavage) must be used for toxicity.

Client Education

- Excessive use of adrenergic bronchodilators can cause paradoxical bronchoconstriction.
- Take theophylline (Theo-Dur) with food or a full glass of water to decrease gastrointestinal irritation.
- Shake the container thoroughly immediately before use.
- Allow at least one minute between inhalations of an aerosol medication; wait 5 minutes between different medications.
- Do not take more than 12 doses of ipratropium (Atrovent) in a 24-hour period.
- Do not chew or crush long-acting oral forms of theophylline (Respbid, Theo-Dur).
- Avoid caffeinated beverages.

Decongestants

Overview

Nasal congestion is usually characterized by nasal "stuffiness" and drainage. Nasal congestion is a common manifestation of the common cold and allergic rhinitis. The symptoms of nasal congestion are caused by dilation of blood vessels in the nasal mucosa and increased mucus secretion. The drugs most commonly used as nasal decongestants are topical adrenergics. Nasal decongestants are available as oral tablets, nasal drops, and nasal sprays.

Uses

- Nasal decongestants are most commonly used to relieve nasal congestion.

Adverse Effects

- Oral decongestants have more systemic adrenergic effects than topical preparations.
- Central nervous system (CNS) effects
  - Oral decongestants stimulate the CNS, causing:
    - Restlessness
    - Irritability
    - Anxiety
    - Insomnia
  - Decongestants applied by nasal spray or drops are unlikely to cause CNS effects.

- Cardiovascular effects
  - Oral decongestants can stimulate the heart and constrict cardiac and peripheral blood vessels, causing:
    - Tachycardia
    - Palpitations
    - Cardiac arrhythmias
    - Hypertension
- Gastrointestinal effects
  - Excessive use (> 10 days) of topical agents can lead to chronic nasal congestion and red, edematous mucosa.

Precautions

- Nasal decongestants are generally contraindicated with severe hypertension, coronary artery disease, and narrow-angle glaucoma.
- Use caution in clients who are also taking tricyclic or MAO inhibitor antidepressants.
- Use cautiously in clients with cardiac arrhythmias, hyperthyroidism, diabetes mellitus, and prostatic hypertrophy.
- Excessive or prolonged use can lead to chronic nasal congestion; limit use to 10 days for oral agents.
- The risk of cardiac arrhythmias increases with codeine, digoxin, general anesthetics, MAO inhibitors, other adrenergics, thyroid drugs, and xanthines.
- The risk of hypertension increases with:
  - Antihistamines
  - Epinephrine
  - Ergot alkaloids
  - MAO inhibitors

Important Drugs

- Pseudoephedrine is an active ingredient in decongestant remedies (e.g., Sudafed, Novafed, Afrinol Repetabs).
- Oxymetazoline is used in Afrin solution for nasal spray and drops.
- Phenylephrine is used in Neo-Synephrine.

Therapeutic Nursing Interventions

- Assess client's ability to breathe through nose before and after treatment.
- Note characteristics of nasal discharge: amount, color, and consistency.
- Be sure you have the right strength of phenylephrine because it comes in various strengths.

Client Education

- Blow your nose before instilling nasal decongestant drugs.
- Do not use nasal decongestants more frequently than recommended or for more than 10 days for oral agents. Overuse can cause chronic congestion.

- Do not touch the dropper/spray nozzle to your nostril if possible; cleanse the dropper or nozzle after each use. This may not be practical; however, the client should attempt to use a clean technique.

Expectorants

Overview

Expectorants stimulate the flow of respiratory secretions, which thins mucus, making it easier to clear from the respiratory tract by coughing. Some experts question the effectiveness of expectorants.

Uses

- The purpose of using expectorants is to make cough more productive so that mucus will be cleared from the airways.

Adverse Effects

- CNS effects
  - Guaifenesin may cause dizziness and headache.
- Gastrointestinal effects
  - Adverse gastrointestinal effects of guaifenesin include stomach pain, vomiting, nausea, and diarrhea with large doses.
- Dermatological effects
  - Rashes and urticaria have been reported with guaifenesin.

Precautions

- Preparations that contain alcohol, such as some cough syrups, can cause severe symptoms in clients who are taking naltrexone (ReVia).

Important Drugs

Guaifenesin (Robitussin, Anti-Tuss, and other brands) is the primary expectorant.

Therapeutic Nursing Interventions

- Assess lung sounds, note the frequency and type of cough, and document the characteristics of expectorated secretions.
- To help thin secretions, encourage fluid intake of 1500-2000 mL/day unless contraindicated.
- Institute safety measures if dizzy.

Client Education

- Drink at least eight 8-ounce servings of fluids each day to make it easier to expectorate mucus.
- Follow each dose of guaifenesin with a full glass of water.
- If a sustained-release form is prescribed, swallow the capsule or tablet whole.
- This drug may cause you to feel dizzy.
- Notify your primary care provider if your cough is not relieved within one week.

Inhaled Corticosteroids

Overview

Inhaled corticosteroids suppress inflammation in the airways, which decreases mucus secretion, decreases edema in the mucosa of the airway, and helps repair damaged epithelium. Inhaled corticosteroids also increase the number and sensitivity of $beta_2$- adrenergic receptors, which improves the response to beta2-adrenergic bronchodilators. The systemic absorption of corticosteroids is much less when given by inhalation than when given systemically; therefore, clients have fewer side effects with the inhalation route. Drug combinations used to treat asthma often include inhaled corticosteroids, a bronchodilator, and a mast cell stabilizer.

Uses

- Reduces the frequency and severity of acute bronchoconstriction
- Prevents lung damage with chronic asthma

Adverse Effects

- Compared to oral corticosteroids, inhaled corticosteroids are very safe.
  - Recent studies have shown that inhaled steroids cause side effects, such as impaired growth in children at normal doses.
- Musculoskeletal effects
  - Beclomethasone (Beclovent) 600 mcg/day predisposes the client to osteoporosis by promoting calcium loss from bones and decreasing the amount of calcium deposited in bones.
  - Budesonide (Pulmicort) can cause back pain.
  - Fluticasone (Flovent) can cause muscle soreness.
- CNS effects
  - Fluticasone (Flovent) can cause headache, agitation, depression, fatigue, insomnia, and restlessness.
  - Budesonide (Pulmicort) can cause headache.
- Nose and throat
  - All inhaled corticosteroids can cause hoarseness, dysphonia, cough, oropharyngeal fungal infections, and cataracts.
  - Nasally inhaled fluticasone can cause nasal stuffiness and sinusitis.
- Eyes
  - Use of inhaled corticosteroids over a long period of time may increase the risk of cataracts.
- Growth
  - Daily use of inhaled corticosteroids by children and adolescents may decrease their growth by a small amount.

Precautions

- These drugs are contraindicated for people with systemic fungal infections who have persistently positive sputum cultures for candida albicans.

- The change from oral to inhaled corticosteroids must be done gradually.
- Inhaled corticosteroids are contraindicated in acute asthma attacks.

Important Drugs

Beclomethasone (Beclovent, Vanceril) suppresses inflammation

Budesonide (Pulmicort)

Triamcinolone (Azmacort)

Fluticasone (Flovent)

Flunisolide (AeroBid)

- All drugs listed above are administered by oral inhalation.
  - Beclomethasone, fluticasone, and flunisolide are also available as a nasal spray.
- Prednisone and prednisolone are corticosteroids given orally or intravenously to clients who do not respond to topical therapy.
  - Long-term systemic therapy has many serious adverse effects.

Therapeutic Nursing Interventions

- Instruct client in proper use of inhaler.
- Assess oral cavity for irritation and for white patches typical of candidal infection.
- A spacer is often used for children to assist in obtaining a complete dose and minimize the taste factor that can interfere with compliance.

Client Education

- Inhaled corticosteroids are used to prevent acute bronchoconstriction, not to treat an acute attack.
- If taking a corticosteroid and a bronchodilator, use the bronchodilator first, then wait 5 minutes before using the corticosteroid.
- Gargling after inhaling these drugs will decrease oral irritation and the risk of fungal infection.
- Small children should be taught to brush their teeth after taking the inhalant medication.

Leukotriene Modifiers

Overview

Leukotrienes are natural chemicals that promote bronchoconstriction, mucus production, airway edema, and eosinophil infiltration. Leukotriene modifiers prevent symptoms of asthma by suppressing synthesis of leukotrienes or blocking their receptors. These drugs are often used in combination with inhaled corticosteroids and bronchodilators.

Uses

- These drugs are used to prevent acute asthma attacks, not to arrest them.

Adverse Effects

- Central nervous system effects
  - Leukotriene modifiers may cause headache, dizziness, and fatigue.
- Gastrointestinal effects
  - Leukotriene modifiers can cause gastrointestinal distress, such as heartburn and abdominal pain.
  - Montelukast (Singulair) is the only current leukotriene modifier that does not appear to harm the liver.
- Miscellaneous effects
  - The potentially fatal Churg-Strauss syndrome has occurred with zafirkulast (Accolate) and montelukast (Singulair). The syndrome is characterized by flu-like symptoms, weight loss, cardiac complications, neuropathy, and inflammation of pulmonary blood vessels.
- Drug allergy
  - There is a risk of hypersensitivity to leukotriene modifiers.

Precautions

- Zafirkulast (Accolate) increases the blood levels of theophylline (Theo-Dur) and warfarin (Coumadin).
- To prevent toxicity, the theophylline and warfarin dosages should be reduced.

Important Drugs

Zafirkulast (Accolate)

Montelukast (Singulair)

Therapeutic Nursing Interventions

- Promptly report cardiac, respiratory, or neurologic symptoms that may indicate Churg-Strauss syndrome.
- Check list of client's medications to detect potential interactions.
- Monitor lab results for liver function studies. Report elevations to the primary care provider.

Client Education

- While taking zafirkulast (Accolate), it is necessary to keep regular appointments for blood studies to evaluate your liver function.
- Take this medication one hour before or two hours after meals for best absorption.
- If the leukotriene modifier causes gastrointestinal distress, take it with 8 ounces of water or after eating.
- Leukotriene modifiers are not effective in treating acute asthma attacks.

Mast Cell Stabilizer

Overview

Mast cells are located in many body tissues. During the inflammatory response, mast cells release histamine. Effects of histamine are to:

- Constrict bronchioles
- Dilate blood vessels
- Produce mucus
- Increase capillary permeability

The effects of histamine account for many of the symptoms of upper respiratory infections and allergic responses, including nasal discharge, congestion, and increased mucus. Mast cell stabilizers decrease the release of histamine from mast cells, thereby reducing allergic symptoms.

Uses

- Mast cell stabilizers are used on a regular basis to prevent asthmatic attacks, not to terminate an asthma attack.
- Mast cell stabilizers may be used before exercise to prevent exercise-induced bronchospasm.
- Symptoms of allergic rhinitis may respond to intranasal cromolyn.

Adverse Effects

- Drug allergy
  - Clients who are allergic to mast cell stabilizers may have anaphylactic reactions.
- Central nervous system effects
  - Headache, dizziness, and difficulty speaking sometimes occur.
  - Eyes, ears, nose and throat (EENT) effects
  - Mast cell stabilizers may cause cough, rhinitis, throat irritation with inhalation, and nasal irritation with intranasal use.
- Gastrointestinal effects
  - Nausea, vomiting, anorexia, dry mouth, and a bitter taste have been reported.
  - Nedocromil (Tilade) has an unpleasant taste that some clients cannot tolerate.
- Respiratory effects
  - Mast cell stabilizers occasionally cause bronchospasm.

Precautions

- Mast cell stabilizers are contraindicated during acute asthma attacks because they may actually worsen the symptoms.
- Safety during pregnancy and lactation has not been established.

Important Drugs

Cromolyn sodium (Intal) is available as a metered nasal spray, capsules for inhalation, nebulization solution, aerosol, and in an oral form.

Nedocromil (Tilade) is administered with a metered dose inhaler.

Therapeutic Nursing Interventions

- Instruct the client in proper use of the prescribed form of the drug.
- Monitor respiratory status at intervals to assess effects.

Client Education

- Effective use of mast cell stabilizers requires regular administration.
- This drug will help prevent acute asthma attacks, but will not stop an attack that is in progress.
- Gargling or drinking water after using inhaled forms will decrease oral irritation.
- Effects may not be apparent until the drug has been used regularly for as long as four weeks.
- If a mast cell stabilizer is used to prevent exercise-induced bronchospasm or reactions to specific antigens before exposure, use the drug 10-60 minutes prior to activity.

Mucolytics

Overview

Mucolytics are agents that react directly with mucus to make it thinner and more easily expectorated.

Uses

Mucolytics may be used to promote mucus clearing in:

- Bronchitis
- Pneumonia
- Cystic fibrosis
- Chronic obstructive pulmonary disease (COPD)
- Tuberculosis
- Atelectasis
- Complications of cardiovascular or thoracic surgery
- Diagnostic procedures to obtain a mucus specimen

Acetylcysteine, taken orally or instilled per oroduodenal tube, is also used to treat acetaminophen (Tylenol) overdose.

Adverse Effects

- Drug allergy
  - Clients who are sensitive to mast cell stabilizers may have allergic reactions, including anaphylaxis.
- Central nervous system effects
  - Acetylcysteine (Mucomyst) can cause:
    - Dizziness
    - Drowsiness

        - Headache
        - Fever and chills
- Gastrointestinal effects
    - Nausea and vomiting
    - Stomatitis
    - Constipation
    - Anorexia
    - Hepatotoxicity
- Eyes, ears, nose and throat (EENT) effects
    - Acetylcysteine (Mucomyst) may cause rhinorrhea and tooth damage.
- Cardiovascular effects
    - Hypertension may develop with acetylcysteine use.
- Respiratory effects
    - Mucolytic agents can trigger bronchospasm and hemoptysis.
- Integumentary effects
    - Urticaria and rash have been reported with acetylcysteine.

Precautions

- Acetylcysteine (Mucomyst) is contraindicated in clients with hypersensitivity, status asthmaticus, and increased intracranial pressure.
- Do not mix acetylcysteine (Mucomyst) with certain antibiotics. Consult pharmacist.
- Do not use acetylcysteine (Mucomyst) with iron, copper, or rubber.

Important Drugs

Acetylcysteine (Mucomyst) is available in forms for oral use and inhalation.

Therapeutic Nursing Interventions

- Have bronchodilators available in case bronchospasm occurs.
- Have suction equipment available in case client is unable to clear mucus from airway.
- Assess lung sounds before and after treatments.
- Document respiratory status and effects of treatment.
- Schedule inhalation treatments before meals.
- Prepare fresh dilutions and use within one hour.

Client Education

- Unpleasant taste will diminish with repeated treatments.
- Gum, hard candy, or frequent liquid intake will help relieve dryness of the mouth.

Critical Thinking Exercise: Drugs Affecting the Respiratory System

Note: *It is recommended that the following exercises be reviewed with a partner or in a small group to achieve maximum student interaction and to enhance critical thinking skills.*

1. With which condition are antihistamines generally considered safe? Provide rationale as to why.

2. Discuss the difference between antitussives and expectorants. What are the indications for the use of each type of medication?

3. Discuss the advantages and disadvantages of using inhaled corticosteroids.

Situation: S.S. is a 32-year-old woman with a long history of bronchial asthma. She is currently maintained on theophylline (Theo-Dur) 200 mg twice a day. She uses a fluticasone (Flonase) inhaler, one puff, twice a day. When respiratory wheezing increases, she uses an albuterol (Proventil) inhaler, two puffs every four hours, until her breathing improves.

4. What clinical manifestations would you expect to see in S.S. if her serum theophylline level was >20 mcg/mL?

5. Because albuterol (Proventil) is a $beta_2$ agonist drug, you would expect to see what kind of a response related to adrenergic receptors?

After an acute attack of asthma during which S.S. was treated with aerosolized albuterol and systemic corticosteroids, her primary care provider is considering adding an additional medication she hopes will prevent future attacks.

6. What medications would you expect the primary care provider to consider?

CHAPTER 9

Drugs Affecting the Renal System

Key Points

- Diuretics increase the renal excretion of water, sodium, and other electrolytes.
  - The exact mechanism by which they work remains unknown.
- Diuretics are the mainstays in the treatment of hypertension.
  - Generally produce the same effects as strict dietary sodium restriction
  - Often first drugs prescribed for older clients with hypertension
- For all clients on diuretic therapy, monitor fluid intake and output (I & O), serum electrolyte levels, blood pressure, heart rate and rhythm, and muscle strength.
- Daily weights are the best measure of fluid loss or retention. Clients should report any significant weight change to their primary care provider.
- Administer diuretics in the morning or early afternoon (if ordered twice a day) to decrease nighttime voiding.
- There are several classifications of diuretics:
  - **Thiazides** are synthetic drugs that are related to the sulfonamides. Hydrochlorothiazide is among the most popular members of this group. Qualitatively, all the thiazides are identical. They differ only in the doses required to produce diuresis. They are generally considered safe in normal therapeutic doses.
    - Thiazides are often the drug of first choice for treating essential hypertension and fluid retention caused by mild/moderate heart failure, hepatic, or renal disease.
  - **Loop diuretics** act primarily on the ascending loop of Henle to limit water, sodium, and chloride absorption. These are the drugs of choice for rapid diuresis. They promote greater sodium-potassium exchange so potassium excretion is increased. Electrolyte depletion is their major adverse effect.
    - Because loop diuretics are the most effective classification of diuretics, they are the drugs of choice when rapid diuresis is needed.
  - **Potassium-sparing diuretics** are generally prescribed concurrently with other diuretics. They are relatively weak diuretics when used alone. Hyperkalemia is the major adverse effect. These agents are contraindicated for clients with renal failure.
    - A potassium-sparing diuretic may be used concurrently with potassium-wasting diuretics to reduce the risk of hypokalemia.
    - Hypokalemia is the most dangerous adverse effect of all diuretics except potassium-sparing diuretics.
    - Potassium-sparing diuretics are relatively weak; therefore, they are rarely used alone for diuresis.

- The risk of hyperkalemia is increased if the client is given multiple potassium-sparing diuretics or potassium supplements with potassium-sparing diuretics.
- **Carbonic anhydrase inhibitors** decrease reabsorption of water, sodium, potassium, and bicarbonate; raise the seizure threshold; and decrease intraocular pressure.
  - Clients who are allergic to sulfonamides should not take carbonic anhydrase inhibitors or thiazides because they are derivatives of sulfonamides.
  - Dorzolamide (Trusopt) is a newer topical ophthalmic carbonic anhydrase inhibitor used to reduce the formation of aqueous humor, lowering intraocular pressure with open-angle glaucoma.
- **Osmotic diuretics** cause water to be pulled from extravascular sites into the bloodstream, thereby increasing blood volume and decreasing reabsorption of water and electrolytes in the renal tubules.
  - Osmotic diuretics are used to maintain urine output and prevent renal failure, reduce intracranial pressure caused by cerebral edema, reduce intraocular pressure, and promote renal elimination of toxins.
  - To prevent crystals from entering the circulation, warm the mannitol solution to dissolve any crystals seen, cool the solution to body temperature, and use one filter to draw up and a separate filter to infuse the solution.
  - Because mannitol causes excess extracellular fluid to shift into the bloodstream for elimination, the client must be monitored for fluid overload and heart failure.

Carbonic Anhydrase Inhibitors

Overview

The carbonic anhydrase inhibitors are among the most versatile of diuretics. By inhibiting the action of carbonic anhydrase in the renal tubules, these drugs decrease reabsorption of water, sodium, potassium, and bicarbonate. The carbonic anhydrase inhibitors also decrease carbonic anhydrase in the central nervous system thereby raising the seizure threshold, and decrease the formation of aqueous humor in the eye. For various purposes, the drugs are available in IV, IM, PO, and topical (ophthalmic) forms.

Uses

- Open-angle glaucoma
- Epilepsy
- Edema associated with congestive heart failure (CHF)
- Acute mountain sickness (altitude sickness)
- Preoperatively when surgery for narrow-angle glaucoma is delayed

Adverse Effects

- Genitourinary
  - Polyuria
  - Glucosuria
  - Hematuria
  - Uremia
- Central nervous system
  - Drowsiness
  - Paresthesia
  - Convulsions
  - Headache
  - Depression
- Gastrointestinal
  - Nausea and vomiting
  - Anorexia
  - Constipation or diarrhea
  - Hepatic insufficiency
- Eye, Ears, Nose, Throat (EENT)
  - Myopia
  - Tinnitus
- Integumentary
  - Rash, pruritus, urticaria
  - Stevens-Johnson Syndrome
  - Endocrine
  - Hyperglycemia
- Hematological
  - Aplastic anemia, hemolytic anemia
  - Leukopenia, agranulocytosis (a significant decrease in the number of neutrophils)
  - Thrombocytopenia, purpura
  - Pancytopenia
- Fluids and electrolytes
  - Hypokalemia
  - Hyperchloremic acidosis

Precautions

- Carbonic anhydrase inhibitors must be used cautiously with hypercalciuria (increases risk of renal calculi) and during pregnancy.
- Clients who are allergic to sulfonamides should not take carbonic anhydrase inhibitors because they are derivatives of sulfonamides.
- Other contraindications are:
  - Severe renal or hepatic disease

    - Hyponatremia, hypokalemia, hyperchloremic acidosis
    - Addison's disease
    - Chronic obstructive pulmonary disease (COPD)
    - Long-term use in narrow-angle glaucoma
- Drug interactions: carbonic anhydrase inhibitors
    - Increase the effects of anticholinergics, procainamide, and quinidine
    - Increase excretion of lithium
    - Are decreased by methenamine

Important Drugs

Acetazolamide (Diamox, Dazamide) is available in:

- PO, IM, and IV preparations for treatment of glaucoma and prevention of seizures
- IM and IV preparations for edema associated with congestive heart failure
- PO preparations for renal stones and mountain sickness

Dorzolamide (Trusopt) is a topical preparation (opthalmic) used to reduce the formation of aqueous humor to reduce intraocular pressure with open-angle glaucoma.

- The most common side effects are ocular stinging and a bitter taste immediately after application.
- Clients who are allergic develop inflammation of the conjunctiva and eyelids.

Brinzolamide (Azopt) is also an ophthalmic preparation, but has fewer side effects.

Therapeutic Nursing Interventions

- Monitor for excessive diuresis: dehydration and electrolyte imbalances.
- Monitor blood pressure to detect postural hypotension.
- Teach clients with postural hypotension to rise slowly and to avoid prolonged standing in one place.
- Monitor blood glucose, especially if the client has diabetes.

Client Education

- If you miss a dose, do not double up.
- Notify your primary care provider if you experience:
    - A rash, unusual bleeding, or bruising
    - Tremors and abnormal sensations
    - Flank pain
- Eyedrops should be instilled into the conjunctival sac by gently down pulling down the lower lid.
- After instilling eyedrops, gently press the inner corner of the eye to reduce loss of the drug.

Loop (High Ceiling) Diuretics

Overview

Loop diuretics are the most effective of all diuretics. Loop diuretics increase water excretion by blocking reabsorption of sodium and chloride in the loop of Henle, which results in decreased water reabsorption. Because loop diuretics are the most effective classification of diuretics, they are the drugs of choice when rapid diuresis is needed. Loop diuretics are reserved for emergency situations or when less powerful drugs are ineffective.

Uses

- Pulmonary edema with CHF
- Edema that does not respond to less powerful diuretics and is caused by hepatic, renal, or cardiac conditions
- Hypertension that cannot be controlled with other types of diuretics
- A loop diuretic may be used with other types of diuretics to enhance diuresis.

Adverse Effects

- Fluids and electrolytes
  - Hyponatremia
  - Hypochloremia
  - Hypokalemia
  - Hypomagnesemia
  - Hypocalcemia
  - Dehydration
- Cardiovascular
  - Hypotension caused by decreased blood volume and dilation of veins which reduces afterload
  - Increased low-density lipoproteins and decreased high-density lipoproteins
  - Neurologic: ototoxicity
- Other
  - Hyperuricemia
  - Hyperglycemia
  - Photosensitivity

Precautions

- Using loop diuretics with other ototoxic drugs increases the risk of hearing loss.
- A potassium-sparing diuretic may be used concurrently to reduce the risk of hypokalemia.
- Contraindications:
  - Allergy to sulfonamides
  - Anuria, hypovolemia, electrolyte depletion
  - Lactation
  - Infants

Drug Interactions

- Digitalis: Increased risk of digitalis toxicity and potentially fatal dysrhythmias if hypokalemia is present
- Lithium: Excretion is reduced, possible lithium toxicity
- Antihypertensive agents: Additive hypotension
- Nonsteroidal anti-inflammatory drugs (NSAIDs): Decreased effectiveness of loop diuretic

Important Drugs

Furosemide (Lasix) is the prototype loop diuretic.

- Other very similar loop diuretics are:
  - **Ethacrynic acid** (Edecrin)
  - **Bumetanide** (Bumex)
  - **Torsemide** (Demadex)
- Only furosemide and torsemide have U.S. Food and Drug Administration (FDA) approval to treat hypertension.

Therapeutic Nursing Interventions

- Monitor intake and output, serum electrolytes, and blood pressure.
- Particularly, assess for effects of hypokalemia on body systems.
  - Cardiovascular: weak pulse, dysrhythmias
  - Respiratory: weak respirations
  - Digestive: anorexia, nausea, vomiting, abdominal distention, absent or hypoactive bowel sounds
  - Skeletal muscles: weakness
  - CNS: confusion
- Administer in the morning to decrease nighttime voiding.
- Assess dependent body areas for edema; weigh daily.
- Assess lung sounds to evaluate drug effects on pulmonary edema.
- Assess for orthostatic hypotension; institute safety measures to prevent falls.
- Some sources recommend an increased intake of potassium-rich foods (e.g., bananas, orange juice), but the amount of food required to make a difference is not practical (4-6 bananas, 1000 mL of orange juice per day).

Client Education

- Take diuretic in the morning to avoid nighttime voiding.
- Change positions slowly to prevent dizziness and loss of balance.
- Report weakness, confusion, gastrointestinal distress, or palpitations.
- Loop diuretics can be taken with food or milk to decrease gastrointestinal irritation.
- Wear protective clothing or sunscreens when exposed to sunlight.
- Follow directions for fluid intake.

Osmotic Diuretics

Overview

Osmotic diuretics increase the osmotic pressure of the glomerular filtrate, causing water to be drawn into the bloodstream from the extracellular fluid compartment. The increased blood volume causes excretion of water and electrolytes by the kidneys. These drugs can cause rapid diuresis even when renal circulation and glomerular filtration rate are decreased as in shock or dehydration.

Uses

- Maintain urine output and prevent renal failure in conditions such as hypovolemic shock.
- Reduce intracranial pressure caused by cerebral edema.
- Reduce intraocular pressure by drawing fluid from the eye.
- Eliminate toxins through the kidneys.

Adverse Effects

- If mannitol passes through the capillary pores into the tissues, edema results.
- The increased blood volume caused by mannitol can precipitate congestive heart failure and pulmonary edema.
- Other adverse effects include:
    - Headache
    - Nausea and vomiting
    - Fluid and electrolyte imbalances

Precautions

- Mannitol is contraindicated in clients with heart failure or pulmonary edema who develop renal failure.

Important Drugs

- Mannitol (Osmitrol) is the only osmotic diuretic that is used for its diuretic effects.
    - Freely filtered at the glomerulus, but little is reabsorbed
        - It is not metabolized and has no direct effects on the biochemistry or physiology of cells.
    - Does not significantly affect electrolytes

Therapeutic Nursing Interventions

- Be aware that mannitol intravenous solutions are available in several concentrations.
- Determine compatibility with other intravenous fluids.
- The infusion is usually regulated to maintain a urine output of 30-50 mL/hr.
- Check the solution for crystals. If present, warm the solution to dissolve the crystals, then cool the solution to body temperature prior to administration.
- Use a filter needle and an inline filter to reduce the risk of crystals entering the circulation.

- If client is not catheterized, have urinal, bedpan, or bedside commode readily available.
  - Most often clients receiving osmotic diuretics will have an indwelling urinary catheter.
- If allowed out of bed, assist to the bathroom or bedside commode to avoid falls.
- Assess for therapeutic and adverse effects:
  - Monitor fluid intake and output (I&O), serum electrolytes, BUN, creatinine, blood pH, and arterial blood gasses (ABGs).
  - Stop the infusion immediately if urine output ceases.
  - Assess for hypokalemia: postural hypotension, weakness, and tachycardia.
  - Assess for metabolic acidosis: drowsiness, restlessness.
  - Assess mucous membranes, skin turgor, and thirst to detect dehydration.
  - Assess respiratory status (rate, effort, depth, rhythm, lung sounds).

Client Education

- Change positions slowly to prevent dizziness and possible falls.
- Inform the nurse if you have pain in your eyes or blurred vision while receiving this medication.
- Call for help if you need to get up; you may feel dizzy.

Potassium-Sparing Diuretics

Overview

Potassium-sparing drugs induce modest diuresis. The two subcategories of potassium-sparing diuretics are aldosterone antagonists and nonaldosterone antagonists. An aldosterone antagonist blocks the action of aldosterone in the distal tubules. A nonaldosterone antagonist directly inhibits the exchange of sodium and potassium in the tubules so that sodium is eliminated and potassium is retained. Unlike thiazide and loop diuretics, these drugs increase sodium excretion and potassium retention. Potassium-sparing diuretics are relatively weak; therefore, they are rarely used alone for diuresis. Potassium-sparing drugs are often used in combination with a thiazide or loop diuretic to counteract excessive potassium excretion. These drugs have a slower onset of action than other diuretics.

Uses

- Treat hypertension and edema
- Prevent hypokalemia in clients taking thiazide or loop diuretics

Adverse Effects

- Both types of potassium-sparing diuretics can cause hypokalemia.
- Spironolactone (Aldactone), an aldosterone antagonist, also can cause endocrine disorders, including:
  - Gynecomastia
  - Menstrual irregularities
  - Erectile dysfunction

    - Hirsutism
    - Deepening of the voice
- Nonaldosterone antagonists also can cause:
    - Nausea and vomiting
    - Leg cramps
    - Dizziness
    - Blood dyscrasias (rarely)

Precautions

- Hyperkalemia
    - Insulin may be given to promote the movement of potassium into body cells, thereby reducing the serum level if needed.
    - The risk of hyperkalemia is increased if the client is given multiple potassium-sparing diuretics or potassium supplements with potassium-sparing diuretics.

Important Drugs

Spironolactone (Aldactone) is the only aldosterone antagonist approved for use in the U.S.

- The two nonaldosterone antagonists are **triamterene** (Dyrenium) and **amiloride** (Midamor).

Therapeutic Nursing Interventions

- With all potassium-sparing diuretics, assess for hyperkalemia, which is manifested by:
    - Serum potassium level > 5 mEq/mL.
    - Prolonged PR interval, wide QRS complex, peaked T-wave, depressed ST segment.
    - Cardiac dysrhythmias.
- If the client's serum potassium exceeds 5 mEq/mL or if cardiac dysrhythmias occur, potassium-sparing diuretics should be discontinued and potassium intake restricted.
- Monitor I & O (if hospitalized) and weight to assess effects of diuretics.
- Inspect and palpate dependent body parts to detect and evaluate edema.
- Assess for endocrine changes.

Client Education

- Do not use salt substitutes because they provide too much potassium.
- Take your potassium-sparing diuretic in the morning to avoid nighttime voiding.
- Weigh yourself daily or weekly as your primary care provider instructs and report unexplained weight gain.
- Notify your primary care provider if you have palpitations or feel faint.
- For women, report changes in your menstrual period, increased body hair, or deepened voice.

- For men, report breast enlargement or sexual dysfunction.
- Triamterene (Dyrenium) may cause urine to turn blue.

Thiazide and Related Diuretics

Overview

Thiazide diuretics are chemically related to the sulfonamides. A group of drugs with actions identical to the thiazides are referred to as related diuretics. Thiazides and related diuretics decrease reabsorption of sodium, water, chloride, and bicarbonate in the distal convoluted tubules. These drugs have effects similar to the loop diuretics, but produce a lower maximum diuresis than the loop diuretics and are ineffective when urine output is very low. Thiazide and related diuretics are only effective if the client has adequate kidney function.

Uses

- Thiazides are often the drug of first choice in the treatment of essential hypertension, fluid retention caused by mild/moderate heart failure, and hepatic or renal disease.
- For reasons not understood, thiazides significantly reduce urine output in clients with diabetes insipidus.

Adverse Effects

- Hyponatremia, hypochloremia, hypokalemia, hypomagnesemia, hypocalcemia
- Dehydration
- Increased low-density lipoproteins (LDL), total cholesterol (TC), triglycerides
- Hyperglycemia
- Hyperuricemia
- Blood dyscrasias (rarely)
- Photosensitivity

Precautions

- Thiazides are not recommended during pregnancy because they are harmful to the fetus.
- Important drug interactions:
    - Digoxin: Increased risk of digitalis toxicity with hypokalemia
    - Antihypertensives: Enhanced lowering of blood pressure
    - Lithium: Potential for lithium toxicity due to reduced excretion
    - NSAIDs: Reduced diuresis
    - Potassium-sparing diuretics: Less risk of hypokalemia
- Contraindicated with allergy to sulfonamides
- May precipitate an acute attack of gouty arthritis in clients with gout by raising the serum uric acid level
- Dosage of antidiabetic drugs may have to be adjusted to accommodate increased serum glucose.

Important Drugs

Hydrochlorothiazide (HydroDIURIL, and other brands) is the prototype thiazide diuretic.

- Some other thiazides are:
  - Chlorothiazide (Diuril)
  - Bendroflumethiazide (Naturetin)
  - Methyclothiazide (Enduron)
- Related diuretics include:
  - Chlorthalidone (Hygroton, Thalitone)
  - Indapamide (Lozol)
  - Metolazone (Zaroxolyn, Mykrox)
  - Quinethazone (Hydromox)

Therapeutic Nursing Interventions

- Monitor I & O, serum electrolytes, and blood pressure.
- Assess for effects of hypokalemia on body systems:
  - Cardiovascular: weak pulse, dysrhythmias
  - Respiratory: weak respirations
  - Digestive: anorexia, nausea, vomiting, abdominal distention, absent or hypoactive bowel sounds
  - Skeletal muscles: weakness
  - CNS: confusion
- Administer in the morning to decrease night-time voiding.
- Assess dependent body areas for edema; weigh at regular intervals.
- Assess for orthostatic hypotension and confusion; institute safety measures to prevent falls.
- Some sources recommend an increased intake of potassium-rich foods (bananas, orange juice), but the amount of food required to make a difference is not practical (4-6 bananas, 1000 mL of orange juice).
- Monitor clients with diabetes for hyperglycemia.
- Monitor clients for gouty arthritis.

Client Education

- Take your diuretic in the morning to avoid nighttime voiding.
- Change positions slowly to prevent dizziness and loss of balance.
- Report weakness, confusion, gastrointestinal distress, or palpitations to your primary care provider.
- Wear protective clothing or sunscreens when exposed to sunlight.
- Follow primary care provider's directions for fluid intake.

Critical Thinking Exercise: Drugs Affecting the Renal System

Note: *It is recommended that the following exercises be reviewed with a partner or in a small group to achieve maximum student interaction and to enhance critical thinking skills.*

Situation: L.L. is a 72-year-old female who has had chronic CHF (congestive heart failure) for five years. She currently takes sustained-release diltiazem (Cardizem) 180 mg po qd for hypertension and digoxin (Lanoxin) 0.25 mg q a.m. to improve her cardiac function. She is admitted to the hospital after reporting increasing dyspnea and edema in her ankles and feet. On admission, she was started on oxygen per nasal cannula and intravenous fluids through a peripheral line. Your assessment reveals crackles in the lower lobes of both lungs. Her respiratory rate is 22, pulse 100, and BP 170/92.

1. A new order is written for furosemide (Lasix) 20 mg IV push now.

    a. What is the action of furosemide (Lasix)?

    b. Describe two benefits of furosemide (Lasix) for this client.

2. Identify at least two drug interactions among the drugs L. L. is taking.

3. A blood sample is drawn to measure serum electrolytes.

    a. Which electrolytes are influenced most by furosemide (Lasix)?

    b. Explain why electrolytes must be closely monitored when clients are receiving loop diuretics and digoxin (Lanoxin).

4. If L.L. is discharged on furosemide (Lasix), list three important client teaching points.

5. L.L. is discharged home with prescriptions for diltiazem (Cardizem), digoxin (Lanoxin), and furosemide (Lasix). One month after discharge she tells the home health nurse she feels weak and nauseated. She also says she feels like her heart is skipping beats. The home health nurse should immediately suspect ________________.

CHAPTER 10

Drugs Affecting the Digestive System

Key Points

- All antacids are not the same.
  - Magnesium-based antacids:
    - Are not given to clients with renal insufficiency
    - Can cause diarrhea
  - Aluminum and calcium-based antacids can cause constipation.
- Antacids interfere with absorption of many other drugs by binding with them in the gastrointestinal tract.
- Magnesium hydroxide is considered an ideal antacid because it:
  - Acts rapidly
  - Has a high capacity for neutralizing acid
  - Has a long duration of action.
- Drugs commonly used to treat diarrhea include opioids, anticholinergics, and bulk-forming agents.
- Opioids are the most effective agents available to treat diarrhea.
- Clients taking psyllium (Fiberall) must be well-hydrated to prevent hardening of the psyllium in the bowel, which can cause obstruction.
- Antiemetic drugs are those used to treat or to prevent nausea and vomiting in a variety of clinical conditions.
- Selective serotonin antagonists are the most effective antiemetics for clients on chemotherapy.
- Histamine$_2$-receptor antagonists and proton pump inhibitors suppress secretion of gastric acid and decrease pepsin in the stomach.
- Drugs that decrease acid secretion interfere with other drugs that are absorbed in an acidic medium.
- Intravenous potassium supplements must be diluted before administration. Concentrated solutions of potassium can have fatal effects.
- In clients receiving intravenous fluids, monitor:
  - Heart rate
  - Heart rhythm
  - Blood pressure
  - Urine output—to detect fluid volume excess or deficit.
- Gastrointestinal stimulants are used to increase upper gastrointestinal motility in clients with diabetic gastroparesis or other nonobstructive disorders characterized by gastric retention of food and fluids.

- Laxatives and stool softeners produce a soft, formed stool, whereas cathartics act quickly to produce a semi-liquid or liquid stool.
- Laxatives and cathartics are used to treat acute constipation and to empty the bowel for diagnostic or therapeutic procedures.
- Stool softeners and bulk-forming agents are used to treat chronic constipation by increasing stool bulk or moisture. They are used when it is important to prevent straining with defecation.
- Laxatives are contraindicated with undiagnosed abdominal pain, intestinal obstruction, and fecal impaction.
- Even though vitamins do not require a prescription, they can be harmful if taken in excess.
- Vitamin requirements are increased during infancy, pregnancy, lactation, fever, and hyperthyroidism.
- Common antibacterials used to treat ulcers caused by Helicobacter pylori are:
    - Amoxicillin
    - Clarithromycin
    - Metronidazole (Flagyl)
    - Tetracycline
- Misoprostol (Cytotec) is used to prevent peptic ulcers in people who take NSAIDs regularly.
    - Contraindicated in pregnancy because it can cause abortion
- Sucralfate (Carfate) binds to many compounds in the intestinal tract and, therefore, should be administered 2 hours apart from other medications.
- Ipecac can only be administered to an alert individual, and must be followed with at least 8-10 ounces of water for adults (4-8 ounces for children).

Antacids

Overview

Antacids are alkaline compounds that contain aluminum, magnesium, calcium, and/or sodium. The action of antacids is to neutralize acids and to prevent the conversion of pepsinogen to pepsin in the stomach. Antacids are available in various compounds as over-the-counter drugs. The use of these drugs has been reduced since the development of newer drugs that act by other mechanisms to reduce gastric acidity.

Uses

- Antacids are useful in the treatment of peptic ulcer disease) and GERD (gastroesophageal reflux disease (GERD).
- The management of PUD and GERD often employs antacids in combination with other drugs.
- Although there is no strong evidence of efficacy, many people take antacids for heartburn and indigestion.
- Sodium bicarbonate is used to treat acidosis and to promote the excretion of acidic drugs. It is not recommended for treatment of PUD.

Adverse Effects

The adverse effects of antacids depend on the specific compound.

- Magnesium hydroxide retains water in the intestinal lumen, causing diarrhea.
- Aluminum hydroxide can cause constipation.
  - It may also cause hypophosphatemia because it combines with phosphates in the intestines.
- Giving a preparation that contains both aluminum and magnesium minimizes the gastrointestinal effects.
- Calcium carbonate is constipating, increases intestinal gas, and can cause acid rebound.
  - Although a rare occurrence, systemic absorption can cause milk-alkali syndrome (hypercalcemia, metabolic alkalosis, impaired renal function, and soft tissue calcification).
- Sodium bicarbonate is systemically absorbed, so it can aggravate hypertension and heart failure.
  - It can also release carbon dioxide in the intestines, causing increased gas.

Precautions

- Since magnesium stimulates the bowel, it should not be used with undiagnosed abdominal pain.
- With renal impairment, magnesium can accumulate and cause CNS depression.
- Aluminum interferes with absorption of many other drugs including tetracycline, warfarin, and digoxin by binding with them in the gastrointestinal tract.

Important Drugs

- The most commonly used antacids for PUD and GERD are aluminum hydroxide, magnesium hydroxide, and calcium carbonate.
- Magnesium hydroxide is considered the ideal antacid because it acts rapidly, has a high capacity for neutralizing acid, and has a long duration of action.
- Sodium bicarbonate is recognized as an antacid, but its most important uses are based on its systemic effects.

Therapeutic Nursing Interventions

- Assess pain before and after antacid administration.
- Monitor results of electrolyte studies in clients on long-term therapy.
- The goal of antacid therapy is to maintain the pH of gastric fluids above 5.
- Antacids are sometimes administered via nasogastric (NG) tubes with the dosage titrated based on the pH of gastric fluids until the desired pH is attained.

Client Education

- Take antacids as directed, usually one and three hours after meals and at bedtime.
- Do not take antacids within one hour of other medications.
- Shake liquid preparations before pouring.

- Chew tablets thoroughly and follow with a full glass of water.
- Taking antacids on a regular basis, rather than only when pain occurs, may provide better pain control.

Antidiarrheals

Overview

Diarrhea is a protective mechanism that rids the gastrointestinal system of irritants. Persistent diarrhea requires treatment because it can cause significant loss of water and electrolytes. The very young and the very old are at greatest risk for complications from diarrhea. Drugs given to treat diarrhea act by reducing the fluidity and volume of stools or by decreasing peristalsis. Drugs commonly used to treat diarrhea include opioids, anticholinergics, and bulk-forming agents. Examples of bulk-forming agents are psyllium (Fiberall), methylcellulose (Citrucel), and polycarbophil (FiberCon). Antibacterials are not specifically antidiarrheal, but may be used to treat infectious diarrhea. Opioids are the most effective agents available to treat diarrhea. Corticosteroids may be required to treat diarrhea in inflammatory conditions.

Uses

- Non-specific antidiarrheal therapy controls diarrhea without correcting the cause.
- Specific antidiarrheal therapy treats the cause of diarrhea.

Adverse Effects

- All antidiarrheals can cause constipation.
- Other adverse effects depend on the type of drug used:
    - Opioids: Dizziness, nausea, vomiting, hypotension, and bradycardia
    - Anticholinergics: Blurred vision, tachycardia, and urinary retention
    - Combinations of opioids and anticholinergics (diphenoxylate) reduce adverse effects of each type and discourage opioid abuse.
    - Bulk-forming agents: Nausea, vomiting, cramping, and intestinal obstruction

Precautions

- Opioids must be used cautiously with increased intracranial pressure; a history of drug dependence, and severe renal, hepatic, or pulmonary disease.
- Anticholinergics are contraindicated with narrow-angle glaucoma, acute hemorrhage, and tachycardia associated with cardiac insufficiency or thyrotoxicosis.
- Contraindications for bulk-forming agents include dehydration, undiagnosed abdominal pain, nausea, vomiting, serious adhesions, and dysphagia.
- Some bulk-forming agents contain sugar, aspartame, or sodium, which may be undesirable in certain clients.
- Clients taking psyllium (Fiberall) must be well-hydrated to prevent hardening of the stool in the bowel, which can cause obstruction.

Important Drugs

Lomotil is an opioid (diphenoxylate) combined with an anticholinergic (atropine). If taken in excess amounts, the anticholinergic side effects are extremely unpleasant.

Loperamide (Imodium) is related to meperidine (Demerol), but has little or no potential for abuse because it does not cross the blood-brain barrier.

Psyllium (Fiberall) preparations such as Metamucil are most often used to prevent constipation by retaining water in the stool. The absorption of water forms a gel that is also effective in reducing watery diarrhea.

Therapeutic Nursing Interventions

- Assess the abdomen for distention, pain, and bowel sounds.
- Record the number and characteristics of stools.
- With severe or persistent diarrhea, assess for dehydration and electrolyte disturbances.
- With psyllium:
  - Prepare immediately before administering, as the agent will thicken on standing.
  - Monitor blood glucose in clients with diabetes.
  - Dissolve powder or granules in a full glass of water; follow with a second glass of water.

Client Education

- Use antidiarrheals only as directed because excessive intake can cause constipation.
- Notify the primary care provider if diarrhea is severe, persistent, or does not respond to usual doses of antidiarrheals.
- When taking bulk-forming agents, it is vital that you take one glass of water with the drug and follow it with a second glass of water.

Antiemetics

Overview

Nausea and vomiting are common symptoms of many illnesses and are common adverse effects of many drugs. If severe or prolonged, vomiting can cause dehydration and pH and electrolyte imbalances. Infants and the elderly are at greatest risk for adverse effects of vomiting. Drugs used to treat nausea and vomiting are classified as serotonin receptor antagonists, dopamine antagonists, glucocorticoids, cannabinoids, and benzodiazepines.

Uses

- Antiemetic drugs are those used to treat or to prevent nausea and vomiting in a variety of clinical conditions.
- Antiemetic drugs relieve nausea and vomiting by acting in the vomiting center, chemoreceptor trigger zone, cerebral cortex, vestibular apparatus, or a combination of these sites.
- Antihistamines and scopolamine are used primarily to prevent nausea and vomiting associated with motion sickness.

- The dopamine antagonist metoclopramide (Reglan) is used as an antiemetic for clients on cancer chemotherapy.
    - Also used with histamine2-receptor antagonists and proton pump inhibitors in the treatment of GERD (gastroesophageal reflux disease)
    - Increases lower esophageal sphincter tone and promotes gastric emptying

Adverse Effects

- Drowsiness is a side effect common to many antiemetics. Other side effects are specific to the drug type.
- Serotonin receptor antagonists:
    - Ondansetron (Zofran): Headache, diarrhea, dizziness
    - Granisetron (Kytril): Weakness, diarrhea or constipation, fatigue
    - Dolasetron (Anzemet): Headache, increases or decreases in heart rate and blood pressure, diarrhea, fatigue, dizziness, pruritus
    - Dopamine antagonists
    - Phenothiazines: Extrapyramidal reactions, anticholinergic effects, hypotension, sedation
    - Butyrophenones: Extrapyramidal reactions, hypotension, sedation
    - Prokinetic agents: Sedation and diarrhea with high doses; changes in heart rate and blood pressure; extrapyramidal reactions
- Glucocorticoids: No major side effects with short-term, intermittent use
- Cannabinoids: Tachycardia, hypotension, and subjective CNS effects
- Benzodiazepines: Sedation, CNS depression, tolerance, physical dependence and insomnia when discontinued

Precautions

- Antiemetics that cause dizziness and sedation may put the client at risk for injury.
- Serotonin receptor antagonists must be used cautiously in liver impairment and after abdominal surgery.
- Phenothiazines are contraindicated with narrow-angle glaucoma and severe liver or cardiovascular disease.
- Butyrophenones are contraindicated with narrow-angle glaucoma, bone marrow depression, CNS depression, and severe liver or cardiovascular disease.
- Contraindications for prokinetic agents include gastrointestinal obstruction or hemorrhage, history of seizure disorders, pheochromocytoma, and Parkinson's disease.
- The CNS depressant effects of metoclopramide (Reglan) are enhanced by other CNS depressants.
- Corticosteroids are contraindicated with active untreated infections; lactation or known sensitivity to alcohol.
- Benzodiazepines are contraindicated in uncontrolled severe pain, and narrow-angle glaucoma.
- During pregnancy, non-pharmacologic therapy is preferred. No drugs have been proven absolutely safe.

Important Drugs

Selective serotonin antagonists are the most effective antiemetics for clients on chemotherapy.

- Ondansetron (Zofran)
- Granisetron (Kytril)
- Dolasetron (Anzemet)

Dopamine antagonists used as antiemetics include:

- Phenothiazines: Chlorpromazine (Thorazine), prochlorperazine (Compazine), promethazine (Phenergan)
- Butyrophenones: Haloperidol (Haldol) and droperidol (Inapsine)
- Prokinetic agent: Metoclopramide (Reglan)

Antihistamines used to treat motion sickness and vertigo are meclizine (Antivert) and dimenhydrinate (Dramamine).

Glucocorticoids often used as antiemetics with cancer chemotherapy are methylprednisolone (Solu-Medrol) and dexamethasone (Decadron), even though the U.S. Food Drug Administration (FDA) has not approved them for that purpose.

A **benzodiazepine** that is used as an antiemetic with cancer chemotherapy is lorazepam (Ativan).

Therapeutic Nursing Interventions

- With severe or prolonged vomiting, monitor the client's intake and output, and review laboratory studies of fluid and electrolyte status.
- Position sedated clients on one side to prevent aspiration of vomitus.
- Take safety precautions if client is drowsy or dizzy.
- Administer antiemetics before procedures or treatments that commonly cause nausea because it is easier to prevent nausea than to treat it.
- Complement drug therapy with comfort measures.
- Promptly empty emesis basins; change soiled linens as soon as the client can tolerate the movement.

Client Education

- Call for assistance if you need to get up because this drug may make you drowsy.
- Notify the nurse as soon as you begin to feel nauseated.
- When using oral antiemetics to prevent motion sickness, take drug one hour before travel.
- When using transdermal patches to prevent motion sickness:
  - Apply the patch at least four hours before travel.
  - Place the patch on a clean, dry, hairless area behind the ear and press to secure.
  - The system is waterproof and is effective for 3 days.

Antiflatulents

Overview

Excess gas in the gastrointestinal tract (flatulence) is a common postoperative problem. Flatulence also may result from:

- Swallowing air
- Dyspepsia, peptic ulcer disease, or diverticulitis
- Consuming gas-forming foods
- Some drug effects

Uses

- Drugs used to treat flatulence are called antiflatulents.

Adverse Effects

- Simethicone (Mylicon) has no significant adverse effects.

Precautions

- Simethicone (Mylicon) should be used cautiously with undiagnosed abdominal pain.
- This drug should not be used for infant colic.

Important Drugs

Simethicone (Mylicon) is the effective component of agents used to treat flatulence.

Therapeutic Nursing Interventions

- Assess the abdomen for distention and bowel sounds.
- Note frequency of belching or passage of flatus.
- For best results, administer after meals and at bedtime.
- Shake liquids well before pouring.
- Dilute drops in 30 mL of water.

Client Education

- Chew tablets thoroughly before swallowing.
- Exercise and proper diet can minimize flatulence.
- Avoid gas-forming foods such as cabbage, beans, and large amounts of dietary fiber and fructose.
- To avoid swallowing air, eat slowly, chew with the mouth closed, and do not drink through straws.

Antiulcer Drugs

Overview

Peptic ulcer disease (PUD) is characterized by erosion of the lining in the upper gastrointestinal tract. Most cases of PUD are caused by infection with *Helicobacter pylori*. Treatment of PUD involves various combinations of:

- Antibacterials to eradicate *Helicobacter pylori*
- Proton pump inhibitors to suppress secretion of gastric acid
- Histamine$_2$-receptor antagonists to prevent ulcers in clients with

gastroesophageal reflux disease (GERD)
- Antacids to neutralize gastric acid and relieve pain
- Assorted agents to protect the ulcer and promote healing

Histamine2-Receptor Antagonists

Overview

Histamine$_2$-receptor antagonists suppress the secretion of gastric acid and decrease pepsin in the stomach.

Uses

- Promote healing of erosive esophagitis and peptic ulcer disease
- Prevent recurrence of peptic ulcer disease and esophagitis
- Prevent stress ulcers
- Treat heartburn (with over-the-counter agents)
- Treat Zollinger-Ellison syndrome, a rare disorder in which there is excessive secretion of gastric juice due to high levels of circulating gastrin, which, in turn, cause ulceration of the upper gastrointestinal tract.

Adverse Effects

- CNS effects: Depression (sedation) or stimulation (excitation)
- Antiandrogenic effects: Gynecomastia, reduced libido, and erectile dysfunction
- Gastrointestinal effects: Growth of candida in the stomach; epigastric pain
- Hematologic effects are rare, but include neutropenia, leukopenia, and thrombocytopenia
- Effects of IV bolus: Possible hypotension and dysrhythmias
- Other: Headache, dizziness, malaise, nausea, diarrhea or constipation, rash, pruritus
- Confusion has been reported in older adults taking cimetidine.

Precautions

- Histamine$_2$-receptor blockers must be used cautiously in clients with renal impairment and lower doses are recommended for older adults.
- Cimetidine (Tagamet) inhibits drug-metabolizing enzymes, which can increase the serum levels of other drugs, including warfarin, phenytoin, theophylline (Theo-Dur), and lidocaine.
- Cimetidine (Tagamet) is contraindicated during pregnancy and lactation.
- Ranitidine (Zantac), nizatidine (Axid), and famotidine (Pepcid) have few drug interactions and do not inhibit enzymes.
- Because histamine$_2$-receptor blockers decrease acid secretion, they will interfere with other drugs that are absorbed in an acidic medium.

Important Drugs

Ranitidine (Zantac)

Ranitidine bismuth citrate (Tritec)

Famotidine (Pepcid)

Nizatidine (Axid Pulvules, Axid AR)

Cimetidine (Tagamet): because of its adverse effects and interactions with other drugs, other drugs in the category are usually preferred over cimetidine.

Therapeutic Nursing Interventions

- Assess for epigastric and chest pain.
- Schedule drugs to avoid interactions.

Client Education

- Do not take histamine$_2$-receptor blockers within an hour of other drugs.
- Cimetidine should be taken with meals or at bedtime; famotidine (Pepcid), nizatidine (Axid), ranitidine (Zantac), and ranitidine bismuth citrate (Tritec) can be taken with or without food.
- If you are using over-the-counter drugs to treat epigastric pain, see primary care provider if the pain continues for more than two weeks.

Proton Pump Inhibitors

Overview

Proton pump inhibitors suppress gastric acid secretion by inhibiting the enzyme system in the gastric cells.

Uses

- Proton pump inhibitors are used to treat:
  - Peptic ulcer disease
  - Gastroesophageal reflux disease (GERD)
  - Erosive esophagitis related to GERD
  - Zollinger-Ellison syndrome
- Proton pump inhibitors are also used to prevent recurrence of GERD.
- To eradicate *Helicobacter pylori*, proton pump inhibitors are often used in combination with antibacterials.

Adverse Effects

- Low incidence of adverse effects with short-term therapy: headache, diarrhea, nausea, vomiting
- With long-term therapy, there may be a risk of gastric cancer.
- Stomach colic or pain with omeprazole (Prilosec)
- Diarrhea for lansoprazole (Prevacid)

Precautions

- Cautious use with severe hepatic dysfunction
- Lower doses for older adults

- Be aware that serum levels of phenytoin (Dilantin), warfarin (Coumadin), diazepam (Valium), and other drugs may increase.

Important Drugs

Omeprazole (Prilosec)

Lansoprazole (Prevacid)

Rabeprazole (Aciphex)

Pantoprazole (Protonix)

Therapeutic Nursing Interventions

- Assess for epigastric and chest pain.
- Schedule drugs to avoid interactions.
- Remember that drugs that decrease acid secretion will interfere with other drugs that are absorbed in an acidic medium.

Client Education

- Omeprazole (Prilosec) capsules must be swallowed whole or they will be inactivated in the stomach.
- Lansoprazole (Prevacid) capsules can be opened and sprinkled on soft food for clients who have difficulty swallowing capsules.
- Do not crush or chew the granule form of these drugs.

Sucralfate

Overview

Sucralfate (Carafate) is activated by gastric acid to form a gel that protects the ulcer surface.

Uses

- A 4-8 week treatment with sucralfate is used to treat ulcers.
  - The dosage should be reduced when used long-term to prevent ulcer recurrence.

Adverse Effects

- Constipation and dry mouth are the most common adverse effects of sucralfate (Carafate).
- Other less common side effects include:
  - Dizziness, drowsiness
  - Pruritus, rash
  - Diarrhea, dry mouth, gastrointestinal distress, nausea

Precautions

- If given per nasogastric tube, a bezoar may form if given with food or other medications.
- Do not give antacids with sucralfate. Antacids reduce gastric acid, which is needed to activate sucralfate.

Important Drugs

Sucralfate (Carafate) is broadly classified as an antiulcer drug, or more specifically as a cytoprotective agent.

- There are no other drugs with the exact action as sucralfate.

Therapeutic Nursing Interventions

- Because sucralfate (Carafate) can interfere with the absorption of other drugs, schedule it two hours apart from other drugs.
- Assess for abdominal or chest pain.

Client Education

- Do not take any antacids within an hour of taking sucralfate.
- Sucralfate should be taken at least one hour before meals and at bedtime.
- Swallow tablets whole.
- Shake suspension to mix thoroughly before pouring.
- Do not double up if you miss a dose.
- Increase fluids, exercise, and dietary fiber to prevent constipation.
- Unless healing can be confirmed earlier by endoscopic examination, continue the drug for the period prescribed (even if you begin to feel better).

Prostaglandin

Overview

Prostaglandin E is produced in the stomach and duodenum. The effects of prostaglandin E are to:

- Inhibit acid secretion
- Increase mucus
- Increase mucus and bicarbonate secretion
- Improve mucosal blood flow
- Possibly promote mucosal repair

When prostaglandin E synthesis is inhibited, gastric and duodenal ulcers may form. Aspirin and other NSAIDs are believed to cause ulcers by inhibiting synthesis of prostaglandin E.

Uses

- Prostaglandin E is used to prevent ulcers in clients taking high doses of nonsteroidal anti-inflammatory drugs (NSAIDs).

Adverse Effects

Adverse effects of a common prostaglandin (misoprostol) include:

- Diarrhea (common, and sometimes severe)
- Abdominal pain, nausea, vomiting
- Headache

Precautions

- Prostaglandins induce abortion, so they are contraindicated during pregnancy and in women of childbearing age unless effective contraception is used.
- To prevent giving to pregnant women, a test for pregnancy is performed. If it is negative, the drug is started on the second or third day of the next menstrual period.

Important Drugs

Misoprostol (Cytotec) is a prostaglandin that is used to prevent gastric ulcers in clients taking NSAIDs.

Therapeutic Nursing Interventions

- Assess for epigastric and chest pain, bloody or tarry stools, emesis, or gastric aspirate.
- Administer after meals to reduce incidence of diarrhea.

Client Education

- If you miss a dose, do not double the next dose.
- Misoprostol (Cytotec) causes abortion, so it is very important to take/use contraception.
- If you think you may be pregnant, stop taking the misoprostol (Cytotec) and call your primary care provider.
- Notify primary care provider if you have epigastric or abdominal pain or bloody stools.
- If you have severe diarrhea or diarrhea that lasts more than a week, notify your primary care provider.
- Avoid alcohol and other irritating foods to decrease gastrointestinal distress.

Emetics

Overview

An emetic is a drug that induces vomiting.

Uses

- It is desirable to induce vomiting in conscious clients who have recently ingested drug overdoses or poisoning with non-caustic substances.

Adverse Effects

The most common antiemetic, syrup of ipecac, can cause:

- Sedation
- Diarrhea
- Dysrhythmias
- If absorbed, myocarditis

Precautions

- Safety in infants under 6 months of age has not been established.

- Contraindications to the use of emetics include:
  - Ingestion of caustic substances
  - Diminished consciousness
  - Inebriation
  - Absence of gag reflex
  - Seizures
  - Shock
- The effectiveness of an emetic is reduced if given with antiemetics, activated charcoal, or milk.
- Carbonated beverages given with an emetic will cause abdominal distention.

Important Drugs

- Syrup of ipecac is the only drug commonly used to induce vomiting.
- Do not confuse syrup of ipecac with ipecac fluid extract because the extract is 14 times stronger than the syrup.

Therapeutic Nursing Interventions

- Attempt to find out what substance was ingested.
- Syrup of ipecac usually induces projectile vomiting; if not, the dose may be repeated only once.
- Each dose of syrup of ipecac should be given with 8 ounces of water for adults and 4-8 ounces of water for children.
- Be sure the client is seated upright and turned toward one side to prevent aspiration of vomit.
- Record the characteristics of emesis.
- Monitor the client's heart rate and rhythm.

Client Education

- If possible, contact the Poison Control Center (1-800-POISON1) to determine appropriate treatment before administering syrup of ipecac.
  - Most states also have state-sponsored Poison Control Centers that can also be contacted.
- The Poison Control Center telephone number should be immediately available in every home.
- Do not drink milk or carbonated beverages to dilute poisons; these liquids can interfere with the action of an emetic drug.

Gastrointestinal Stimulants

Overview

Gastrointestinal stimulants increase motility of the upper gastrointestinal tract to accelerate gastric emptying. People who have diabetes may develop gastroparesis, a condition marked by slow gastric emptying. The effects of anesthetic agents also slow the rate of gastric emptying.

Uses

- Increase motility in the upper gastrointestinal tract of clients with gastroparesis
- Reduce esophageal reflux in clients with GERD
- Prevent and treat postoperative nausea and vomiting

Adverse Effects

Adverse effects of metoclopramide (Reglan), the prototype gastrointestinal stimulant, are:

- Drowsiness, restlessness, and extrapyramidal reactions
- Dysrhythmias and changes in blood pressure
- Gynecomastia

Extrapyramidal reactions are more common in older adults and children.

Precautions

- Metoclopramide (Reglan) is contraindicated with Parkinson's disease, pheochromocytoma, and a history of seizures.
- Use cautiously with pregnancy and with diabetes.
- Metoclopramide (Reglan) interacts with many other drugs to cause:
    - Additive hypotension with CNS depressants
    - Increased absorption of cyclosporine (Sandimmune)
    - Decreased absorption of other oral drugs
    - Exaggerated hypotension with general anesthetic agents
    - Hypertension with MAO inhibitors
    - Increased neuromuscular blockade with succinylcholine (Anectine)
    - Decreased effectiveness of levodopa

Important Drugs

Metoclopramide (Reglan) is the prototype gastrointestinal stimulant.

Therapeutic Nursing Interventions

- Assess for bowel sounds, abdominal distention, nausea, and vomiting.
- Monitor for extrapyramidal reactions, tardive dyskinesia, and depression, especially with therapy lasting more than a few weeks.
- Monitor results of liver function tests.
- Administer by correct route; can be given PO, IM, rectally, by direct intravenous injection, or by intermittent intravenous infusion.
- Take safety precautions if drowsy.
- Assess and document effectiveness.

Client Education

- Take metoclopramide (Reglan) 30 minutes before meals and at bedtime.
- Avoid using this medication with alcohol or other drugs that make you drowsy.
- Immediately notify primary care provider if you have involuntary movements of your face, eyes, or limbs.

Laxatives

Overview

Constipation is a common problem that can be caused by inactivity, lack of dietary fiber, inadequate fluid intake, and drugs that affect gastrointestinal motility. Laxatives are drugs used to induce bowel elimination. The terms **laxative** and **stool softener** generally refer to drugs that produce a soft, formed stool. Generally, laxatives have more rapid effects than stool softeners, which often take several days to be effective. Stronger drugs that act quickly to produce a semi-liquid or liquid stool are called cathartics. Various types of laxatives act in different ways:

- Bulk-forming laxatives: Stimulate peristalsis by adding bulk to the stool
- Surfactant laxatives or stool softeners: Decrease surface tension of the fecal mass, allowing water to penetrate the stool
- Saline cathartics: Cause water to be retained, which distends the bowel, leading to increased peristalsis
- Irritant or stimulant laxatives: Irritate the gastric mucosa, thereby increasing motility.
- Lubricant laxatives: Lubricate the intestine and may soften the stool
- Hyperosmotic agents: Cause retention of fluid in the colon via osmotic action
- Miscellaneous:
  - Lactulose: Not absorbed from gastrointestinal tract; decreases production of ammonia in the intestines.
  - Polyethylene glycol electrolyte solution (GoLYTELY, CoLyte) stimulates bowel emptying by distending the intestines.

Uses

- Laxatives and cathartics are used to treat acute constipation and to empty the bowel for diagnostic or therapeutic procedures.
- Stool softeners and bulk-forming agents are used to treat chronic constipation by increasing stool bulk or moisture.
  - This is useful when it is important to prevent straining at stool.
- Mineral oil, a lubricant laxative, may be given orally or used as a retention enema to facilitate defecation.
- Hyperosmotic agents are considered preferred agents for pediatric use.
- Polyethylene glycol electrolyte solution (GoLYTELY, CoLyte) is used to cleanse the bowel in preparation for diagnostic or therapeutic procedures.
  - Because it is isotonic, it does not cause fluid shifts or electrolyte imbalances.

Adverse Effects

- Occasional use of laxatives is generally safe.
  - Frequent or long-term use can lead to dependence.

- Adverse effects vary with the type of laxative:
    - Stimulant saline laxatives: Diarrhea; fluid and electrolyte imbalances if used often
    - Bulk-forming laxatives: Intestinal obstruction, impaction
    - Saline laxatives: Diarrhea, hypermagnesemia, fluid retention, edema
    - Mineral oil: Lipid pneumonitis, decreased absorption of fat-soluble vitamins, leakage through anal sphincter

Precautions

- Laxatives are contraindicated with undiagnosed abdominal pain, intestinal obstruction, and fecal impaction.
- Bulk-forming laxatives are contraindicated in clients who cannot or will not consume adequate fluids.
- Gastrointestinal stimulants increase the effects of laxatives.
- CNS depressants such as opioids and drugs with anticholinergic effects counteract the effects of laxatives.
- Clients who are prone to aspiration should not be given mineral oil.
- Saline and stimulant cathartics should not be given more than once a week.

Important Drugs

Bulk-forming laxatives

- Bran cereals
- Metamucil, the most physiologic laxative, may take up to 3 days for results

Surfactant laxatives: results may take 1-5 days.

- Docusate sodium (Colace)
- Docusate sodium with casanthranol (Peri-Colace)

Saline Cathartics:

- Milk of Magnesia: results within 2-12 hours, depending on dose
- Magnesium citrate

Stimulant laxatives: strongest and most abused; results within 6-12 hours

- Bisacodyl (Dulcolax)
- Castor oil
- Ex-Lax

Hyperosmotic agents

- Glycerin suppositories
- Lactulose (Constulose)

Miscellaneous:

- Lubricant laxative: mineral oil
- Polyethylene glycol-electrolyte solution (GoLYTELY, CoLyte)

Therapeutic Nursing Interventions

- Assess for bowel sounds, abdominal distention, and pain in clients at risk for constipation.

- Record frequency of stools and characteristics.
- Encourage good hydration, high dietary fiber, and exercise as appropriate in high-risk clients.
- Encourage toileting at the same time each day; provide for privacy and comfort.
- Evaluate and record effects of laxatives; report lack of results.
- Assess for fluid and electrolyte imbalances when saline or cathartic laxatives are used.
- When giving polyethylene glycol electrolyte solution (GoLYTELY, CoLyte), be sure the client has ready access to the toilet.
  - Assist as needed.

Client Education

- Frequent laxative use can lead to dependence and disturbances in your body fluids and electrolytes.
- If you are often constipated, try increasing your activity and your intake of fluids and dietary fiber.
- Consult with your primary care provider about the most appropriate laxative for you.
- For long-term use, bulk laxatives are the safest and produce the most normal pattern of elimination.
- If you take bulk laxatives, you must drink 8 cups of water each day. Without adequate fluids, intestinal obstruction can develop.
- When polyethylene glycol electrolyte solution (GoLYTELY, CoLyte) is prescribed:
  - Drink 8 ounces every 10 minutes until all 4 liters are taken.
  - Results may begin before you complete the entire amount.

Vitamins

Overview

Vitamins are organic compounds that are essential for energy transformation and regulation of metabolic processes. Recommended daily allowances (RDAs) represent the average daily intake of vitamins that is sufficient to meet nutritional requirements of most healthy people.

Vitamin classifications

Fat-soluble:

- A
- D
- E
- K

Water-soluble:

- B complex
  - B_1:Thiamin
  - B_2: Riboflavin
  - B_3: Niacin
  - B_5: Pantothenic acid
  - B_6: Pyridoxine
  - B_9: Folic acid
  - B_{12}: Cyanocobalamin
  - Biotin
- C

In a healthy person, a normal diet will meet the recommended daily allowance for most vitamins except:

- Vitamin B_{12} for people over age 50
- Folic acid for women of childbearing age

Water-soluble vitamins are not stored, so they must be consumed regularly to prevent deficiency. Fat-soluble vitamins are stored, which decreases the risk for deficiency, but creates the potential for toxicity. Supplemental vitamins may be indicated to prevent or treat deficiencies in people who are elderly, malnourished, chronically or severely ill, or dependent on alcohol. Vitamin requirements are increased during:

- Infancy
- Pregnancy
- Lactation
- Fever
- Hyperthyroidism

Some drugs (e.g., some NSAIDs and antacids, valproic acid) can deplete specific vitamins. Whenever possible, plan the diet to provide vitamins rather than using supplements.

Adverse Effects

- Adverse effects are rare with recommended doses.
- Vitamin A excess
  - Anorexia and vomiting
  - Irritability, headache, fatigue
  - Skin dryness and peeling
  - Muscle, bone, and joint pain
- Vitamin B complex excess
  - Hypotension
  - With parenteral forms: anaphylaxis
  - With oral niacin: nausea, vomiting, diarrhea, postural hypotension, flushing
- Vitamin C megadoses
  - Diarrhea
  - If stopped suddenly, rebound deficiency

- Vitamin K: with IV phytonadione (AquaMEPHYTON), hypotension and anaphylaxis
- Discontinuing the supplements and allowing the body to use or eliminate the excess usually treats vitamin excess.

Precautions

Be aware of drugs that affect the absorption or effects of vitamins:

- Laxatives and antibiotics can decrease the absorption of fat-soluble vitamins.
- Bile salts increase absorption of fat-soluble vitamins.
- Cycloserine (Seromycin) and isonicotinic acid hydrazide (INH, also called isoniazid), which are used to treat tuberculosis, decrease the effects of B-complex vitamins.
- Drugs that decrease the effects of folic acid:
    - Methotrexate (Rheumatrex, Trexall)
    - Oral contraceptives
    - Phenytoin (Dilantin)
    - Triamterene (Dyrenium)

Important Drugs

- Vitamins are available in individual and combination preparations.
- Many multivitamins are combined with mineral supplements.
- The label will indicate the percent of the RDA that the supplement provides for each vitamin.

Therapeutic Nursing Interventions

- Administer vitamins separately from laxatives, especially mineral oil.
- Assess for signs of vitamin deficiencies and excesses.

Client Education

- Even though vitamins do not require a prescription, they can be harmful if taken in excess.
- There is no evidence that "natural" vitamins are superior to synthetic vitamins.
- Vitamins in food are more available for absorption and have greater biological value than synthetic forms.
- Megavitamins can be dangerous; consult with your primary care provider before taking them.

Critical Thinking Exercise: Drugs Affecting the Digestive System

Note: *It is recommended that the following exercises be reviewed with a partner or in a small group to achieve maximum student interaction and to enhance critical thinking skills.*

Situation: J.L. is a 50-year-old man with ESRD (end-stage renal disease). He was hospitalized when his AV access clotted off. He has been dependent on hemodialysis for several years following a failed renal transplant. J.L.'s past medical history includes hypertension, end-stage renal disease, history of ulcers, ventricular tachycardia and atrial fibrillation, chronic pancreatitis, anemia, Staphylococcus aureus sepsis, and steroid-induced diabetes mellitus. A Tenckhoff catheter was inserted during the current hospitalization and J.L. was placed on continuous cycling-assisted peritoneal dialysis (CCPD) with plans to discharge him on continuous ambulatory peritoneal dialysis (CAPD). His current medications are:

- Ferrous sulfate (Feosol) 325 mg PO bid
- Terazosin (Hytrin) 10 mg PO at HS
- Amiodarone (Cordarone) 200 mg PO QD
- Sucralfate (Carafate) 1g PO qid
- Epoetin alpha (Epogen) 6000 units SC 3x/wk
- Docusate sodium (Colace) 100 mg PO bid
- Calcitrol (Rocaltrol) 25 mcg, 2 tabs PO bid
- Calcium carbonate (Tums) 420 mg, 3 tabs with meals
- Nifedipine (Procardia XL) 120 mg PO bid at 10 a.m. and 10 p.m

1. What antacids are contraindicated in renal clients and why?

2. Identify the reasons J.L. is taking docusate sodium (Colace).

3. In regard to his other medications, when would you give him sucralfate (Carafate) and why?

4. How do you think popular opinion and the media influence the choice of over-the-counter antacids? Discuss some of the positive and negative implications involved.

5. What are some of the nursing implications of self-medication with over-the-counter antacids?

6. Place the corresponding letter of the drug you feel would be most appropriate for the condition listed to the right. There may be more than one correct answer. A list of drugs is located at the bottom of the page for reference.

Peptic ulcers ______________________

Gastric reflux ______________________

Constipation ______________________

Diarrhea ______________________

Nausea and vomiting ______________________

Motion sickness ______________________

Flatulence ______________________

Stress ulcers ______________________

GERD ______________________

Drugs:

A. Aluminum hydroxide
B. Magnesium hydroxide
C. Dramamine
D. Lomotil
E. Psyllium
F. Biscodyl
G. Reglan
H. Antivert
I. Imodium
J. Zantac
K. Tagamet
L. Colace
M. Mylicon
N. Amoxicillin
O. Metamucil

CHAPTER 11

Drugs Affecting the Endocrine System

Key Points

- Normal blood glucose is 90-130 mg/dL.
    - Hypoglycemia occurs when blood glucose is < 60 mg/dL.
    - Hyperglycemia occurs when blood glucose is >120 mg/dL.
- Hypoglycemia requires prompt medical attention.
- Insulin may be ordered as scheduled doses or per a sliding scale.
    - Sliding scale insulin orders consist of specific, prescribed doses of insulin based upon defined blood glucose ranges.
    - Sliding scale insulin may be prescribed independently or in conjunction with scheduled insulin or oral hypoglycemic agents.
- The primary classifications of antithyroid agents are:
    - Thioamides
    - Iodide products
    - Radioactive iodine
- All antithyroid drugs are contraindicated during pregnancy and lactation.
- Physiologic corticosteroid dosages are used for replacement therapy when there is insufficiency, such as Addison's disease.
- Pharmacologic corticosteroid dosages are used to treat:
    - Inflammatory diseases
    - Allergic conditions
    - Neoplastic disease
    - Brain-injury victims
    - Skin conditions
    - Ophthalmic conditions
    - Collagen disorders
    - They also prevent rejection of transplanted organs/tissue.
- Corticosteroid therapy, especially in high doses or for long durations, has multiple serious adverse effects, including:
    - Lowered resistance to infection
    - Risk of peptic ulcers
    - Elevated blood glucose
    - Osteoporosis
- Hormone replacement therapy (HRT) for postmenopausal women prevents:
    - Urogenital atrophy

    - Maintains bone mass
    - May protect against coronary artery disease
    - May protect against colon cancer
    - Suppresses vasomotor symptoms ("hot flashes")
- Estrogen used alone poses a risk of endometrial hyperplasia and carcinoma.
- The use of estrogen with progestins may increase the risk of breast cancer.
- Pharmacologic uses of progesterone include:
    - Oral contraception (most often with estrogen)
    - HRT
    - Treatment of:
        - Endometriosis
        - Dysmenorrhea
        - Uterine bleeding
- The effects of testosterone on males include sexual development and spermatogenesis.
- Virilization is the most common adverse effect of testosterone in males and females.
- Antiandrogens are used, in combination with surgical or chemical castration, to treat advanced prostate cancer.
- In addition to other functions, immunosuppressants are use to treat autoimmune disorders and to prevent transplant rejection reactions.
- All immunosuppressants place the client at risk for:
    - Infection
    - Malignancy, most often lymphoma with long-term therapy
    - Bone marrow suppression
    - Gastrointestinal disturbances
- Immunizations protect people from infection by stimulating the immune system to develop specific antibodies.
- Live virus vaccines should not be given to an immune-suppressed person.
- When giving immunizations, be sure epinephrine 1:1000 is available for immediate treatment of allergic reactions.
- A mild local reaction and low fever are common after immunizations; more serious symptoms should be reported to the primary care provider.
- Thyroid hormones stimulate metabolism and cardiac function and are essential for normal growth and development of the nervous and musculoskeletal systems.
- Manifestations of hypothyroidism in adults include bradycardia, cold dry skin, brittle hair, low body temperature, fatigue, cold intolerance, flat affect, slowed cognition, and weight gain.
- Hypothyroidism is a chronic condition requiring lifelong HRT.
- If the thyroid hormone dosage is too high, the client will develop signs and symptoms of hyperthyroidism.
- Few other classes of drugs produce such profound therapeutic benefits or adverse reactions as the corticosteroids.

Antiglycemics

Overview

Blood Glucose Regulation is controlled by insulin. Insulin is a hormone produced by the beta cells in the pancreas. Insulin is responsible for:

- Facilitating the passage of glucose into cells for energy
- Suppressing excess production of sugar in the liver and muscles
- Suppressing the breakdown of fat for energy

Hyperglycemia may result from three main abnormalities:

- Excessive glucose production in the liver
- Absent or impaired insulin production and secretion by the pancreas
- Peripheral insulin resistance

Antiglycemics prevent hyperglycemia by decreasing insulin resistance and decreasing glucose production in the liver.

- These agents can be used as monotherapy in the treatment of Type 2 diabetes.
- May be used in combination therapy with insulin in the treatment of Type 1 diabetes

Biguanides

Overview

An anti-hyperglycemic agent that primarily reduces hepatic production of glucose by inhibiting glycogenolysis (the formation of glycogen from non-carbohydrates); decreasing the intestinal absorption of glucose; and improving lipid profile.

Uses

- Monotherapy in the treatment of Type 2 diabetes or secondary diabetes where there is capacity for pancreatic insulin production
- Combination therapy in the treatment of Type 2 diabetes

Adverse Effects

- Abdominal discomfort and diarrhea
- Metallic taste, agitation, sweating, and headache
- Lactic acidosis (rare)

Precautions

- Safety during pregnancy, lactation, or in children is not established.
- Contraindicated in clients with hepatic or renal dysfunction, a history of alcoholism, binge alcohol ingestion, or congestive heart failure (CHF) requiring pharmacologic treatment.
- Should be temporarily withheld in situations that predispose to acute renal dysfunction or hypoperfusion.
- Not recommended for individuals > 80 years old unless renal function is sufficient.

- Use cautiously in persons with dehydration, hypoxia, or pituitary or thyroid dysfunction.
- Contraindicated in clients with renal dysfunction manifested with a serum creatinine = 1.4 mg/dL in females; 1.5 mg/dL in males.

Important Drugs

Metformin (Glucophage, Glucophage XR)

Therapeutic Nursing Interventions

- Monitor for therapeutic and adverse effects.
- Assess renal and liver function on regular basis.
- If taken as combination therapy, monitor for hypoglycemia.
- Insulin is the drug of choice for controlling blood sugar during pregnancy.

Client Education

- Take before meals or with food to decrease adverse effects.
- Inform your doctor you are taking metformin (Glucophage) before any surgical procedure or diagnostic procedure using a contrast dye.
- Adhere to other regimens prescribed to control your diabetes, such as nutrition and exercise plan.
- Perform self blood-glucose testing regularly to monitor therapeutic benefit.
- A slight weight loss may occur when you first take this drug.
    - This is normal and this weight loss can help you control your diabetes.
- Carry emergency identification that identifies you as a diabetic.
- Carry a form of sugar in case of hypoglycemia.
- Metformin may cause a transient metallic taste.

Alpha-Glucosidase Inhibitors

Overview

Anti-hyperglycemics act primarily by inhibiting alpha-glucosidase enzymes in the small intestine and alpha-amylase in the pancreas. This decreases the rate of complex carbohydrate metabolism. The result is a reduced rate of glucose absorption postprandially (following a meal).

Uses

- Most effective in clients with Type 2 diabetes mellitus who demonstrate a significant post-meal hyperglycemia

Adverse Effects

- Flatulence, bloating, and diarrhea
- Reductions in hematocrit have been observed, but are not associated with concurrent change in hemoglobin.

Precautions

- Not intended for use during pregnancy, lactation, or by children

- Contraindicated in clients with inflammatory bowel disease, chronic intestinal disorders, or obstructive bowel disorders
- Contraindicated in clients with cirrhosis of the liver
- Use with caution in clients with renal dysfunction manifested by a serum creatinine > 2.0 mg/dL.
- Hypoglycemia may occur if taken in combination with other hypoglycemic agents.

Important Drugs

Acarbose (Precose)

Miglitol (Glyset)

Therapeutic Nursing Interventions

- Monitor for drug's therapeutic and adverse side effects.
- If taken as combination therapy, treat any occurring hypoglycemia with glucose, such as glucose tablets or milk in the conscious client.
- Not effective when taken on an empty stomach
- Assess for signs of hypoglycemia (sweating, tremors, dizziness, hunger, tachycardia, and irritability).

Client Education

- Take with food.
- Adhere to other regimens prescribed to control your diabetes, such as nutrition and exercise plan.
- Perform self blood-glucose testing regularly to monitor therapeutic benefit.
- Carry emergency identification that identifies you as a diabetic.
- Avoid taking other mediation without consultation with your primary care provider.

Thiazolidinediones

Overview

Anti-hyperglycemic agent that functions primarily by enhancing insulin action at the cell receptor and post-receptor site and decreases insulin resistance.

Uses

- Monotherapy in the treatment of Type 2 NIDDM (non-insulin dependent diabetes mellitus) or secondary diabetes where there is capacity for pancreatic insulin production
- Combination therapy in the treatment of Type 2 NIDDM

Adverse Effects

- Can cause injury to the liver
- Weight gain may occur
- Lower extremity edema
- Gastrointestinal discomfort

- Increase in plasma volume with associated decrease in hemoglobin and hematocrit

Precautions

- Not intended for use during pregnancy, lactation, or by children.
- May inhibit effectiveness of oral contraceptives, increasing risk for pregnancy.
- May cause an increase in high-density lipoprotein (HDL) and low-density lipoprotein (LDL); however, the ratio remains unchanged.
- At risk for hypoglycemia if taken in combination with other diabetes medications.
- When used in combination with insulin, the insulin dose is usually reduced by 10-20% when blood glucose reaches levels of <120 mg/dl.

Important Drugs

Pioglitazone (Actos)

Rosiglitazone (Avandia)

Therapeutic Nursing Interventions

- Monitor for drug's therapeutic and adverse side effects.
- Particularly monitor liver function.
- Give with or without food.
- Caution women of childbearing age of the increased risk of pregnancy if taking oral contraceptives.

Client Education

- Report any signs of liver disease (nausea, vomiting, stomach pain, lack of appetite, yellowing of skin or eyes, dark colored urine) to your primary care provider immediately.
- Report any change in energy level.
- Perform self blood-glucose testing to monitor therapeutic benefit.
- Carry emergency identification that identifies you as a diabetic.
- Adhere to other regimens prescribed to control your diabetes, such as nutrition and exercise plan.

Antithyroid Agents

Overview

Hyperthyroidism is the abnormally increased secretion of thyroid hormone. The two primary types of hyperthyroidism are Grave's disease (an autoimmune disorder) and toxic nodular goiter. Manifestations of hyperthyroidism include tachycardia, dysrhythmias, restlessness, insomnia, weak skeletal muscles, increased body temperature, and weight loss despite increased food intake. Extremely high serum levels of thyroid hormone can cause thyroid crisis (or "storm") characterized by hyperthermia, tachycardia, and profound weakness. Thyroid crisis is life-threatening, as it can lead to heart failure and coma. One cause of thyroid crisis is the escape of excess hormones into the bloodstream during subtotal thyroidectomy, which can be averted by suppressing hormone secretion preoperatively. Hyperthyroidism can be treated surgically or with antithyroid drugs. The primary classifications of antithyroid agents are:

- Thioamides
- Iodide products
- Radioactive iodide (^{131}I)

Uses

- Antithyroid drugs suppress thyroid hormone synthesis and prevent the conversion of T4 (triiodothyronine, which contains 3 atoms of iodine) to T3 (thyroxine, which contains 4 atoms of iodine).
- Specific uses for thioamides in the treatment of hyperthyroidism include the:
  - Treatment of Grave's disease
  - Suppression of thyroid hormone synthesis until radiation therapy destroys thyroid tissue
  - Suppression of thyroid hormone synthesis before thyroid surgery to reduce the risk of thyroid crisis
  - Treatment of thyroid crisis
- Radioactive iodine (^{131}I) is used to:
  - Destroy part of the thyroid tissue in Grave's disease
  - Treat some types of thyroid cancer
  - Diagnose various thyroid disorders
- Iodide preparations are used to:
  - Suppress thyroid function before surgery for hyperthyroidism
  - Treat Grave's disease
  - Treat thyroid crisis
  - Prevent thyroid damage resulting from exposure to radiation (as in a nuclear accident)
- Combinations of the various antithyroid agents are used in some situations.

Adverse Effects

- The primary adverse effects of antithyroid drugs occur when excessive suppression of hormone secretion causes hypothyroidism.
- The most common adverse effects of thioamides are:
  - Rash
  - Nausea
  - Muscle aches
  - Headache
  - Dizziness
  - Paresthesia
- The most harmful adverse effects of the thioamides are blood dyscrasias, including agranulocytosis (a significant decrease in the number of neutrophils).
  - Occurrence is rare.

- Usually occurs in the first two months of therapy
- Early symptoms: fever and sore throat
- Reversible when propylthiouracil (PTU) is discontinued

- Adverse effects of ^{131}I (radioactive iodine) depend on the dose.
  - Dosage used for diagnostic purposes have no adverse effects.
  - The dosage required to treat cancer is much larger and may cause:
    - Radiation sickness
    - Leukemia
    - Bone marrow depression
- Adverse effects of oral iodide preparations
  - Iodism: Metallic taste, burning sensation in mouth and throat, sore teeth and gums, headache, cold symptoms, salivation, skin lesions
  - Toxicity: Abdominal pain, vomiting, diarrhea, and edema of the glottis
  - Sodium iodide: Potentially fatal hypersensitivity reaction

Precautions

- Antithyroid agents are generally contraindicated during pregnancy and lactation because the thyroid function of the fetus/infant will be suppressed.
- With thioamides, periodic blood counts are necessary to detect agranulocytosis.
- Radioactive agents are contraindicated during pregnancy and lactation because of the risk to the fetus/infant.
- Radiation precautions must be followed for clients given high doses of ^{131}I (radioactive iodine) for thyroid cancer.

Important Drugs

Thioamides

- The two thioamides in use are:
  - Propylthiouracil (PTU)
  - Methimazole (Tapazole): may carry slightly less risk of agranulocytosis

Radioactive iodine: ^{131}I

- Iodide products
- Potassium iodide (SSKI)
- Strong iodine solution (Lugol's solution)
- Sodium iodide

Therapeutic Nursing Interventions

- Monitor weight, heart rate, and laboratory studies of thyroid hormones.
- Assess for iodism and iodine toxicity.
- Mix iodide solutions in full glass of water, fruit juice, or milk. Administer after meals.
- Discard brownish iodide solutions.
- If crystals form in iodide solutions, warm and shake the solution to dissolve the crystals.

Client Education

- Report excessive fatigue and weight gain that could indicate hypothyroidism.
- Effects of antithyroid drugs make take up to two weeks with thioamides and several months with ^{131}I.
- Thioamides should be taken at regular intervals around the clock.
- Females who are sexually active should use contraception when taking antithyroid drugs.
- The radiation dose used for diagnostic purposes is very small with no adverse effects.
- Report symptoms of iodism and iodine toxicity (provide written list).

Corticosteroids

Overview

Corticosteroids are necessary for life. The rate of secretion changes according to need. It accelerates rapidly in response to stress. Stress causes the hypothalamus to secrete corticotropin-releasing hormone that stimulates the anterior pituitary to secrete adrenocorticotropic hormone (ACTH). In response to stress, ACTH increases rapidly. Shortly after ACTH is released, corticosteroids, particularly hydrocortisone, are released.

Hydrocortisone secretion is subject to variation at certain times of the day. (High levels are found in early morning hours and low levels in the evening.) People who work nightshift peak shortly after arising and drop again before going to bed.

Corticosteroids are hormones produced by the adrenal cortex. These hormones and their physiologic functions follow:

Glucocorticoids

- Maintain adequate serum glucose for brain metabolism by:
  - Stimulating gluconeogenesis
  - Promoting glycogen storage
  - Reducing peripheral glucose use
- Promote breakdown of fats
- Inhibit synthesis of protein
- Maintain normal capillary permeability and vasomotor tone
- Maintain function of skeletal muscle
- Affect excitability of the CNS and mood
- Increase RBCs and polymorphonuclear leukocytes

Mineralocorticoids

- Maintain fluid and electrolyte balance by:
  - Increasing the renal reabsorption of sodium and water
  - Promoting the excretion of potassium

Cortisol is the primary glucocorticoid, while aldosterone is the primary mineralocorticoid. Disorders related to altered production of adrenal hormones are:

- Cushing's syndrome: adrenocortical hormone excess
- Addison's disease: adrenocortical hormone deficiency

Corticosteroid preparations differ in the amount of mineralocorticoids present.

Uses

- Corticosteroid therapy is given in physiologic or pharmacologic dosages, depending on the diagnosis.
    - A physiologic dose is relatively low and intended to restore normal levels.
    - A pharmacologic dose is high and is used to treat a variety of nonendocrine disorders.
- Physiologic dosages of corticosteroids are used for replacement therapy when there is insufficiency, such as Addison's disease.
- Pharmacologic dosages are used to treat:
    - Inflammatory diseases:
        - Rheumatoid arthritis
        - Chronic ulcerative colitis
        - Ocular inflammations
        - Nephrotic syndromes
        - Liver disorders
    - Allergic conditions:
        - Status asthmaticus
        - Bronchial asthma
        - Allergic reactions
    - Neoplastic disease:
        - Leukemias
        - Hodgkin's disease
    - Brain-injury victims (suppress edema)
    - Skin conditions:
        - Psoriasis
        - Dermatitis
    - Prevent rejection in transplant clients
    - Ophthalmic conditions (topical ophthalmic preparations):
        - Allergic conjunctivitis
        - Corneal injury
        - Suppression of graft rejection
        - Prevention of postoperative inflammation
    - Collagen diseases:
        - Systemic lupus erythematosus
        - Scleroderma

- Unlabeled uses:
  - Acute spinal cord injury
  - Antiemetic with chemotherapy
  - Stimulation of lung maturation in premature infants (drug administered to mother shortly before delivery)
  - Reduction of inflammation in proximal and terminal airways of babies and children with chronic lung disease

Adverse Effects

- Corticosteroids are relatively safe for short-term treatment of self-limiting conditions.
- Sometimes corticosteroids are given every other day to reduce adrenal suppression and other adverse effects.
- Topical corticosteroids can have systemic effects, and even toxicity, with significant absorption through skin or mucus membranes.
- Adverse effects of pharmacologic doses (risk increases with dosage and duration of therapy):
  - Adrenal insufficiency
  - Increased risk of infection
  - Increased blood glucose
  - Muscle weakness
  - Cataracts and open-angle glaucoma
  - Osteoporosis
  - Abnormal fat distribution ("buffalo hump," "moon face," "potbelly")
  - Mood swings, hallucinations (rare)
  - Increased gastric acid and pepsin; decreased gastric mucus and blood flow
  - Fluid and electrolyte imbalances
    - Water and sodium retention: edema and increased blood pressure
    - Hypokalemia: muscle weakness, cardiac dysrhythmias
- Adverse effects of topical corticosteroids are most likely to be local and may include:
  - Skin rash
  - Burning and dryness
  - Increased hair growth
  - Loss of pigmentation

Precautions

- Corticosteroids are contraindicated with active untreated infections.
- If corticosteroid therapy is stopped abruptly, the client may develop acute adrenal insufficiency.
- During times of stress such as surgery or trauma, the client with adrenal insufficiency may die if not given supplemental glucocorticoids.
- Clients taking corticosteroids should be given vaccinations with caution.
  - The vaccine may be ineffective because the client cannot manufacture adequate antibodies.

- Live-virus vaccines may cause the infection they were intended to prevent.
- Corticosteroids must be used cautiously with:
  - Pregnancy
  - Lactation
  - Children
  - Clients at high risk for infection
  - Osteoporosis, peptic ulcer disease, cardiac or renal failure, diabetes mellitus, hypertension, and myasthenia gravis
  - Immunocompromised persons
- Significant drug interactions include:
  - Increased risk of hypokalemia with potassium-depleting diuretics
  - Increased risk of digitalis toxicity with hypokalemia
  - Increased risk of gastric ulcers with NSAIDs
- Do not use ophthalmic preparations with fungal or viral eye infections.

Important Drugs

Systemic

- Cortisone (Cortone) is a short-acting corticosteroid.
- Prednisone (Deltasone) is an intermediate-acting corticosteroid.
- Betamethasone (Celestone) is a long-acting corticosteroid.
- Fludrocortisone (Florinef Acetate) is a potent mineralocorticoid used to treat adrenal insufficiency states.
- Dexamethasone (Decadron) is a glucocorticoid used to treat allergic and inflammatory conditions. Dexamethasone is also administered at the beginning of a supression test that is used to diagnose and evaluate Cushing's syndrome. The client takes dexamethasone orally in the evening to suppress the secretion of corticotropin-releasing hormone. A plasma cortisol blood sample is drawn the next morning. Normally there is a 50% decrease in the production of cortisol. An increase in cortisol levels indicates Cushing's syndrome or disease.
- Note: Corticosteroids typically have both glucocorticoid and mineralocorticoid activity.

Topical: Hydrocortisone

Inhaled: Beclomethasone (Vanceril)

Ophthalmic: Prednisolone (AK-Pred)

Therapeutic Nursing Interventions

For all clients on corticosteroid therapy:

- Corticosteroids come in many preparations for various routes of administration; be careful to select the correct preparation.
- Assess for adverse effects, although serious systemic effects are not expected with physiologic doses.

For clients receiving pharmacologic dosages:

- Monitor the effects of the corticosteroids on the condition being treated.
- Assess for subtle signs of infection.

- Implement safety measures to prevent falls and fractures.
- Monitor clients with diabetes for hyperglycemia.
- Monitor growth in children.
- Assess for psychologic disturbances.
- Assess for fluid and electrolyte imbalances.
- Monitor clients taking digitalis for toxicity.
- Assess stools for melena.

For parenteral corticosteroids:

- Be certain you have the correct preparation.
- Shake suspensions to mix thoroughly.
- Do not give suspensions intravenously.
- Do not dilute with other solutions.

Client Education

All clients on corticosteroid therapy

- Always wear a medical alert tag noting that you take corticosteroids.
- Always have an emergency supply of medication with you.
- Never stop taking this medication without medical supervision.
- Take oral medications with food or milk to minimize gastrointestinal irritation.
- Your resistance to infection is low, so you should avoid people with active infections.
- Notify your primary care provider of the following:
    - Any sign of infection
    - Weight gain, edema
    - Blurred or cloudy vision
    - Pregnancy
    - Dark or tarry stools, abdominal pain

Clients receiving physiologic dosages

- For Addison's disease:
    - It is important to take two-thirds of the daily dosage in the morning, and the remainder in the afternoon.
    - Lifelong corticosteroid therapy will be required.
    - You will require increased dosage during times of stress (surgery, trauma, infection).

Clients receiving pharmacologic doses

- Avoid activities that could cause bone fractures.
- Do not take NSAIDs (aspirin, ibuprofen, etc.) unless directed by your primary care provider.
- Approve with primary care provider before receiving any vaccinations.
- Increase dietary intake of protein, calcium, and potassium; reduce intake of sodium and carbohydrates; avoid alcohol.

Hormones

Overview

The neurologic and endocrine systems maintain homeostasis. Neurologic responses are generally rapid in onset and brief in duration, whereas the endocrine system responds more slowly and produces more long-lasting effects. The hypothalamus receives information from the nervous system and responds by secreting, stimulating or releasing factors that act on the anterior pituitary.

Hormones which are secreted by the anterior pituitary produce the following effects:

- Growth hormone: Stimulates growth of body tissues
- Corticotropin: Stimulation of adrenal cortex
- Thyroid-stimulating hormone: Stimulation of thyroid gland
- Luteinizing hormone: Stimulation of hormone production by gonads
- Follicle-stimulating hormone: Stimulates growth of ovarian follicles
- Prolactin: Plays a role in milk production
- Melanocyte-stimulating hormone: Affects skin pigmentation

Hormones stored and released by the posterior pituitary produce the following effects:

- Antidiuretic hormone: Plays a role in water balance
- Oxytocin: Initiates uterine contractions and causes milk to move to the nipples

Hypothalamic hormones are given in very limited clinical situations. The primary clinical use for pituitary hormones is to replace or supplement deficient hormones. This section will address estrogen, progesterone, testosterone, androgens, and antiandrogens.

Estrogen

Overview

Estrogens are ovarian hormones that:

- Promote the development and maintenance of sexual characteristics in females.
- Influence growth of female reproductive tissue.
- Influence the menstrual cycle.
- Help maintain bone mass by blocking bone resorption.
- Elevate blood level of high-density lipoproteins and lower blood levels of low-density lipoproteins.

There are several estrogens, but estradiol is the most common.

Uses

- Hormone replacement therapy for postmenopausal women:
  - Prevents urogenital atrophy
  - Maintains bone mass
  - May protect against coronary artery disease and colon cancer

    - Suppresses vasomotor symptoms ("hot flashes")
- Promotion of normal sexual development and function in girls with estrogen deficiency
- Androgen suppression in men with prostate cancer
- Oral contraception by inhibition of ovulation

Adverse Effects

- Risk of endometrial hyperplasia and carcinoma if used without progestins
- The use of estrogen with progestins may increase the risk of breast cancer.
- The most common adverse effects of estrogen therapy are nausea, fluid retention, and breast tenderness.
- Less common adverse effects associated with high dosages:
    - Headache
    - Dizziness
    - Depression
- Adverse effects of combination estrogen/progestin oral contraceptives include:
    - Hypertension
    - Thromboembolic disorders
    - Endometrial cancer (low risk)
    - Teratogenic effects (causing a malformation of an embryo or fetus)
    - Abnormal uterine bleeding
    - Other less common effects:
        - Benign liver tumor
        - Multiple births
        - Glucose intolerance
        - Gallbladder disease

Precautions

- A woman who has not had a hysterectomy should be given estrogen only in combination with progestins to reduce the risk of uterine cancer.
- Estrogens are contraindicated with:
    - Pregnancy and lactation
    - Undiagnosed vaginal bleeding
    - Previous or active thrombophlebitis or thromboembolic disorders
    - Estrogen-dependent cancers
    - History of cerebrovascular accident
    - Coronary artery disease
    - Breast carcinoma
    - Liver tumors
    - Undiagnosed abnormal genital bleeding
- Combination oral contraceptives must be used cautiously by clients with diabetes and by women who smoke.
- Many common antimicrobials decrease the effectiveness of oral contraceptives.

Important Drugs

- Various estrogen preparations are available for PO, IM, IV, transdermal, and intravaginal use.
- Some common forms of estrogens used for HRT are:
  - Conjugated estrogens, equine
  - Conjugated estrogens, synthetic
  - DES (diethylstilbestrol)
  - Estradiol
  - Estrone
  - Estropipate
  - Ethinyl estradiol
- There are many estrogen/progestin combinations used for oral contraception.

Therapeutic Nursing Interventions

- Counsel women to have annual breast and pelvic examinations.
- Teach clients how to do breast self-examinations.

Client Education

- Notify the primary care provider if you have persistent or recurrent vaginal bleeding.
- Perform breast self-examination every month; have annual mammograms.
- If you suspect you are pregnant, stop taking estrogen immediately.
- Instructions for using the estradiol transdermal system:
  - Apply the patch to clean, dry skin on the trunk, avoiding the breasts and waistline.
  - Rotate application sites to avoid skin irritation.
  - Replace patches once or twice weekly, as prescribed.
  - A patch that falls off can be reapplied or replaced with a fresh one.
- If using an intravaginal cream or tablet, use the applicator provided to insert the medication high into the vagina.
- If one dose of an oral contraceptive is missed, take it with the next scheduled dose.
- For two missed doses of your oral contraceptive, take two doses each for the next two days.
- For three or more missed doses, start a new cycle seven days after the last dose taken. Use another birth control method for the first two weeks of the new cycle.

Progesterone

Overview

Progesterone is a progestin that plays a vital role in reproduction. Progestins are predominately ovarian hormones; however, the adrenal glands and testes also produce small amounts of progestins. Progesterone is secreted by the corpus luteum after ovulation and prepares the endometrial lining to receive the fertilized ovum. If fertilization occurs, progesterone maintains the uterine lining. It promotes the development of milk-producing cells in the breasts.

Uses

- Oral contraception (most often with estrogen)
- Hormone replacement therapy (HRT)
- Ovarian suppression to treat endometriosis, dysmenorrhea, or uterine bleeding

Adverse Effects

- Irregular ("breakthrough") vaginal bleeding
- Teratogenic during first four months of pregnancy
- Nausea
- Impaired glucose tolerance (especially in people with diabetes)
- Depression
- Drowsiness
- Insomnia
- Edema
- Weight gain

Precautions

Progesterone is contraindicated with:

- Pregnancy
- Undiagnosed vaginal bleeding
- Previous or active thrombophlebitis or thromboembolic disorders
- Cancer of the breast or reproductive organs
- Severe liver disease
- Undiagnosed abnormal genital bleeding

Many antimicrobials interfere with the effects of progestins.

Important Drugs

Medroxyprogesterone acetate (Provera)

Prometrium micronized capsules

Crinone micronized vaginal cream

Progesterone injectable (IM)

Norethindrone (combined with estradiol) **transdermal**

Therapeutic Nursing Interventions

- Monitor weight, blood pressure, liver function studies, and mental/emotional state.
- Administer IM preparation deeply in large muscle mass; rotate sites.
- Monitor blood glucose in people with diabetes mellitus.

Client Education

- Take oral progesterone with food or milk to decrease nausea.
- If pregnancy is suspected, stop taking progesterone and notify primary care provider.
- Report:
  - Weight gain
  - Pain and tenderness in legs
  - Chest pain
  - Mental depression
- Have periodic blood studies, as well as breast and pelvic exams.

Androgens

Overview

Androgens are male sex hormones that are produced by the testes, the ovaries, and the adrenal cortex. There are three classes of androgens:

- Testosterone and testosterone esters
- 17-alpha alkylated androgens
- Others: Nandrolone decanoate, stanozolol, etc.

Testosterone is the most important androgen. The effects of testosterone in males include:

- Enlargement of testes, penis, and scrotum
- Increased body hair
- Growth of bone and skeletal muscle
- Enlargement of the larynx
- Increased number of sebaceous glands
- Beard development
- Spermatogenesis

In females, testosterone may:

- Influence clitoral growth
- Maintain normal libido
- Have masculine effects (virilization), but only in the presence of ovarian or adrenocortical dysfunction, or when it is given for therapeutic purposes

Anabolic steroids are synthetic drugs that have more anabolic (tissue building) and less androgenic effects than testosterone.

Uses

In males to treat:

- Hypogonadism
- Cryptorchidism
- Erectile dysfunction
- Oligospermia

- Delayed puberty
- Muscle wasting with acquired immune deficiency syndrome (AIDS)

In females to treat:

- Endometriosis
- Fibrocystic breast disease
- Hereditary angioedema
- Some menopausal symptoms
- Advanced breast cancer (palliative)

Anabolic steroids are widely abused to promote tissue building and growth with minimal virilization.

Adverse Effects

Virilization is the most common adverse effect of testosterone.

- Adult males with normal testosterone secretion may experience:
  - Increased sexual desire
  - Reduced sperm count
  - Prostate enlargement
  - Priapism
- Women may experience:
  - Deepening of the voice
  - Increased hair growth
  - Menstrual irregularities
  - Women being treated with androgens for breast cancer receive high doses; so virilization is common.
    - Are also at risk for hypercalcemia
- In prepubertal boys:
  - Premature sexual development may occur
  - Premature epiphyseal closure may occur, decreasing adult height
- Masculinization of a female fetus

Decreased high-density lipoproteins; increased low-density lipoproteins.

Hepatotoxicity (jaundice, hepatitis, liver cancer) has occurred with some androgens, but not with testosterone.

Edema

Gynecomastia in males

Precautions

- Contraindicated during pregnancy and with prostate enlargement
- Children must have bone growth evaluated every six months.
- Because anabolic steroids have the potential for abuse by athletes seeking to enhance athletic performance, they are classified as Schedule III controlled substances.
- Androgens enhance the effects of oral anticoagulants, oral anti-glycemics, and insulin.

Important Drugs

There are many **testosterone preparations**. Examples are:

- **Testosterone cypionate** (Depo-Testosterone, and other brands)
- **Testosterone enanthate** (Andro LA, and other brands)
- **Testosterone propionate** (Testex, and other brands)
- **Testosterone transdermal** (Androderm, Testoderm)

Danazol (Danocrine) is primarily used to treat endometriosis, to palliate fibrocystic breast disease, and to prevent hereditary angioedema.

The most commonly used anabolic steroids are **nandrolone decanoate** (Deca-Durabolin) and **stanozolol** (Winstrol).

Therapeutic Nursing Interventions

- Advise women to avoid pregnancy while taking androgens.
- Monitor for virilizing effects in women, girls, and boys. Effects can be minimized if drug is stopped early.
- Emphasize the importance of growth assessments every 6 months for children.
- Monitor for the following adverse drug effects:
    - Boys: precocious puberty
    - Adult males: breast enlargement, persistent erections, difficulty urinating
    - Women: deep voice, unusual hair growth or loss, menstrual irregularities, acne, clitoral enlargement
    - Women with breast cancer: hypercalcemia (nausea, polyuria, weakness, lethargy)
- Administration of IM injection:
    - Warm and shake vial to dissolve crystals, if present.
    - Administer deep into gluteal muscle.

Client Education

- Report weight gain, edema, and difficulty voiding to your primary care provider.
- Virilizing effects may be reversible if reported promptly to the primary care provider.
- Continue medical supervision while taking androgens.
- Children must have growth assessments every 6 months.
- Transdermal patches
    - Apply testosterone (Testoderm) patches once daily to the scrotum. Apply two testosterone (Androderm) patches each night to the back, abdomen, upper arms, or thighs.
    - Apply to clean, dry, hairless (shaved) site.
    - If skin irritation occurs, apply corticosteroid cream to site as ordered.
    - Patches can be reapplied if they loosen during bathing, swimming, etc.
- Buccal tablets
    - Place tablet between the cheek and gum and allow it to dissolve.
    - Do not eat, drink, or smoke while the tablet is in the cheek.

- Oral tablets: take before or with meals.
- The use of anabolic steroids for bodybuilding is inappropriate, potentially dangerous, and illegal if not prescribed by a primary care provider.

Antiandrogens

Overview

Tumor cells in prostate cancer are dependent on androgenic stimulation. Antiandrogens block the receptors in tumor cells, which deny the cells of androgenic stimulation. To be effective, antiandrogens must be used in combination with other therapies that prevent or suppress androgen secretion. This can be achieved by:

- Orchiectomy (surgical castration)
- Gonadotropin-releasing hormone agonists which inhibit the testes from producing androgens

Uses

- Antiandrogens are used in combination with surgical or chemical castration to treat advanced prostate cancer.
- In addition to prostate cancer, nilutamide is used after tamoxifen to treat advanced breast cancer in postmenopausal women.

Adverse Effects

- Gynecomastia can occur with all androgen receptor blockers.
- Although rare, flutamide can also cause nausea, vomiting, diarrhea, and toxic hepatitis.
- Bicalutamide is more likely to cause serious diarrhea. When combined with leuprolide, it often causes hot flashes.
- Nilutamide is not tolerated as well as other antiandrogenics. Additional adverse effects include:
  - Hot flashes
  - Visual disturbances and delayed adaptation to dark
  - Constipation
  - Nausea
  - Interstitial pneumonitis (rare)
  - Hepatitis (rare)
- Bicalutamide and nilutamide may cause loss of hair.

Precautions

- Flutamide is contraindicated with severe liver impairment and should be used cautiously with severe cardiovascular disease.
- Bicalutamide is contraindicated during pregnancy.
- Nilutamide is contraindicated with severe liver impairment or severe respiratory impairment.
- Bicalutamide and nilutamide enhance the effect of warfarin.
- Liver toxicity can be fatal.

Important Drugs

Flutamide (Eulexin)
Bicalutamide (Casodex)
Nilutamide (Nilandron)

Therapeutic Nursing Interventions

- Monitor for signs of liver toxicity: jaundice, dark urine, abdominal pain, and abnormal liver enzymes.

Client Education

General information related to anti-androgenic drugs:

- It is vital that you keep follow-up appointments for liver function tests.
- This drug may cause you to experience loss of libido and erectile dysfunction.

Flutamide

- This drug must be taken with leuprolide.
- If you miss a dose, do not double up.

Bicalutamide

- Notify the primary care provider if you have severe or persistent diarrhea.

Nilutamide

- If you miss a dose, do not double the next dose.
- Be aware that it will take longer for your eyes to adapt to changes in lighting.
- This drug can be taken with or without food.

Hyperglycemic Hormones

Overview

Hyperglycemic hormones are produced in the alpha cells of the pancreas. Serum blood glucose level is raised by breaking down stored glycogen in the liver and muscles and synthesis of glucose. The hormones are secreted normally in response to hypoglycemia, the concurrent release of insulin, and catecholamines.

Uses

The emergency treatment of severe hypoglycemia when:

- The client is unconscious or uncooperative
- It is not possible for emergency personnel to treat hypoglycemia with 50% dextrose
- IV access is not available and a client is unconscious

Adverse Effects

- Nausea and vomiting
- Generalized allergic reaction manifested as urticaria, respiratory distress, and hypotension

Precautions

- Safety during pregnancy and lactation undetermined

- May interact with oral anticoagulants and thus increase risk of bleeding
- Generally contraindicated in clients with pheochromocytoma
- Protect the airway of the unconscious client
- Dosage is dependent on age and clinical condition

Important Drugs

Glucagon

Therapeutic Nursing Interventions

- May be given subcutaneously or intramuscularly.
- Monitor blood glucose for response, generally in 5-20 minutes, additional dose may be given as needed.
- When the client is conscious, provide oral glucose to restore liver glycogen stores.
- Provide education to the diabetic client and family on how to avoid hypoglycemia.

Client Education

- Report repeated episodes of hypoglycemia to primary care provider and work with diabetes education team to adjust medication or other regimen activities to prevent hypoglycemia.
- Carry emergency identification that identifies you as a diabetic.
- Perform blood glucose testing on a regular basis.

Sulfonylureas

Overview

Classified as first or second generation, sulfonylureas act to increase insulin secretion from the pancreas. They enhance performance and the number of insulin receptors on muscle and fat cells. Sulfonylureas facilitate glucose transport into cells and decrease hepatic glucose production.

Uses

- Monotherapy or combination therapy in the treatment of Type 2 diabetes
- Treatment of secondary diabetes if there is a potential for insulin secretion

Adverse Effects

- Hypoglycemia
- Skin rash
- Weight gain
- Gastrointestinal disturbances
- Photosensitivity
- Agranulocytosis

Precautions

- Not intended for use during pregnancy, lactation, or by children

- Not recommended in the treatment of diabetic ketoacidosis (DKA), or postsurgical glycemic management
- First-generation agents are not recommended in the elderly or those with hepatic and renal dysfunction.

Important Drugs

First-generation agents (rarely used)

Tolbutamide (Orinase)

Acetohexamide (Dymelor)

Tolazamide (Tolinase)

Chlorpropamide (Diabinese)

Second-generation agents

Glipizide (Glucotrol, Glucotrol XL)

Glyburide (DiaBeta, Glynase PresTab, Micronase)

Glimepiride (Amaryl)

Therapeutic Nursing Interventions

- Monitor for drug's therapeutic and adverse side effects.
- Teach clients and family the symptoms, prevention, and treatment of hypoglycemia.

Client Education

- Perform self blood glucose testing to monitor therapeutic benefit.
- Adhere to other regimens prescribed to control client's diabetes, such as nutrition and exercise plan.
- Carry emergency identification that identifies self as diabetic.
- Do not ingest alcohol when taking this medication.
- Wear long sleeves and hats to avoid photosensitivity side effect.

Meglitinides

Overview

A nonsulfonylurea, which facilitates the pancreas to produce more insulin right after a meal.

Uses

- Monotherapy in treatment of type 2 diabetes mellitus or secondary diabetes when the pancreas is capable of insulin production
- Combination therapy in the treatment of type 2 diabetes mellitus

Adverse Effects

- Hypoglycemia
- Weight gain
- Gastrointestinal disturbances
- Headache

- URI (upper respiratory infection) or symptoms
- Arthralgia or back pain

Precautions

- Not intended for use during pregnancy, lactation, or by children
- Not recommended in the treatment of diabetic ketoacidosis, or post-surgical glycemic management
- Elderly, debilitated, or malnourished clients are more susceptible to hypoglycemic effects.
- Use with caution in clients with hepatic dysfunction.

Important Drugs

Repaglinide (Prandin)

Therapeutic Nursing Interventions

- Monitor for drug's therapeutic and adverse side effects.
- Teach clients and families the symptoms, prevention, and treatment of hypoglycemia.
- Dosing is "meal-based," with maximum dose not to exceed 16 mg daily.

Client Education

- Perform self blood-glucose testing to monitor therapeutic benefit.
- Adhere to other regimens prescribed to control your diabetes, such as nutrition and exercise plan.
- Carry emergency identification that identifies you as a diabetic.
- Take 15 minutes before each meal with maximum dose to not exceed 16 mg daily.
- Do not take if you skip a meal.

D-phenylalanine Derivatives

Overview

A nonsulfonylurea, which facilitates the pancreas to produce more insulin right after a meal.

Uses

- Monotherapy in the treatment of type 2 diabetes mellitusand secondary diabetes when the pancreas has the capacity to produce and secrete insulin
- Combination therapy in the treatment of type 2 diabetes mellitus

Important Drugs

Nateglinide (Starlix)

Adverse Effects

- Hypoglycemia

Precautions

- Not intended for use during pregnancy or lactation

- Not intended for the treatment of diabetic ketoacidosis (DKA)

Therapeutic Nursing Interventions

- Monitor for drug's therapeutic and adverse side effects.
- Teach clients and families the symptoms, prevention, and treatment of hypoglycemia.

Client Education

- Perform self blood-glucose testing to monitor therapeutic benefit.
- Adhere to other regimens prescribed to control your diabetes, such as nutrition and exercise plan.
- Carry emergency identification that identifies you as a diabetic.
- Take 30 minutes before each meal.
- Do not take if you skip a meal.

Combination Oral Medicines

Overview

Two medicines are combined to provide enhanced therapeutic benefit. They stimulate the pancreas to make more insulin and decrease production of glucose

Uses

- Monotherapy in the treatment of type 2 diabetes

Adverse Effects

- Hypoglycemia
- Gastrointestinal disturbances including diarrhea, nausea and upset stomach
- Photosensitivity
- Skin reaction and dark-colored urine

Precautions

- Not recommended in clients with chronic kidney or liver problems
- Not intended for use during pregnancy
- Should not be taken by clients who drink alcohol excessively

Important Drugs

Glyburide/metformin (Glucovance)

Therapeutic Nursing Interventions

- Monitor for therapeutic and adverse side effects.
- Teach clients and families the symptoms, prevention, and treatment of hypoglycemia.

Client Education

- Notify your primary care provider you are taking Glucovance and are scheduled for surgery or a diagnostic procedure using a contrast dye.
- Take with meals.
- Perform self blood-glucose testing to monitor therapeutic benefit.

- Adhere to other regimens prescribed to control your diabetes, such as nutrition and exercise plan.
- Carry emergency identification that identifies you as a diabetic.

Hypoglycemics

Overview

Hypoglycemics are naturally occurring hormones, such as insulin or oral medications, aimed at lowering blood glucose levels. Insulin is produced and secreted from the beta cells in the Islets of Langerhans in the pancreas. Elevated blood glucose levels stimulate the secretion of insulin.

Insulin

Overview

Insulin facilitates the passage of glucose into cells for energy. It suppresses excess production of sugar in the liver and muscles, as well as the breakdown of fat for energy.

Uses

- All individuals with type 1 diabetes mellitus
- Some individuals with type 2 diabetes mellitus
- Women with gestational diabetes if dietary therapy is not effective
- Some clients receiving parenteral nutrition therapy
- Treatment of:
    - Diabetic ketoacidosis (DKA)
    - Hyperosmolar hyperglycemic nonketotic syndrome (on occasion)
- Clients with diminished functioning of the pancreas secondary to other diseases, such as pancreatitis

Adverse Effects

- Hypoglycemia
- Weight gain

Precautions

- Insulins vary by species and sources and thus, may have antigenic properties.
- Only regular insulin may be given intravenously.
- Some clients may develop urticaria at the injection site.

Important Drugs

Insulins are classified by their effect and duration.

Rapid-acting

- Insulin lispro (Humalog)
- Insulin aspart (NovoLog)
    - Starts working in 10-20 minutes
    - Peaks in 30 minutes to 3 hours
    - Therapeutic duration of 3-5 hours

Short-acting

- Regular (R)
    - Starts working in 30-60 minutes
    - Peaks in 1-5 hours
    - Therapeutic duration of 6-10 hours

Intermediate-acting

- NPH (N)
- Lente (L)
    - Starts working 1-3 hours
    - Peaks in 6-10 hours
    - Therapeutic duration up to 24 hours

Long-acting

- Ultralente (U)
    - Starts working in 4-6 hours
    - Peaks in 18-20 hours
    - Therapeutic duration of 24-28 hours

Premixed

- NPH and Regular insulin mixed together in one bottle (70/30 & 50/50)
    - Starts working in 30 minutes
    - Peaks in 8-12 hours
    - Therapeutic duration of 14-18 hours

Therapeutic Nursing Interventions

- Teach clients using insulin the symptoms, prevention, and treatment of hypoglycemia.
- Teach clients to routinely carry a source of carbohydrate.
- Teach the proper method for storing, preparing, and injecting insulin.
- Monitor for drug's therapeutic and adverse side effects.
- When administering insulin intravenously, monitor blood glucose levels at least every hour.
- Teach client principles of sick-day management.

Client Education

- Perform self blood-glucose testing to monitor therapeutic benefit.
- Adhere to other regimens prescribed to control your diabetes, such as nutrition and exercise plan.
- Carry an emergency source of carbohydrate to treat hypoglycemia.
- Carry emergency identification that identifies you as a diabetic.
- To reduce local irritation, never inject cold insulin.
- Carry insulin and supplies when traveling and do not check with baggage.
- Inject insulin SC and rotate injection sites.
- Do not massage injection sites.
- If mixing insulins, draw up regular (R) insulin first.

Immunosuppressants

Overview

The role of the immune system is to protect the body against internal and external threats. Autoimmune disorders occur when the immune system reacts to normal body tissue as if it were foreign. These inappropriate immune responses can have devastating effects on affected tissues. Examples of autoimmune disorders include rheumatoid arthritis, systemic lupus erythematosus, and inflammatory bowel disease. It is necessary to suppress the immune system when clients receive transplanted organs; without immune suppressants, they will probably reject the organ. Immunosuppressants include corticosteroids, cytotoxic antineoplastic drugs, antirejection drugs, antibody preparations, and others. Corticosteroids are discussed earlier in this chapter. The prototypes are the cytotoxic antineoplastic agents methotrexate and azathioprine.

Uses

- Treatment of autoimmune disorders
- Prevention of transplant rejection reactions

Adverse Effects

All immunosuppressants place the client at risk for

- Infection
- Malignancy, most often lymphoma with long-term therapy

Adverse effects of methotrexate include:

- Bone marrow suppression
- Oral and gastrointestinal ulcers
- Pulmonary infiltrates and fibrosis
- Nausea and vomiting
- Nephrotoxicity with high dosage
- Fetal malformation

Adverse effects of azathioprine include:

- Gastrointestinal distress
- Hepatotoxicity
- Bone marrow suppression
- Serum sickness
- Fever
- Chills

Precautions

- These drugs are contraindicated during pregnancy and lactation.
- Clients should not receive live virus vaccinations because of the risk of contracting the disease.

Important Drugs

Cytotoxic agents

Azathioprine (Rheumatrex, Trexall) is used primarily to prevent rejection reactions. It may also be used for rheumatoid arthritis.

Methotrexate (Imuran) is used to treat some autoimmune disorders, such as rheumatoid arthritis and psoriasis, as well as some types of cancer.

Conventional antirejection agents

Cyclosporine (Sandimmune) is used to treat rejection reactions.

Mycophenolate (CellCept) is used to prevent rejection of cardiac and renal transplants.

Tacrolimus (Prograf) is used to prevent rejection reactions.

Antibody preparations

Polyclonal antibody

Monoclonal antibodies

Other

Etanercept (Enbrel)

Leflunomide (Arava)

Therapeutic Nursing Interventions

- Monitor for any sign of infection. They may be subtle due to the effects of immunosuppressants.
- Be alert for allergy and anaphylaxis.
- Carefully follow directions for reconstitution of IV preparations.
- Azathioprine: Monitor renal, hepatic, and hematologic function.
- Methotrexate: Monitor respiratory, hepatic, and hematologic function.

Client Education

- Avoid contact with people who have active infections.
- Do not take over-the-counter drugs unless approved by primary care provider.
- Avoid pregnancy during therapy and for a prescribed time thereafter.
- Protect your skin from excessive sun exposure.
- Notify the primary care provider of:
    - Any signs of infection (e.g., fever, cough, sore throat)
    - Unusual bleeding or bruising
- **Drugs**
    - Methotrexate (Rheumatrex, Trexall)
        - Do not double up if you miss a dose.
        - Do not drink alcohol or take NSAIDs while on this drug.
        - You may have hair loss while taking this drug.
    - Azathioprine (Imuran)
        - If you take the drug only once a day and miss a dose, do not double up.

- If you take this drug several times a day, you can take the missed dose with the next dose.
- Take oral drug with or after meals to reduce gastrointestinal symptoms.
- Lifelong therapy will be needed to prevent rejection.
- After kidney transplant: Immediately report fever or chills, back or side pain, urinary symptoms, severe diarrhea, black stools, and bloody urine to primary care provider.

Immunizations

Overview

The immune system responds to some infectious organisms by developing antibodies that protect the client from being infected again by that organism. The person who has protective antibodies against a particular infection is said to be immune to that infection. Immunizations protect people from infection by:

- Providing antibodies from immune people or animals (passive immunity)
- Administering antigens that stimulate the immune system to develop antibodies against that antigen (active immunity)

Whereas immunizations carry some risk, the benefits far outweigh those risks in the population as a whole. Vaccines are the preparations used to administer whole or fractional microorganisms. Killed vaccines are made of whole, killed organisms or isolated components. Live (attenuated) vaccines are made of live organisms that have been weakened so they cannot cause disease, but can still evoke antibody production.

Toxoids are nontoxic preparations made from bacterial toxins. When administered, they evoke the production of antitoxins, which protect against the bacterial toxins. They do not kill the bacteria. The discussion in this section will be confined to the measles, mumps, rubella (MMR), diphtheria, tetanus, pertussis (DTP), and hepatitis B virus (HBV) immunizations.

Uses

Prevention of:

- Diphtheria
- Tetanus
- Pertussis
- Measles
- Mumps
- Rubella
- Invasive *Haemophilus Influenzae* type B (Hib)
- Hepatitis B
- Polio
- Varicella
- Invasive pneumococcal disease

Adverse Effects

Common mild reactions include:

- Swelling, redness, and warmth at the injection site
- Fever

Serious reactions are rare, but can include:

- Anaphylaxis with MMR
- Acute encephalopathy with DPT

Precautions

Contraindications:

- A vaccine should not be given to a person who has had a previous anaphylactic reaction to that vaccine or any others containing that immunizing agent.
- A vaccine should not be given to a person who has an allergy to eggs.
- Vaccines should not be given to a person who has a moderate or severe illness with or without a fever.
- Live virus vaccines should not be given to an immunosuppressed person.

Important Drugs

MMR (measles, mumps, and rubella) vaccine

DTP (diphtheria, tetanus, and pertussis)

DTaP (diphtheria, tetanus, acellular pertussis)

HBV (hepatitis B virus) vaccine

Therapeutic Nursing Interventions

- Check expiration dates on all vaccines.
- Always aspirate before giving a parenteral vaccine to prevent accidental intravenous injection.
- Be sure epinephrine 1:1000 is available for immediate treatment of allergic reactions.
- Have the client remain in the office/clinic for 30 minutes after receiving a vaccine.
  - If an allergic reaction occurs, it is usually within 30 minutes.
  - Signs and symptoms include difficulty breathing, collapse, shock, and urticaria.
  - Treatment: subcutaneous epinephrine 1:1000 0.5 mL for adults, 0.01 mL/kg for children.
- MMR
  - Reconstitute exactly as directed by manufacturer.
  - Use within 8 hours of reconstitution.
  - Give subcutaneously.
- Give infant DTP vaccine in lateral thigh muscle.
- Administer HBV intramuscularly.
  - Infants and young children: anterolateral thigh
  - Adults and older children: deltoid
- Maintain accurate records.

Client Education

- A mild local reaction and low fever is common.
- If you have more serious symptoms, notify your primary care provider.
- Keep your vaccination record, as you may have to present it to your school or employer.

Thyroid Agents

Overview

Thyroid hormones stimulate metabolism and cardiac function, and are essential for normal growth and development of the nervous and musculoskeletal systems. Hypothyroidism is the abnormally decreased secretion of thyroid hormone. In adults, it is caused by:

- Chronic autoimmune thyroiditis
- Insufficient dietary iodine
- Thyroidectomy
- TSH (thyroid stimulating hormone) deficiency
- TRH (thyroid releasing hormone) deficiency. A hormone secreted by the hypothalamus, stimulates the pituitary gland to secrete TSH.

Cretinism is hypothyroidism in infants. Unless treated early, the infant will be short in stature and delayed in mental and physical development. Infants of untreated hypothyroid women also demonstrate some effects of hypothyroidism. Manifestations of hypothyroidism in adults include bradycardia, cold dry skin, brittle hair, low body temperature, fatigue, cold intolerance, flat affect, slowed cognition, and weight gain. Extremely low serum levels of thyroid hormone can cause myxedema coma. Myxedema coma is life-threatening, as it can lead to severe fluid and electrolyte imbalances, acidosis, hypoglycemia, water intoxication, adrenal insufficiency, and severe hypothermia.

Uses

- Thyroid hormone replacements are used to treat hypothyroidism.
- Hypothyroidism is a chronic condition requiring lifelong replacement therapy.
- Thyroid hormones are usually given orally: however, an intravenous levothyroxine is available to treat myxedema coma or for clients who cannot take PO medications.

Adverse Effects

- In appropriate doses, thyroid hormones are unlikely to have adverse effects.
- If the dosage is too high, the client will develop signs and symptoms of hyperthyroidism:
    - Tachycardia and angina
    - Heat intolerance, increased body temperature, perspiration
    - Nervousness, insomnia, tremor
- Extremely high doses can cause thyroiditis crisis.

Precautions

- Older adults must be started on low doses of thyroid hormones to prevent excessive cardiac stimulation; dosage is gradually adjusted until blood studies are normal.
- Important drug-drug interactions include:
  - Calcium, aluminum-based antacids, iron, and cholestyramine impair absorption of thyroid hormones. Give these drugs several hours apart.
  - Thyroid hormones enhance the anticoagulant effects of warfarin.
  - Thyroid hormones given with catecholamines can cause excess cardiac stimulation.
  - Thyroid hormone therapy may require increased dosages of insulin and digoxin.

Important Drugs

Levothyroxine (Synthroid, Levoxyl, Levothroid), the most commonly used replacement, is a synthetic agent that is identical to the natural thyroid hormone.

Liothyronine (Cytomel), a synthetic triiodothyronine (T3) is useful in treating myxedema coma because it has a rapid onset of action.

- Liothyronine is more expensive and has a shorter duration of action than levothyroxine.
- Effects are monitored by measuring T3 and thyroid stimulating hormone (TSH) in serum.

Therapeutic Nursing Interventions

- Monitor pulse and blood pressure, mental status, activity tolerance, tolerance of heat and cold, and weight.
- If heart rate is greater than 100 bpm, withhold, and notify primary care provider.

Client Education

- Take your thyroid hormone every morning before breakfast.
- Do not take this medication with calcium or iron supplements.
- Count your heart rate each day; notify your primary care provider if it is more than 100 bpm (instruct in counting pulse).
- Notify your primary care provider if you have palpitations, chest pain, diarrhea, or excessive nervousness.
- Keep follow-up appointments to evaluate drug effects; dosage adjustments are sometimes needed.
- Do not stop taking your hormone unless instructed by the primary care provider; most people require lifelong replacement therapy.

Critical Thinking Exercise: Drugs Affecting the Endocrine System

Note: *It is recommended that the following exercises be reviewed with a partner or in a small group to achieve maximum student interaction and to enhance critical thinking skills.*

Situation: : S.L. is an 80-year-old woman with a history of hypertension and adult onset diabetes mellitus. She has just moved to the area and has come for an initial visit. S.L. has had hypertension for 20 years and diabetes for 10 years. Until eight months ago, the diabetes was treated with diet and an oral hypoglycemic agent. However, she began to lose weight, her thirst and urine output increased, and her blood sugar increased substantially, despite increasing doses of the hypoglycemic agent. She was then started on subcutaneous insulin injections. S.L. monitors her blood glucose at home twice a day. Five years ago, she had a left radical mastectomy performed for breast cancer and now has bone metastatis. S.L.'s current medications are:

- Enalapril (Vasotec) 5 mg bid
- Hydrochlorothiazide and triamterene (Dyazide) 50 mg qd in a.m.
- Tamoxifen 20 mg bid
- NPH insulin 20 IU before breakfast, 5 units before supper
- Humalog Insulin 5 IU before breakfast, 2 units before supper
- Oxycodone (OxyContin) 10 mg q 12 hrs

1. Hydrochlorothiazide (HCTZ) is one of the drugs ordered for S.L.'s hypertension. Given she has diabetes, what teaching should be done for this client?

2. If S.L. takes her NPH insulin at 7 a.m., during what time period should the drug peak?

3. S.L. is complaining about severe hot flashes. She has a bottle of unused estrogen in her medicine cabinet, and she says she is going to start taking it. How would you respond?

4. S.L.'s family knows to be alert to a possible hypoglycemic reaction around supper time related to her NPH insulin, but they are uncertain if they should anticipate a similar reaction to the Humalog insulin. What is the nurse's best response?

Discussion questions:

5. Discuss the role of the estrogen in the body.

6. What kind of symptoms would the nurse expect to see in a client with hypothyroidism?

7. Discuss client teaching considerations the nurse should address with the client who has type 2 diabetes mellitus.

CHAPTER 12

Drugs Affecting Reproduction

Key Points

- Drugs that affect the female and male reproductive systems include synthetic and natural substances.
- Synthetic hormones provide the same action in the body as the natural substances made by the body.
- Females produce gonadotropin-releasing hormone (GRH), female sex hormones, (estrogen and progestin), and use synthetic agents such as oral contraceptives and ovulatory stimulants.
- Drugs that affect female reproductive systems are divided into two categories: ovulation suppressants and ovulation stimulants.
- Oral contraceptives provide a high degree of protection against pregnancy if taken on a regular basis.
- Oral contraceptives are less effective in women who smoke and are over 35.
- Ovulation stimulants such as Clomid require a strict compliance to be effective.
    - These also have many side effects that must be monitored closely in follow-up visits.
- Estrogen is used to help maintain bone mass in postmenopausal clients.
    - If a client on estrogen therapy develops DVT (deep vein thrombosis) or cardiac complications, the estrogen therapy must be discontinued.
- Women who require androgen therapy must use a non-hormonal form of birth control.
- Oxytocin (Pitocin) should not be used to induce labor if less than 37 weeks gestation, if multiple birth is suspected, or if cephalocaudal disproportion is present.
- Lactation inhibitors are rarely used now with the increased risk of serious adverse effects.
- Normal male development and maintenance of sex characteristics depends on androgens, primarily testosterone.
    - Testosterone and its derivatives, plus synthetic agents, are commonly used when the normal processes are hindered.
- Male clients using estrogen therapy must be informed that side effects will go away when the therapy is stopped.
- Endometriosis is an important cause of infertility and is sometimes treated using bromocriptine (Parlodel), danazol (Danocrine), and leuprolide acetate (Lupron).

Ovulation Suppressants

Overview

Oral contraceptives are the most common drugs used to inhibit reproduction. Oral contraceptives consist of a synthetic estrogen and/or progestin. These prevent ovulation by blocking follicle-stimulating hormone (FSH) and luteinizing hormone (LH). They also increase uterine mucous viscosity. This results in decreased sperm movement and fertilization of the ovum and possible inhibition of implantation of a fertilized egg.

Uses

- Inhibit reproduction (prevent pregnancy)
- Treat endometriosis and excessive bleeding during menstruation
- Migraine headaches (hormone regulation)

Important Drugs

Loestrin
Lo-Ovral
Nordette
Ovral
Ortho-Novum
Micronor and many others

Precautions

- Oral contraceptives are safest when used by women under 35 who don't smoke.
- CNS effects
  - Dizziness
  - Headache
  - Migraines
  - Depression
  - Stroke
- Cardiovascular effects
  - Hypotension
  - Thrombophlebitis
  - Edema
  - Pulmonary embolism
  - Myocardial infarction
- Gastrointestinal effects
  - Nausea
  - Vomiting
  - Diarrhea
  - Anorexia
  - Cramps
  - Increased appetite

    - Weight gain
- Genitourinary effects
    - Amenorrhea
    - Cervical erosion
    - Breakthrough bleeding
    - Breast changes

Therapeutic Nursing Interventions

- Interactions with these drugs are numerous.
- Further instruction is needed when taking antibiotics, anticonvulsants, anticoagulants, antihypertensive agents, caffeine, corticosteroids, and analgesics.

Client Education

- Teach the client how to take the medication.
- Missing a dose may result in pregnancy.
- Encourage monthly breast self-exams.
- Monitor monthly cycle to notice any abnormalities.
- Instruct the client to use alternate forms of birth control in addition to the oral ovulation suppressant during an antibiotic course.
- Emphasize the importance of avoiding smoking because of the increased risk of heart attack and blood clots.
- Teach the signs and symptoms of blood clots and inform the client about the need to report the any leg or calf pain immediately.
- Teach the client to report abnormal bleeding or excessively heavy menstrual flow.
- If pregnancy is suspected, the client must stop taking the medication immediately.
- Educate the client about the need to report weight gain of more than 10 lbs (4.5 kg).

Ovulation Stimulants

Overview

Ovulation stimulants are the most common drugs used to enhance/enable reproduction. A variety of drug therapies are used to treat infertility because there are many causes. Ovulation stimulants are used when the ovaries are normal, but the process that stimulates ovulation is absent or altered. These drugs stimulate the growth and maturation of ova and increase the release of gonadotropins (luteinizing hormone, and follicle-stimulating hormone). The effects of ovulation stimulants are the same as the effects of natural hormones. By manipulating these drugs in various ways, they can be made to mimic the natural effects of these hormones. They may also stimulate spermatogenesis (sperm production) in men.

Uses

- Treat female infertility
- Treat various menstrual abnormalities in women and hormonal abnormalities in men

Important Drugs

Clomiphene citrate (Clomid) is used to treat female infertility.

Bromocriptine mesylate (Parlodel) is used to treat various menstrual abnormalities in women and hormonal abnormalities in men.

Leuprolide (Lupron) and menotropins treat female infertility, as well as various menstrual abnormalities in women and hormonal abnormalities in men.

Precautions

CNS effects

- Dizziness
- Headache
- Flushing
- Depression
- Restlessness
- Anxiety
- Fatigue

Cardiovascular effects

- Tachycardia
- Phlebitis
- Deep vein thrombosis
- Hypovolemia

Gastrointestinal effects

- Nausea
- Bloating
- Constipation
- Abdominal pain
- Anorexia

Other effects

- Urticaria
- Ovarian hyperstimulation
- Multiple pregnancies
- Blurred vision
- Breast pain

Nursing Interventions

- Monitor compliance carefully, follow-up visits are necessary.

- Contraindicated in women with history of breast cancer, thromboembolic disorders, malignancies of the reproductive tract, or abnormal vaginal bleeding.
- Use with caution during pregnancy and lactation or in clients with a history of hypertension, asthma, diabetes, congestive heart failure (CHF), or depression.
- Gather baseline blood pressure, weight, blood glucose levels, liver function tests, and urinary output.
- Assess for signs of ovarian hyperstimulation syndrome, which can occur in as many as 20% of women treated with menotropins.
- Report severe pelvic pressure, marked weight gain or ascites, and dyspnea immediately.

Client Education

- Report any symptoms or unusual findings, such as weight gain of more than 5 lbs/week, abdominal pain, vaginal bleeding, or shortness of breath.
- Report any abdominal or side pain, which may indicate an ectopic pregnancy.
- Maintain routine and regular pap smears and breast self-exams.
- May use precautions against phlebitis, such as support hose and regular walks.
- Discuss the possibility of multifetal pregnancy.

Estrogen, Progestins, and Androgens

Overview

Other drugs used to enhance reproduction are the synthetic female and male sex hormones. Estrogen, progestins and androgens are used frequently. The gonads and adrenal cortices of both men and women produce these. When they are given from exogenous sources such as drugs for therapeutic purposes, their effects are the same as naturally-occurring ones. These are synthesized from cholesterol and have the basic structure of a steroid. They are sometimes referred to as steroid hormones.

Estrogen

Overview

Estrogen binds with estrogen receptors and stimulates the synthesis of deoxyribonucleic acid (DNA) and ribonucleic acid (RNA) and proteins. Estrogen is necessary for female reproductive organs, maintenance of the menstrual cycle, growth of the ducts and nipples of the mammary glands and support of secondary sex characteristics, such as soft skin and female voice.

Uses

Estrogens are used in the treatment or prevention of an assortment of disorders, including:

- Menopause
- Osteoporosis
- Menstrual disturbances
- Acne in females
- Lactation suppression

- Oral contraceptives
- Prostate cancer treatment in men

Important Drugs

Steroidal

Conjugated estrogens (Premarin)
Estradiol (Estrace)
Estropipate (Ogen)

Nonsteroidal

Chlorotrianisene (TACE)
Diethylstilbestrol (DES)

Precautions

- Side effects increase in women over age 35 and in persons who smoke.
- Use of estrogen may be contraindicated if taking antihyperglycemic and anticoagulant drugs.
- CNS effects
    - Headache
- Cardiovascular effects
    - Thromboembolic events
    - Hypertensions
    - Hyperlipidemia
- Gastrointestinal effects
    - Nausea
    - Vomiting
    - Loss of appetite
- Endocrine effects
    - Breast tenderness
    - Fluid retention
    - Hyperglycemia
    - Female characteristics for men

Therapeutic Nursing Interventions

- Monitor blood pressure on a monthly basis.
- Estrogens may alter lab results.
- Monitor for calf/leg pain.
- Monitor weight gain and edema.
- Emphasize compliance.
- Estrogen products are not for use during lactation.
- Administer at the same time every day.
- Give oral form with food or milk if nausea occurs.
- Vaginal applications are best given before sleep for best absorption.
- Transdermal application is best using alternating sites.

Client Education

- Inform male clients receiving estrogen therapy that the female characteristics usually disappear when therapy is stopped.
- Instruct on proper use of the form prescribed: oral, intravaginal, transdermal (sites must be rotated weekly).
- Have yearly pap smears and cholesterol screening.
- Perform monthly self-breast exams.
- Use precautions against phlebitis: support hose and regular walks.
- Emphasize the importance of avoiding smoking because of the increased risk of heart attack and blood clots.
- Teach the signs and symptoms of blood clots and inform the client about the need to report the findings immediately.
- For vaginal application of estrogen product, instruct the woman to remain recumbent for at least 30 minutes and not to use tampons.
- Teach the client to report abnormal bleeding or excessively heavy menstrual flow.
- If pregnancy is suspected, the client must stop taking the medication immediately.

Progestins

Overview

When exogenous progestins are given, physiologic production and the release of progestins is reduced. These progestins in the blood stream signal the pituitary gland to inhibit gonadotropin. They are also known to decrease endometrial tissue proliferation.

Uses

- Prepare the uterus and maintain the pregnancy.
- Develop the mammary gland duct during pregnancy.
- Reduce spontaneous contractions. It is also used in the treatment of functional uterine bleeding caused by a hormonal imbalance, fibroids, or uterine cancer.
- Use in oral contraceptives

Important Drugs

Medroxyprogesterone injections (Provera, Depo-Provera)

Progesterone intrauterine (Progestasert)

Megestrol acetate (Megace)

Levonorgestrel implants (Norplant)

Precautions

- Contraindicated in clients with epilepsy, migraine headaches, cardiac disorders, and asthma.
- CNS effects
  - Dizziness
  - Headache

    - Decreased libido
    - Depression
- Endocrine effects
    - Increased vaginal bleeding
    - Acne
    - Fluid retention
    - Vaginitis
    - Breast discharge
- Cardiovascular effects
    - Thromboembolic events
- Gastrointestinal effects
    - Nausea
    - Vomiting
    - Weight gain
- Other effects
    - Muscle pain

Therapeutic Nursing Interventions

- Monitor:
    - Homans' sign and calf pain
        - Although caution must be used with dorsiflexion, as this may dislodge a clot. This is an uncommon clinical finding.
    - Blood pressure
    - Weight
    - Fluid retention
- Assess for decreased libido.
- Levonorgestrel implants (Norplant) is a set of silastic capsules that are implanted under of the skin on the inside of the upper arm. The progestin is released at a constant rate for approximately 5 years. At that time, it must be removed and if continued contraception is desired, a new set of capsules is implanted. Fertility will occur shortly after the removal of the progestin.
- Intrauterine progesterone is inserted into the uterus for one year of contraception. This method is designed for use in a woman who has previously delivered, and has no history of pelvic inflammatory disease (PID).
- Medroxyprogesterone IM (Depo-Provera) is given every three months for contraception.

Client Education

- Report breakthrough bleeding, signs of phlebitis, skin outbreaks, and depression.
- Report any indication that conception has occurred.
- Maintain wellness checks (including Pap smears and breast self-exams), regular exercise, and a low-fat diet; avoid smoking.

Androgens

Overview

Androgens, such as testosterone, stimulate the synthesis of ribonucleic acid (RNA). The increased synthesis of protein aids in the formation and maintenance of muscular and skeletal proteins. Synthetic replacement therapy can be given orally, topically, subcutaneous, or intramuscularly.

Uses

- Testosterone is needed for the normal development of male sex organs and structures, secondary sex characteristics (male voice, body structure), and the synthesis of sperm.
- Replacement therapy is used to treat hypogonadism, delayed puberty, impotence, oligospermia, and can also be used to treat women with endometriosis and metastatic breast cancer.

Important Drugs

Fluoxymesterone (Halotestin)

Testosterone (Depo-Testosterone)

Danazol (Danocrine)

Precautions

- Athletes and weight lifters often misuse anabolic steroids (androgens). They should be advised not to use without a primary care provider's direction.
- Endocrine: Females may show signs of masculinization: hirsutism, acne, deepening of the voice, menstrual irregularities, and regression of the breasts.
- CNS effects
  - Increased libido
- Cardiovascular effects
  - May also see fluid retention
  - Potential heart failure
- Other effects
  - Decreased thyroid function, hypercalcemia, and decreased liver function

Therapeutic Nursing Interventions

- Monitor weight gain.
- Emphasize compliance.
- Obtain baseline weight, height, vital signs, and serum electrolyte levels.
- Assess lab results for renal, cardiac, and liver function

Client Education

- Teach female client about potential side effects.
- Recommend use of nonhormonal contraception.
- Encourage positive body image.
- Maintain normal activity levels during therapy.

- Maintain routine wellness care, exercise, and a low-fat diet.
- Complete prescribed therapy.
- Encourage verbalization of feelings and concerns.

Critical Thinking Exercise: Drugs Affecting Reproduction

Note: *It is recommended that the following exercises be reviewed with a partner or in a small group to achieve maximum student interaction and to enhance critical thinking skills.*

Situation: A 19-year-old woman who recently married schedules an appointment for the first time in the women's clinic. She is here for a follow-up visit after her wedding to evaluate how she is doing on her newly prescribed birth control pills. She was prescribed a 6-month supply of Ortho-Novum prior to her wedding date. She is upset and describes the following: The first two months went well. Then, upon realizing she would have her period on her wedding night, she adjusted her dose to prematurely have her period "out of the way" of her wedding night. This was successful, but ever since then, she has had breakthrough bleeding all month long. She has also experienced severe leg cramping, and this last month she has had feelings of anxiety over a "racing heart." She "hates these pills," but doesn't want to get pregnant yet in her marriage. She verbalizes wanting to stop the pill until she and her husband can decide on an alternative form of birth control. You also discover in your history taking that she has just refilled a prescription for her Accutane because, after all this stress, her acne has returned.

1. What do you need to advise the client about her birth control options? What do you do about the Accutane and these birth control options?

2. What are some of the uses for estrogen?

Matching Question:

3. Match each drug listed in the right column to its action listed in the left column.

Table 1

Drug	Therapeutic Action
Depo-Testosterone	Supresses ovulation
Pitocin	Increases protein synthesis
Progesterone	Ovulation stimulant
Nordette	Decreases endometriosis
Estrogen	Induces labor

CHAPTER 13

Drugs Affecting the Integumentary System

Key Points

- If a wound is weepy and wet, it typically requires a drying agent whereas dry, flaky conditions will need a moisturizing agent.
- **Antiseptics** are chemicals applied to living tissue to kill pathogens that may cause illness to the host.
- **Disinfectants** are chemicals used to destroy organisms present on objects.
- Antiseptics and disinfectants are adequate cleansers as skin preparation, but must be washed off thoroughly before a procedure.
- **Bacteriostatic** agents reduce the growth of organisms or prevent replication without killing the entire population.
- **Bactericidal** agents kill bacterial organisms, although not viral, fungal, or spore populations.
- Most soap provides a substance that breaks down particles to be washed away. Soaps are not antibacterial by nature.
- Skin agents should be applied to a cleansed area and often have side effects, including irritation and rash.
- Sunscreens are only effective when allowed to dry before exposure and are reapplied frequently with sustained exposure to sun and water.
- Steroids can mask superinfections when used in conjunction with antibiotic creams or ointments.
- Antiparasitics must be used with caution and with precise instructions for young children and the elderly due to the risk of CNS toxicity.
- Accutane is often used to treat acne in teenagers.
    - This is a very effective drug
    - Screening about sexual activity and birth control is imperative due to the high risk of fetal toxicity and death when becoming pregnant while taking Accutane.
- The first line of treatment for burns is cold water. Next, pharmacologic agents that provide cooling and debridement are used in conjunction with anti-inflammatories and antibiotics.

Overview

Disorders, infections, disruptions or eruptions of the skin are common and numerous. The agents used to treat these can generally be applied directly to the affected skin surface. A general rule in dermatology is that wounds/abrasions that are weeping or wet need agents to help dry them out. A dry, flaking area needs lubrication or emollients.

General Dermatologic Preparations

Overview

Debriding enzymes are used to clean wounds. They denature protein on skin surfaces, reduce surface tension, and may interfere with processes of bacterial cell growth. Compounds such as iodine, alcohol, hexachlorophene, biguanides, oxidizing agents, and surface active agents have been shown effective for wound cleansing or surface skin cleansing in preparation for surgery or procedures.

Antiseptics and Disinfectants

Uses

- Preoperative cleaning of the skin
- Treating minor wounds
- Irrigants
- Cleaning wounds or abrasions
- Cleaning equipment in medical offices, hospitals, and dental offices
- Hexachlorophene (pHisoHex) has bacteriostatic (slows the growth of organisms) properties against staphylococcal organisms.
  - The residue left is not easily removed by soap or detergent products with repeated uses.
- Chlorhexidine (Hibiclens) is effective against a wide spectrum of gram-positive and gram-negative organisms.
- Benzalkonium (Benza) is rapid-acting for a long duration against a wide variety of bacterial, fungal, protozoal, and viral organisms.
  - Has bacteriostatic and bactericidal (kills organisms) properties, depending on the concentration.
- Iodine solutions are also effective against bacteria, fungi, viruses, yeasts, and protozoa.

Important Antiseptics and Disinfectants

- Iodine tincture, Iodine topical
- Betadine solution
- Triclosan (Septi-Soft, Septisol)
- Benzalkonium Chloride (Benza)
- Chlorhexidine Gluconate (Hibiclens, Peridex)
- Hexachlorophene (pHisoHex, Septisol)
- Glutaraldehyde (Cidex)
- Formaldehyde
- Silver nitrate
- Hydrogen peroxide
- Thimerosal (Mersol)

Precautions

Some general rules to follow:

- Iodine solutions stain skin and clothing.
- Avoid occlusive dressings.
- Benzalkonium chloride (Benza) solutions can be used to disinfect skin areas to prep for procedures, but should be thoroughly rinsed from skin before procedure begins.
- Do not use pHisoHex with open wounds or burns, or as routine bathing agent for infants as it is readily absorbed in significant amounts.
- Most of the agents should avoid eye contact.

Therapeutic Nursing Interventions

- Assess for hypersensitivity reactions, including redness, rash, itching, drying, excoriation, and local swelling. Report skin findings and document in the medical record.
- For preoperative use of betadine solution, avoid pooling beneath the client because of skin irritation or more severe skin reactions.
- Betadine solution should be used with extreme caution in preterm infants. Topical application can be absorbed systemically. Betadine solution can cause skin irritation or even burn injury in low birthweight infants.
- Replace hard-to-read or stained labels to ensure proper identification of the solution.
- Do not keep these solutions at the bedside of any client with confusion, delirium, or alteration in sensorium because the solution may be mistaken for water or another beverage.
- Benzalkonium chloride (Benza) is incompatible with iodine, nitrate, peroxide, oxide, and aluminum solutions. It is ineffective in the presence of soap.
- Chlorhexidine (Hibiclens) should not be used near the eyes or ears.
- Formaldehyde and glutaraldehyde (Cidex) are for use on inanimate objects only.
- PHisoHex has been shown to have systemic absorption and should be used cautiously in children, elderly, and persons with burn injury.
- Thimerosal (Mersol) may cause hypersensitivity reaction.
  - Allow skin to dry thoroughly following application before the dressing is adhered to the skin.
- Silver nitrate was commonly used in newborn eyes shortly after birth to prevent ophthalmic infections.
  - Causes chemical conjunctivitis and is rarely used today.
- Silver-containing products (Silvadene) are effective for the treatment of burns.

Client Education

- Provide client education regarding use, dose, application, length of treatment and potential side effects of agent for home use.
- Iodine solutions and silver-containing products often stain skin and clothing.
- Avoid contact with eyes and mucous membranes.

- Allow hydrogen peroxide to bubble; this is an expected reaction.
- Benzalkonium chloride (Benza) should not be stored on cotton balls or gauze pads because antiseptic properties will be reduced. It is not to be used with an occlusive dressing. It is inactivated by soap; therefore, thorough washing before application of Benza is necessary.

Soaps and Cleansers

Overview

Ordinary soaps are potassium or sodium salts of fatty acids. These help dissolve fats and in turn remove foreign particles from the skin. The pH of bar soaps varies. Cleansers can be soap-free or have a modified pH.

Uses

- Ordinary soaps dissolve fats and remove foreign particles from the skin.
- Cleansers can be soap-free.

Important Soaps/Cleansers

- Neutrogena, Zest, Dove, Cold Cream, Lanolin, Caress, Ivory, pHisoderm, Aveeno, Nivea

Precautions

- These do not have antibacterial action. Persons with sensitive skin can have reactions, including increased drying, rash, and irritation.

Therapeutic Nursing Interventions

- Obtain a skin history for any past reactions to cleansing agent(s); document the description of the lesion, location, distribution, and timing related to the offending agent.

Client Education

- Rinse the skin thoroughly after use of soaps/cleansers to avoid skin irritation.
- Avoid contact with eyes and mucous membranes.
- Soaps containing perfumes and dyes can be irritating to the skin. Non-perfumed, hypo- allergenic soaps and cleansers are preferred for sensitive skin.
- Lotions and emollients after skin cleansing may be useful to prevent drying.
- Avoid use of irritating agents and those causing skin reactions.

Emollients and Protectants (Excluding Sunscreen)

Overview

These agents provide comfort either by their anti-inflammatory capabilities or by their lubricating properties. These are considered over-the-counter (OTC) drugs.

Uses

- Provide lubrication and/or protection to the skin surface to prevent irritation or rash.
- Treat diaper rash, dry or chafed skin, abrasions, minor burns, hemorrhoids or acne.

- Emollients aid with the insertion of catheters or tubes.
- Most emollients contain oil, waxes, fats, or urea to enhance the skin's ability to retain moisture.
  - Active ingredients often include mineral oil, aloe, glycerin, petrolatum, lanolin, and vitamins A, D, and E.

Important Emollients and Protectants

Aluminum Sulfate (Domeboro)

Tucks

Aquaphor

Eucerin Cream

Lubriderm

A&D Ointment

Lanolin

Petroleum Jelly

Benzoin

Desitin

KY products

Precautions

- Discontinue use if skin irritation occurs.
- Adverse reactions are rare.

Therapeutic Nursing Intervention

- Cleanse skin thoroughly before application of the agent.
- Apply emollients or other skin barriers to dry skin. Barrier creams and other protectants can trap moisture on the surface of the skin and prevent healing.
- Assess skin for signs of adverse reaction or hypersensitivity, such as increased induration of the skin, rash, or excoriation.
- Provide instructions regarding preparation of the site, application method, dosage, timing, and duration of treatment.

Client Education

- Watch for signs of hypersensitivity or adverse reaction, such as redness, itching, swelling, rash, or excoriation.
- Wash hands thoroughly prior to application of the emollient or skin protectant.

Wet Dressings, Soaks, Rubs, and Liniments

Overview

Wet dressings and soaks can contain astringents to treat inflammatory skin conditions such as insect bites, ivy-type rashes, acne, or pustular infections. These soothing preparations can contain an insoluble powder, mild acid, or alkaline base solutions. Rubs and liniments provide pain relief for intact skin that may be irritated from muscle aches, sprains, arthritis, or neuralgias. These products can contain analgesias, anti-inflammatories, local anesthetics, or antiseptics.

Uses

- Provide soothing relief for insect bites, ivy-type rashes, minor burns (rash/prickly heat), acne, and muscle aches from sprains, arthritis, gout, and other neuralgias.

Important Wet Dressings, Soaks, Rubs and Liniments

- Calamine lotion or Calamine with phenol
- Diphenhydramine hydrochloride (Benadryl) lotion and cream
- Aluminum acetate solution (Burow's Solution)
- Aluminum sulfate (Domeboro)
- Vlemasque, Aspercreme, Bengay ointments, and Vicks

Precautions

- Discontinue use if irritation continues or worsens.
- Call primary care provider if continued, appropriate use does not alleviate irritation.
- Adverse reactions are rare.
- Use product only as directed.

Therapeutic Nursing Interventions

- Assess the site for condition of skin, signs of secondary infection, or skin hypersensitivity reaction.
- Discontinue treatment if adverse reaction occurs; document the finding on the medical record.
- Soaks are generally preferred using warm water because of a vasodilatation effect for increased circulation for healing. Warm soaks are more soothing as well.

Client Education

- Avoid repeated or continued exposure to the causative agent.
- Maintain good hygiene of the unaffected skin areas and treat the affected area only as directed.
- Avoid touching affected area with other body parts or clothing.
- Apply prescribed agent to affected area(s) only and continue application as directed even if results are not immediate.
- Include rest periods throughout the day with repeated application of agent if needed for pain relief.

Prophylactic Agents

Overview

These agents can be soothing and cooling and form a protective coating on the skin. To be useful, they must not cause any skin breakdown or drying of the skin. They must also keep out light, air, and dust. The most common skin prophylactic agent is sunscreen.

Uses

- Used to block ultraviolet A (UVA) and ultraviolet B (UVB) sun rays to prevent sunburns that can lead to skin cancers. Also used to treat and coat minor skin irritations and rashes.

Important Protectives and Sunscreens

Benzoin

Kerodex

Hawaiian Tropic

Coppertone

Sundown

Lipkote by Coppertone

PreSun Lip Protector

Precautions

- Sunscreens are only effective if applied generously and allowed time to absorb and dry before exposure to sun and water.
- They must also be re-applied at least every 2-3 hours, especially if sun protection factor (SPF) is less than 10.

Therapeutic Nursing Interventions

- These agents are only effective if used properly.
- Apply skin barriers as directed.
- Assess the client's medication regime to identify any medications that may make the client hypersensitive to sunlight exposure (e.g., tetracyclines, etc.).

Client Education

- Apply agent generously.
- Pick an SPF number according to skin type and length of exposure (if skin burns easily, use an SPF of 15 or greater).
- Allow agent to dry and absorb before exposure.
- Re-apply every two hours throughout exposure.
- Avoid exposure between 10 a.m. and 2 p.m. if hypersensitive to sunlight.
- Agents should not be used on infants less than 6 months old. Infants less than 6 months of age should be kept from direct sunlight exposure.
- Agents available for lips should be used as directed and reapplied frequently.
- Avoid getting agent into eyes. If exposure to eyes, rinse thoroughly with water and contact a primary care provider if irritation and burning persist.

Anti-Infectives

Overview

Topical antibiotics interfere with bacterial growth by interrupting their cell wall function.

Antibiotics

Uses

- Treat acne vulgaris
- Impetigo, cellulitis, folliculitis and carbuncles, other wounds and minor burns caused by or infected with streptococcus or staphylococcus organisms.

Important Drugs

Bacitracin (Baciguent)
Polymyxin (Polysporin)
Chlortetracycline hydrochloride (Aureomycin)
Clindamycin phosphate (Cleocin T)
Erythromycin (Erygel, EryDerm)
Mafenide acetate (Sulfamylon)
Mupirocin (Bactroban)
Neomycin sulfate (Mycifradin Sulfate Topical)
Silver sulfadiazine (Silvadene)

Precautions

- Be sure the antibiotic used is effective against the bacteria pathogen.
- Clients may also become hypersensitive to the antibiotic.
- If used in combination with steroids, certain other infections may be masked.

Therapeutic Nursing Interventions

- Assess the skin for change in condition (improvement or worsening of the infection) and signs of secondary complications (cellulites).
- Document the assessment in the medical record; report pertinent findings to the primary care provider.
- Skin culture or scrapings may be necessary for proper diagnosis.
- If used in combination with topical or systemic steroids, the normal signs of infection may be masked.

Client Education

- Cleanse the site thoroughly prior to application of the anti-infective product.
- Complete the full course of treatment for maximum effectiveness.
- Report signs of worsening site, joint pain, increased swelling, redness, tenderness, itching or pain.

Antivirals

Overview

Interfere with viral growth by inhibiting replication within the cell.

Uses

- Treat herpes simplex and zoster, and varicella viruses.

Important Drugs

Acyclovir (Zovirax)

Docosanol (Abreva)

Penciclovir (Denavir)

Precautions

- Side effects include stinging, itching, and rash.
- Hypersensitivity may also occur.

Therapeutic Nursing Interventions

- Assess for signs and symptoms of healing or a secondary infection.
- Skin scrapings may be needed for proper diagnosis.
- Clean affected area before applying medication.
- Apply with gloves on or with an applicator, such as a swab or tongue blade.

Client Education

- Do not use other OTC creams, lotions, or ointments because they may delay healing and cause spread of cutaneous lesions.
- Do not use in eyes.
- Use condoms during sexual contact while prodromal symptoms or active lesions are present.
- Understand that topical antiviral creams for the treatment of herpes is not curative, nor will it prevent the spread of infection.
  - The virus affects the nerve ganglion and is not cured cutaneously.
- Have a yearly Pap smear and gynecologic examination.
  - A higher risk of cervical cancer exists with genital herpes infection.
- Consult a health care professional if improvement does not occur within 5-7 days of treatment.
- Wear loose, dry clothing to prevent further irritation.

Antifungals

Overview

Interrupts continued growth of fungus after long periods of use.

Uses

- Athletes foot
- Jock itch
- Ringworm
- Yeast
- Candidal dermatitis
- Candidal vaginitis
- Oral candidiasis (thrush)

Important Drugs

Amphotericin B (Fungizone)
Butoconazole (Femstat)
Ciclopirox olamine (Loprox)
Clioquinol (Vioform)
Clotrimazole (Gyne-Lotrimin, Mycelex)
Haloprogin (Halotex)
Miconazole nitrate (Micatin, Monistat Derm)
Nystatin (Nilstat, Mycostatin)
Terbinafine HCL (Lamisil)
Tolnaftate (Tinactin)

Precautions

- Side effects include stinging, itching, and rash. Local irritation, scaling, and blistering may occur.
- Hypersensitivity may also occur.

Therapeutic Nursing Interventions

Oral

- Brush teeth before application of oral suspension.
- Soak partial or full dentures in oral suspension to eliminate the fungal infection.
- Shake oral suspension well prior to use to ensure consistency in dosing.
- Protect the suspension from freezing.
- Lozenges (troches) should not be given to children under 5 years of age.

Client Education

Oral

- Continue taking the prescribed drug for the full course.
- Report to the prescribing practitioner if symptoms persist.
- Treatment is needed for a full 48 hours after improvement of symptoms to prevent relapse.
- Good oral hygiene is important.
- Encourage yearly or biyearly dental exams to maintain optimum dental and periodontal health.
- Swish the solution through the mouth and maintain it for as long as possible before swallowing. Gargling is another good way to ensure contact with buccal membranes in the oropharynx.
- Lozenge forms (troches) should be retained in the mouth for at least 15-20 minutes and should not be chewed.

Topical

- Tight-fitting clothing should be avoided. For infants, diapers should be secured snugly without friction. Plastic diaper covers are not recommended because aeration can facilitate the healing process.

- Cotton socks instead of polyester blends are recommended for persons with fungal lesions on the feet.

Antiparasitics

Overview

Attacks the nerve cells causing seizure, paralysis, and death of the offending parasite.

Uses

- Most commonly used to treat scabies and lice.

Important Drugs

Lindane (Kwell, Scabene, G-Well: in cream, lotion, or shampoo)

Permethrin (Elimite, Nix)

Malathion (Ovide)

Crotamiton (Eurax: lotion and cream)

Pyrethrins (RID)

Precautions

Contraindications:

- Pregnant women or nursing mothers
- Use with caution in infants, small children, and elderly because of CNS toxicity

Side effects:

- Stinging, itching, and rash
- Renal and hepatic failure
- Seizures
- Local irritation
- Hypersensitivity may also occur

Therapeutic Nursing Interventions

- Assess the site for signs of secondary infection, including purulent drainage, increased induration, warmth to touch, or increased swelling.
- Obtain a thorough history of home environment, household and other close contacts, and presenting symptoms.
- Excessive use may cause systemic effects on the CNS.
- Antipruritic medication may be needed for scabies infestation.

Client Education

- Wear gloves for application.
- Skin irritation can occur even with proper application.
- All members of the household will need treatment as well as other persons who are close contacts with household members.
- Wash bed linens, towels, and clothing in hot water.
    - Dry in hot dryer.

- Do not share hats.
- Trim nails short and keep them clean.
- Handwashing after toileting is important.

Topical Corticosteroids

Overview

Complete action is unclear. These agents partially or totally block the inflammatory and allergic process at a cellular level. There is a vasoconstrictive mechanism as well as providing an antipruritic benefit.

Actions

- Anti-inflammatory effect
- Antipruritic effect

Uses

- Dermatitis
- Psoriasis
- SLE (systemic lupus erythematosus)
- Acne cysts
- Contact dermatitis
- Minor skin irritations

Important Drugs

Dexamethasone (Topicort)
Fluocinolone acetonide (Derma-Smoother)
Hydrocortisone (Cortaid, Lanacort)
Betamethasone (Valisone)
Mometasone (Elocon)

Precautions

- Adverse effects of topical steroid therapy include:
  - Acne eruptions
  - Allergic skin reaction
  - Hypopigmentation or hyperpigmentation
  - Hirsutism
  - Alopecia
  - Immunosuppression
  - Candidal superinfection
  - Local burning and itching

Therapeutic Nursing Interventions

- Monitor serum cortisol periodically with long-term use; report results.
- Use occlusive dressings with caution.
- Assess condition of skin for change with therapy: healing or secondary infection.

- Apply medication using gloves.
- Penetration of the medication depends on the integrity of the skin and thickness. Medication applied to skin of a younger person tends to be absorbed more readily than transdermal application on an older person.

Client Education

- Instruct client regarding proper use and application of product.
- Provide education regarding side effects of topical corticosteroid therapy. Most often the side effects are transient and will resolve after discontinuation of the medication.
- Typical adult dosing is once or twice daily, as directed.

Debriding Agents and Keratolytics

Overview

Keratolytics soften and loosen the outer layer of skin. They remove excess growth of the epidermis. This allows other medical treatments to be absorbed into the skin layers.

Uses

- Dandruff
- Dermatitis
- Psoriasis
- Warts
- Acne
- Corns
- Calluses
- Debride severe wounds
- Burns

Important Keratolytics

Salicylic acid (Occlusal)
Tretinoin (Retin-A)
Anthralin (Dithocreme)
Sulfur (Sebulex)
Granulex
Collagenase (Santyl)
Tazarotene (Avage)

Precautions

- Hypersensitivity
- Increased irritation at the site
- Severe redness
- Itching
- Burning or swelling

- Allergic reaction

Therapeutic Nursing Interventions

- Assess for signs of healing.
- Assess for signs of photosensitive reactions.
  - Caution client about sun sensitivity when using many of these products.
- Advise client to debride skin carefully so as not to tear underlying skin.
- Avoid applying the product to healthy or healing skin.

Client Education

- Apply debriding agents and keratolytics to clean skin.
- Report signs of hypersensitivity to health care provider.
- Wear protective clothing, sunglasses, and sunscreen during sun exposure because of photosensitivity. Minimize time in direct sun.

Acne Agents

Overview

Acne products are used for treatment of acne vulgaris, which is a skin disorder characterized by comedones, pustules, and nodules that can result in scarring. The face, neck, and shoulders are common sites. Acne begins in puberty with changes in estrogen-androgen balance. Some causative factors include family tendencies, stress, food allergies, endocrine factors, vitamin deficiency, and bacterial overgrowth.

Uses

- Soften and loosen the outer layer of skin
- Remove keratin plugs
- Reduce the bacterial colonization with Propionibacterium acnes (P. acnes)
- Decrease sebum production
- Improve the surface and appearance of the skin

Therapeutic Nursing Interventions

- Obtain a history regarding skin sensitivity to food, drugs, and other allergen sources.
- Discuss previous treatments and the outcome of therapy.
- Persons at risk for cardiovascular disease, family history of high cholesterol, obesity, or diabetes may avoid isotretinoin (Accutane) because of the increase in plasma triglyceride levels.
- Isotretinoin (Accutane) is hazardous to a developing fetus; therefore, women of childbearing age must commit to taking two forms of contraception.

Client Education

- Pregnancy prevention is imperative during isotretinoin (Accutane) treatment because of the risk to the fetus. Therapy is initiated after two negative pregnancy tests.

- When receiving isotretinoin (Accutane), you should not donate blood during or for 30 days after completion of therapy because of the risk to the fetus of a pregnant woman who may receive the blood.
- Erythromycin and tetracycline should not be used near the eyes or mucous membranes.
- Tetracycline should be avoided during pregnancy because the medication may result in abnormal enamel formation in the fetal dental structures.
- Sun sensitivity may occur with the use of many acne products.
- Careful exfoliation is necessary to prevent injury to new epidermal tissue.
- Improvement in the skin is usually noted after 4-6 weeks of treatment.

Important Drugs

Benzoyl peroxide

Tretinoin (Retin-A)

Isotretinoin (Accutane)

Tetracycline (Acfhromycin V, Actisite)

Erythromycin (E-mycin, Ilotycin)

Clindamycin (Cleocin)

Adverse Effects

- Hypersensitivity
- Increased irritation at the site
- Severe redness
- Itching and peeling
- Burning or swelling
- Allergic reaction
- Hyperlipidemia with isotretinoin (Accutane) therapy

Burn Agents

Overview

The first line treatment for burns is to immediately apply cold water or a cold compress to the burned area. Never apply butter, lard, greasy ointments, or dressings to burned skin. Once the burn injury is maintained, the next line of treatment is to apply antimicrobial agents, which act on cell walls and cell membranes to control and kill burn wound flora. Topical medications can penetrate the eschar and prevent wound infection. Systemic antibiotics are usually not administers (especially after 48 hours) because the burn eschar receives little or no blood, and consequently a systemic antibiotic is not able to circulate to the burn site. The client will require systemic antibiotic therapy if invasive burn wound sepsis develops or the client is diagnosed with a pulmonary infection such as pneumonia.

Uses

- Most commonly used on second and third-degree burns.

Important Drugs

Silver sulfadiazine (Silvadene) is a wide-spectrum antibacterial agent, and is fast, painless and easy to apply.

Mafenide acetate (Sulfamylon) is a wide-spectrum antibacterial agent that penetrates eschar and cartilage. This agent may be used to treat ear and electrical burns.

Mupirocin (Bactroban) is effective against many organisms that are resistant to silver sulfadiazine.

Gentamycin sulfate (Garamycin) is used to treat serious burn wound infections.

Precautions

- Pain, burning, or stinging at application site
- Bacterial resistance (most common with Garamycin)
- Possible allergic reaction to sulfa (most common with silver sulfadiazine)
- Renal toxicity if applied over large area (mupirocin)
- Superinfection with prolonged use or repeated therapy

Therapeutic Nursing Interventions

- Maintain clean environment for client at high risk for infection.
- Apply topical medications with a sterile gloved hand.
- Encourage and provide distractions for client up to one hour after application to decrease pain.
- Monitor for signs of pain; provide analgesia if necessary.
- Observe client for signs of respiratory alkalosis.

Client Education

- Teach client that topical agents are applied to the burn site to prevent infection.
- Client should maintain a clean environment and apply medications with a sterile gloved hand.
- Client should report any adverse reactions such as itching or pain to the health care provider.

Antipruritics

Overview

Antipruritics contain antihistamines that stop or decrease itching. Combined therapy with an anti-inflammatory is common.

Uses

- Short-term relief of moderate or severe itching

Important Drugs

Antipruritic:

Diphenhydramine hydrochloride (Benadryl)

Doxepin (Zonalon)

Anti-inflammatory:

Dexamethasone (Topicort)

Fluocinolone acetonide (Derma-Smoothe/FS)

Hydrocortisone (Cortaid, Lanacort)

Betamethasone (Valisone)

Wet dressings, soaks, rubs, and liniment agents:

Calamine lotion or **Calamine with phenol**

Diphenhydramine hydrochloride (Benadryl) lotion and cream

Aluminum acetate solution (Burow's Solution)

Aluminum sulfate (Domeboro)

Aspercreme, Bengay ointments, Vicks, Banalg liniment

Other:

Cornstarch

Oatmeal baths (Aveeno)

Precautions

- Hypersensitivity
- Burning
- Increased Itching
- Dermatitis

Therapeutic Nursing Interventions

- Assess skin for decreased redness.
- Assess for cause of irritant.
- Assess for decreased itching.

Client Education

- Clean area before applying agent.
- Wash hands and clean affected area prior to application.
- Avoid exposure to sunlight.
- Report signs of infection or hypersensitivity reaction to health care provider.

Critical Thinking Exercise: Drugs Affecting the Integumentary System

Note: *It is recommended that the following exercises be reviewed with a partner or in a small group to achieve maximum student interaction and to enhance critical thinking skills.*

Situation: A 17-year-old mother brings her 18-month-old son in the clinic for the second time this month for what she describes as "the bugs are back." Upon assessment, you find the youngster has a thick head of lice. You also notice nits on the blanket he is carrying and in the seams of his clothing. After reviewing his chart, you find he was diagnosed with head lice approximately two weeks prior and sent home with a bottle of Nix shampoo from your sample stock. Instructions were provided to the mother. You begin to question the mother of her understanding of the previous visit and how she used the shampoo. You find out she did shampoo the head of the youngster, but upon further questioning, you discover the young mother's roommate also has a 3-year-old who is a constant playmate; they even sleep together in the same bed. The physician makes a diagnosis of lice and orders Kwell be administered to all exposed family members, household members, and playmates.

1. What is your next course of action?

2. What directions should be given regarding pretreatment?

Situation: You also discover upon closer examination of the child his scalp is reddened and he has areas of excoriations with pustules scattered randomly over the reddened areas. You suspect these may be infected areas because of the scratching. You confirm with your clinic's primary care provider that the child does have a secondary infection, probably impetigo.

3. What should be prescribed?

4. What other instructions would you want to provide for this mother?

Matching Question:

5. Match the medication listed on the left to its appropriate therapeutic action on the right.

Table 1

Medication	Appropriate Therapeutic Action
Emollients and protectants	Applied to living tissue in order to kill pathogens that may cause illness to the host
Cold water	Reduce the growth of organisms or prevent replication without killing the entire population
Prophylactic agents	A substance that breaks down particles to be washed away; not antibacterial by nature
Bactericidals	Must be used with caution and with precise instructions for young children and the elderly due to the risk of CNS toxicity
Keratolytics	Can mask superinfections when used in conjunction with antibiotic creams or ointments
Antiparasitics	The first line of treatment for burns
Bacteriostatic agents	Provides comfort either by their anti-inflammatory capabilities or by their lubricating properties
Steroids	Soothing and cooling; form a protective coating on the skin to keep out light, air and dust
Soaps	Kill bacterial organisms, except for viral, fungal or spore populations
Prophylactic agents	Soften and loosen the outer layer of skin; remove excess growth of the epidermis

Critical Thinking Exercise Answer Keys

Critical Thinking Exercise: CHAPTER 1

Basic Pharmacologic Principles Answer Key

Note: *It is recommended the following exercises be reviewed with a partner or in a small group to achieve maximum student interaction and enhance critical thinking skills.*

---

1. The traditional "five rights" of medication administration include the following:

    a. Medication, client, dose, room number, route of dosage
    b. Medication, dose, strength, route of administration, location
    c. Client, medication, dose, route of administration, time
    d. Client, medication, dose, time, location

    Correct answer: c
    Rationale: Room number is not an identifying criteria. Documentation, though essential, is not officially part of the five rights. Location is ambiguous.

2. A nurse should provide which appropriate intervention when administering an intramuscular injection?

    a. Inject needle at a 45-degree angle
    b. Inform client not to massage the site
    c. Select a 25 to 27-gauge needle
    d. Aspirate prior to injection

    Correct answer: c
    Rationale: All of the sites mentioned are suitable for an intramuscular injection. The trapezius is not an appropriate location.

3. The client's willingness to follow drug therapy is called:

    a. Cooperation
    b. Active participation
    c. Dynamic partnership
    d. Compliance

    Correct answer: d
    Rationale: "Cooperation" is close, but not the same as compliance. "Dynamic partnership" and "active participation" are not terms used to describe a client's willingness to follow drug therapy.

4. A cream or ointment that is applied to the skin for a therapeutic purpose is classified as a ______________ agent.

    a. Cholinergic
    b. Statin
    c. Dermatologic
    d. Cathartic

    Correct answer: c. Creams and ointments can be classified as dermatologic agents; however, not every dermatologic agent is topical. For example, one treatment for acne is ingestion of tetracycline, an oral antibiotic. Answer "a" is an incorrect because cholinergics cause either receptor activation (agonist) or receptor blocking (antagonist) on structures such as the heart, exocrine glands, and smooth muscle structures of the GI tract, bladder or eye. These types of drugs are normally given topically (e.g., in the eye), by mouth (PO) or subcutaneously. Answer "b" is incorrect because statins are given PO to help lower cholesterol levels. Answer "d" is incorrect because cathartics are medications used relieve constipation and are given either orally or rectally.

Situation: S.S. is a 78-year-old who has been admitted to the ED with severe respiratory distress. After determining the cause of her distress to be pulmonary edema resulting from severe heart failure, the primary care provider orders furosemide (Lasix) 40 mg and then another 40 mg after 30 minutes. As the physician gathers the client's history, he learns the client was diagnosed and treated for breast cancer five years ago and now has metastatic disease, involving her thoracic spine. She has been in chronic pain, taking morphine in the form of morphine sulfate (Roxanol) 30 mg several times per day. In addition, the client takes morphine sulfate (MS Contin) 120 mg HS (at bedtime). The physician then adds the following order: morphine 5 mg IV q 3-4 hrs prn pain.

---

5. By which route would you expect the furosemide (Lasix) to be ordered?

    Most likely furosemide would be administered IV to obtain rapid results.

6. What lab work do you anticipate the doctor will be ordering? Why?

    Anticipate that electrolyte studies will be ordered, specifically potassium. Furosemide is a non-potassium-sparing diuretic and it is important to monitor the level of serum potassium as long as the client is taking this medication.

7. Are there any other medications you might anticipate the doctor will order? Why?

    It is common to see potassium ordered in combination with furosemide to counteract the potassium-depleting effect of this medication.

8. Why would the doctor order morphine for S.S.?

Morphine is an opiate analgesic that is used for severe pain. S.S. is suffering from metastatic bone disease and has been taking morphine to manage this pain, so it is prudent to continue the same medication to provide adequate pain control.

9. What kinds of nursing implications are involved with a client who is taking morphine?

- **The client may develop tolerance which may necessitate an increase in dosage to obtain the same level of pain relief.**
- **The client's vital signs, including blood pressure and respiratory rate, should be monitored regularly since morphine causes hypotension and respiratory depression.**

Situation: R.T. is a 76-year-old admitted to the ED with dehydration related to a gastrointestinal infection that resulted in copious diarrhea for the last 2 days. He has had severe abdominal cramping and can only tolerate small amounts of fluid.

---

10. Which of the following would be the most appropriate pharmacological intervention? Please provide a rationale for your answer.

a. IV infusion with 0.45% normal saline at 125 cc/hr
b. Copious amounts of liquid po to replace depleted body fluids
c. IV infusion with 0.9% normal saline at 300 cc hr x 3 hrs, then reduce to 150 cc/hr continuously
d. IV infusion of D5NS with 40 meq KCL/liter to run at 100 cc hr

Correct answer: C
Rationale: Solutions with approximately the same osmolarity (concentration) as plasma are used to replace extracellular fluid losses or without causing fluid shifts between extra- and intracellular compartments. Drinking water, though important, may not supply sufficient fluid replacement in an appropriate time. In addition, the client is only able to tolerate small amounts of fluid. D5NS is a hypertonic solution and would tend to cause a fluid to shift away from the intracellular compartments. 0.45% normal saline is a hypotonic solution.

11. You anticipate R.T. will most likely demonstrate the following labs (explain the nursing principle on which you base your answer):

   a. Elevated sodium and potassium
   b. Increased magnesium and decreased sodium
   c. Elevated BUN and elevated potassium
   d. Decreased potassium levels and elevated urine specific gravity

   Correct answer: D
   Rationale: Potassium is often lost during bouts of severe diarrhea. Dehydration related to persistent diarrhea would result in an elevated urine specific gravity.

12. The physician examines the lab results and recommends potassium 40 meq be added to each liter of IV solution. What is the rationale for ordering this medication?

   Potassium is often depleted in cases of severe diarrhea.

Situation: B.J. is 43 years old. He has worked in construction since he was 16. He was recently admitted to the hospital to treat a herniated disk. Prior to admission, he had been undergoing physical therapy and had been taking oral Vicodin for the last three months as well as muscle relaxants and anti-inflammatories. After surgery to correct the ruptured disk, the physician ordered 75 mg of Demerol with 25 mg Vistaril q 4-6 hours for pain. You have been giving the medication as ordered, but B.J. states he is receiving only minimal pain relief.

---

13. What is the most likely explanation for this situation? Discuss the reason for your answer.

   a. B.J. has developed a tolerance to the effectiveness of the analgesics and a larger dose of analgesics may be needed to provide adequate pain relief.
   b. B.J. has developed psychological dependence on the analgesics.
   c. B.J. is anxious and his perception of pain is much more acute.
   d. B.J.'s dose of Vicodin needs to be decreased.

   Correct answer: A
   Rationale: Tolerance is a progressive decrease in a drug's effectiveness resulting from a physiological adaptation in which the body requires more medication to obtain the same pain relief as the original dose. Anxiety and psychological dependence do not adequately account for the pain Mr. Johnson is experiencing. Decreasing the dose of Vicodin would not be beneficial at this time.

Critical Thinking Exercise: CHAPTER 2

Drugs Used to Treat Infection Answer Key

Note: *It is recommended that the following exercises be reviewed with a partner or in a small group to achieve maximum student interaction and to enhance critical thinking skills.*

Situation: A 26-year-old female comes to the community clinic complaining of a fever, sore throat, and cough. Her posterior pharynx is reddened with patches of purulent exudate and she experiences pain with swallowing. Her cervical lymph nodes are enlarged and tender to touch. The client's vital signs are: temperature, 101.4 orally; pulse, 96; respirations, 22; BP, 122/84. Based on the symptoms and physical examination, the primary care provider suspects a streptococcal infection which is confirmed by a quick strep test performed in the clinic. The client is started on amoxicillin-clavulanate (Augmentin) 500 mg PO q 8h for 10 days.

1. Before administering the first dose of amoxicillin-clavulanate (Augmentin), what additional assessment data do you feel the nurse should collect?

    The nurse needs to inquire if the client has ever had a reaction to a previous antibiotic, especially if the antibiotic was a penicillin product.

2. What teaching do you consider most important for the client taking amoxicillin-clavulanate (Augmentin)?

    Be sure to take the medication with food to avoid gastrointestinal discomfort.

    Finish taking all the medication as ordered, even if condition improves. Failure to complete a course of antibiotics can result in development of resistant strains of organisms.

    The client should be advised to never share this medication because some individuals may be allergic to penicllin and may develop a serious reaction.

    Report any signs or symptoms of allergic reaction to the primary care provider.

3. After the first two doses, the client calls and states she is experiencing an itchy rash. What would be your best response and what is your rationale?

    Assess if the client has any other adverse symptoms or is experiencing any difficulty breathing. If so, advise the client to call 9-1-1 immediately.

    If symptoms are not life threatening, advise the client to stop taking the medication immediately and come to the clinic for further evaluation.

Situation: The client returns to the clinic and the physician discontinues the Augmentin and starts the client on cephalexin (Keflex), 250 mg PO q 6h for 10 days. The physician provides samples so the client can begin taking the medication immediately.

---

4. What would be your best nursing intervention? Explain your rationale.

    The client should take the first dose and then sit in the waiting room for approximately 30 minutes so you can assess for any possible allergic responses.

    Cephalosporins have a cross-sensitivity with penicillin drugs so you want to ensure the client is safe.

    You would carefully document the client's condition prior to sending the client home and consider making a follow-up call to see how the client is doing.

    Instruct the client to report any further signs or symptoms of allergic reaction immediately to the primary care provider.

5. As a nurse, you have particular knowledge about cephalexin (Keflex). List as much information as you can about the drug below.

    It is the oral form of a first-generation cephalosporin.

    It is effective against gram-negative infections.

    Cephalosporins are used as a second-line therapeutic agent in the treatment of strep throat.

    Cephalosporins primarily act to inhibit bacterial cell wall synthesis.

    Hypersensitivity reaction is the most frequent adverse effect and is similar to that observed with the penicillin.

    Superinfections may manifest as fungal infections of the mouth or vagina.

Situation: Mrs. J, a 46-year-old woman comes to your clinic, stating she has been taking trimethopin-sulfamethoxazole (Bactrim) for a bladder infection, but is concerned because she has developed intense perineal client and a whitish, cheesy appearing vaginal discharge. She is visiting an out-of-state relative and would prefer to see her own doctor, but can't wait because the itching is unbearable.

6. How should the nurse respond to the client's concern?

 Inform her that this is a common side effect of antibiotics. The normal bacteria in the body has been altered by the antibiotic, allowing a superinfection to develop.

7. What action do you anticipate from the physician?

 Most superinfections are fungal in nature, so the physician will most likely order an antifungal agent, either prescription or over the counter.

Situation: Mr. R comes to the clinic complaining of frequency and burning for the past two days. A preliminary urinalysis reveals the urine is cloudy with moderate sediment and increased white blood cells. The specimen is sent to the lab for a culture and sensitivity. The primary care provider orders nitrofurantoin (Furadantin).

8. Why did the doctor choose this particular medication?

 Nitrofurantoin (Furadantin) is an antimicrobial agent that achieves good concentration in the urine and is effective against common bacterial pathogens.

9. What are some of the nursing considerations when giving nitrofurantoin?

 Warn the client who is taking nitrofurantoin that the medication may cause a rust-brown discoloration of the urine.

 Drink an adequate amount of fluids in order to maintain a urine output of at least 1200 to 1,500 mL daily to prevent crystalluria and stone formation.

 To prevent photosensitivity reactions, avoid direct sunlight and ultraviolet light, and use a sunscreen and protective clothing when going outdoors.

 If skin rash, fever, sore throat, mouth sores or unusual bleeding or bruising develop, notify the primary care provider.

Critical Thinking Exercise: CHAPTER 3

Drugs Affecting the Immune System Answer Key

Note: *It is recommended the following exercises be reviewed with a partner or in a small group to achieve maximum student interaction and enhance critical thinking skills.*

Situation: R.G. is a 22-year-old pregnant female who has been diagnosed with advanced acquired immunodeficiency syndrome (AIDS). Her CD4 cell count is 145. Her primary care provider has prescribed zidovudine (AZT) (Retrovir) 200 mg tid to be administered with zalcitabine (Hivid) 0.75 mg PO tid. Before starting R.G. on combination therapy, the nurse performed a neurologic assessment. Throughout her course of therapy, the nurse continued to closely monitor R.G.'s neurologic status, and CBC and CD4 count.

1. Why is it important to monitor the CD4 cell count in clients who are being treated for HIV infection?

    This is a critical monitoring parameter that determines the client's response to the drug.

2. Why do you want to closely monitor the CBC of clients taking zidovudine (AZT)?

    Clients are at risk of infection because they are in an immunocompromised state.

    The CBC can be used to identify if there is bone marrow suppression.

3. The client informs you she is experiencing burning and tingling in her fingers and toes. What might this indicate?

    These symptoms may indicate peripheral neuropathy.

4. What are some of the important nursing considerations related to this client?

    Advise the client to continue with regularly scheduled prenatal care.

    Advise the client to avoid crowds to decrease the possibility of contracting an infection.

AZT treats AIDS and HIV infections by slowing the progression of the disease and decreasing complications.

The drug is excreted through the kidneys so the client should drink adequate amounts of water to maintain good hydration.

Take precautions to avoid transmission to others.

R	M	H	T	B	O	J	M	X	B	M	J	C	B	J	K	J	J	N	T	P	Z	A	G	D
K	M	C	I	Y	T	B	Q	I	T	E	I	I	K	Z	L	A	Q	R	V	W	O	S	Y	U
W	Q	D	N	X	E	A	V	V	M	H	H	K	V	A	C	C	I	N	A	T	I	O	N	G
I	X	I	F	S	V	P	I	M	M	U	N	O	S	U	P	P	R	E	S	S	A	N	T	S
A	A	G	E	I	M	M	U	N	O	S	T	I	M	U	L	A	N	T	S	P	K	D	R	V
X	Q	P	C	W	B	Y	M	B	I	V	N	S	Q	D	L	O	I	X	S	J	C	D	N	D
L	Q	L	T	A	J	L	S	A	X	O	G	L	A	I	N	N	A	T	E	Q	R	N	Y	G
W	A	K	I	Q	C	G	D	F	P	V	F	G	S	W	U	L	I	C	Q	G	C	E	K	L
G	Q	A	O	J	G	Q	P	P	R	E	F	R	I	G	E	R	A	T	E	R	R	Z	L	N
J	O	C	N	E	F	Q	U	Z	I	N	O	E	Q	H	R	H	A	P	G	V	V	K	M	T
Y	X	T	H	P	Q	N	C	I	D	L	Y	S	B	C	N	L	P	Q	C	R	L	O	U	L
Q	X	I	V	K	C	R	K	L	R	C	O	K	D	K	R	X	O	T	K	Z	F	I	Q	J
E	X	V	M	C	B	B	Z	T	W	E	E	P	B	Q	M	P	O	V	J	C	K	N	V	X
L	G	E	D	I	C	E	P	P	Y	U	D	U	G	L	P	E	F	Y	D	P	M	L	W	E
U	Q	V	F	L	D	T	R	V	D	O	U	E	E	Y	R	J	A	X	Y	N	V	L	Q	N
U	I	M	L	U	N	O	S	S	P	P	R	E	S	S	A	N	T	S	D	N	H	I	W	K
M	Y	L	W	V	O	U	P	X	I	B	B	E	Z	W	P	G	L	P	E	Q	R	S	A	M

1. ____________________ act to suppress the immune response. [**Immunosuppressants**]
2. Drugs that activate or enhance a person's own immune system: [**Immunostimmulants**]
3. Most vaccines and toxoids are kept in the ______________. [**Refrigerator**]
4. Involves the injection of killed or weakened (attenuated) microorganisms into the body via vaccines and toxoids. [**Vaccination**]
5. All immunosuppressants place a client at risk of _______________. [**Infection**]
6. What kind of immunity is the second line of defense against infectious agents? [**Aquired**]
7. The first line of defense present at birth. [**Innate**]
8. What kind of immunity is produced by the person's own immune system? [**Active**]
9. The nurse should ask a client who is receiving a vaccine if they have an allergy to ___________. [**Eggs**]
10. MMR is an example of a _______________ vaccine. [**Live**]
11. Bone marrow suppression would be most easily measured by this test. [**CBC**]

Critical Thinking Exercise: CHAPTER 4

Drugs for Pain and Inflammation Answer Key

Note: *It is recommended that the following exercises be reviewed with a partner or in a small group to achieve maximum student interaction and to enhance critical thinking skills.*

Situation: D.S. is a 76-year-old woman who had a total hip replacement yesterday. Her pain is managed by patient-controlled analgesia (PCA). She has an epidural catheter in place and is receiving fentanyl (Duragesic) and bupivacaine (Marcaine) via the PCA.

1. D.S. is very worried she will give herself too much medication and become addicted. What do think would be an appropriate nursing intervention? Provide a rationale for your answer?

   The PCA pump is designed to provide optimal analgesia without overdosing. In addition, D.S. is being carefully monitored and will only take the medication until the doctor can wean her to a less potent analgesic. Most likely, she will be on the medication for such a short time that there is little chance that addiction could occur.

2. What are the most important assessment parameters for any client who is receiving narcotic analgesics?

   Respiratory rate
   Blood pressure
   Level of consciousness

3. The plan is to discontinue the epidural catheter in 48 hours and order oxycodone/acetami¬nophen (Percocet 7.5/500), 1 tab q 6h PRN pain management. Your nursing knowledge pro¬vides you with important information regarding the side effects of this medication. Discuss some of the implications this has in relation to your nursing assessments and interventions.

   Constipation
   Nausea

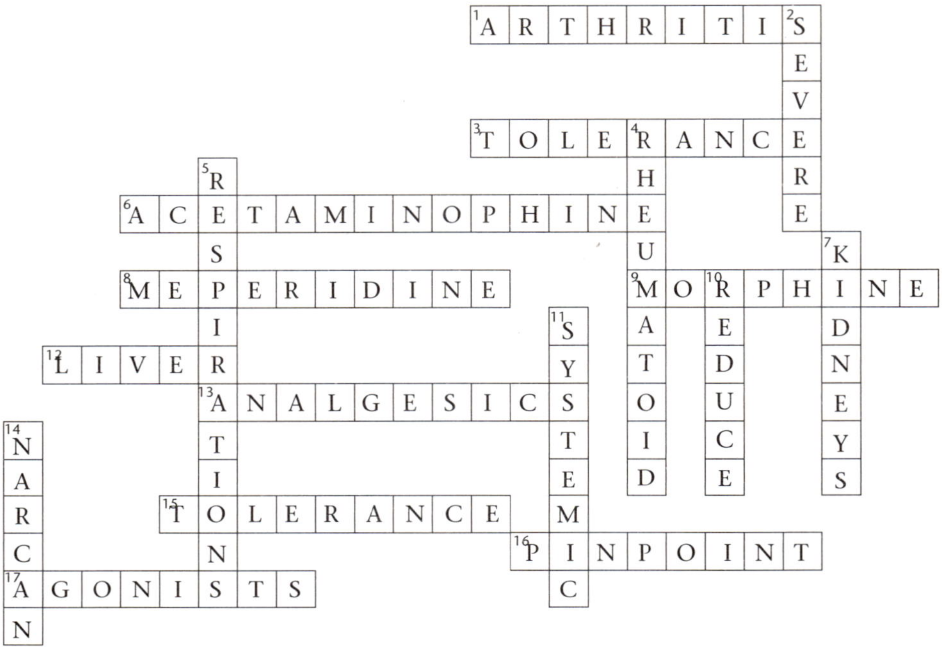
1 ARTHRITIS
2 SEVERE
3 TOLERANCE
4 RHEUMATOID
5 RESPIRATION
6 ACETAMINOPHINE
7 KIDNEYS
8 MEPERIDINE
9 MORPHINE
10 REDUCE
11 SYSTEMIC
12 LIVER
13 ANALGESICS
14 NARCAN
15 TOLERANCE
16 PINPOINT
17 AGONISTS

Critical Thinking Exercise: CHAPTER 5

Drugs Affecting the Nervous System Answer Key

Note: *It is recommended that the following exercises be reviewed with a partner or in a small group to achieve maximum student interaction and to enhance critical thinking skills.*

Situation: M.M., a 32-year-old mother of three, was brought to the hospital by her husband for increasingly erratic behavior. She has been staying up nights "cleaning the house," sleeping only a few hours a day for the last four days. Her husband informs you she has been eating very little, stating she doesn't have time, yet she spends many hours shopping during the day and has spent large amounts of money. More seriously, she has left the children, ages 3, 5, and 8, alone several times stating, "I have important work to do." You do a quick head-to-toe assessment and note the following: She is unkempt, dressed inappropriately with multiple layers of clothes of differing fabrics and patterns. She is wearing a pair of old tennis shoes with mismatched socks. Her mood is euphoric, her speech pressured, and you note she does not seem to be able to stay on topic as you interview her. When she does answer, she demonstrates flight of ideas and erratic thinking patterns. She can't understand what "the fuss" is all about and sees no reason to come to the hospital.

Her husband tells the doctor that M.M. has a long history of manic and depressive episodes, but it was only during this last year that she was formally diagnosed with bipolar disorder and started on lithium. Since then, her mood has been relatively stable and she has been able to function normally.

You learn M.M.'s current dose of lithium carbonate (Lithobid) is 200 mg po tid and she has been taking it regularly and tolerating it well until this last week. The physician orders stat lithium levels and admits M.M. for further evaluation.

1. Based on your nursing knowledge, what information do you know about lithium that is pertinent to this client?

   Lithium is the drug of choice for the long-term management of bipolar disorder, also called manic-depressive disorder. Bipolar disorder is characterized by mood swings or cycles of acute mania, followed by acute depression, with periods of normalcy. The manic phase is characterized by an elevated mood and irritability. The exact mechanism by which lithium stabilizes mood swings is not clear.

   Serum lithium levels should be monitored 2-3 times per week for at least 2 months to ensure lithium levels are within the therapeutic range. After therapeutic levels are established and stable. levels should be checked every 1 to 3 months.

   Monitor client for signs and symptoms of lithium overdose or toxicity, and immediately report manifestations to the primary care provider.

2. The lithium levels come back and are found to be 0.45 mEq/L. The physician views the lab results and writes an order for chlorpromazine hydrochloride (Thorazine) IM stat and prn q 6-8 hours for agitation, and increases the lithium to 300 mg of lithium po tid. Why do you think Thorazine has been ordered? What are some of the most important nursing considerations involved in administering this drug?

   Until therapeutic levels (0.6 to 1.2 mEq/L) of lithium are attained, symptoms of mania and agitation may be controlled with chlorpromazine (Thorazine). The client's mental status should be closely monitored. Additionally, dry mouth, blurred vision and photophobia are common adverse effects so client education and nursing interventions to address these needs are imperative.

3. After four days, M.M.'s condition stabilizes and she is being prepared for discharge home on 300 mg lithium po tid. What discharge teaching is most important for this client and her family?

   Closely follow the prescribed dosage schedule because the range of therapeutic effectiveness for this drug is very narrow.

   Never double the dosage if a dose is missed.

   Take lithium with food or milk to lessen gastrointestinal symptoms.

   Drink at least 2-3 quarts of water per day to prevent dehydration, which can precipitate drug toxicity.

   Carry an identification card that states you are taking lithium medication.

   Be sure to keep all follow-up appointments so blood can be drawn to ensure the drug is being maintained at a therapeutic level.

4. **Exercise**: In the table below, match the drug in the left-hand column to its appropriate category or classification in the right-hand column.

Drug	Classification
Chlorpromazine	Antipsychotic
Lithium	Mood stabilizer
Metoclopramide	Cholinergic
Epinephrine HCL	Adrenergic
Ergotamine tartrate	Anti-adrenergic
Baclofen	Skeletal muscle relaxant
Nembutal	Barbiturate
Xanax	Benzodiazapine
Fluoxetine	Antidepressant
Phenobarbital	Barbiturate

Critical Thinking Exercise: CHAPTER 6

Drugs Affecting the Cardiovascular System Answer Key

Note: *It is recommended that the following exercises be reviewed with a partner or in a small group to achieve maximum student interaction and to enhance critical thinking skills.*

1. Heart failure develops when the following occurs:

    a. The cardiac and pulmonary vessels become occluded with plaque.
    b. When the pulse pressure drops too rapidly.
    c. When the heart muscle fails to pump effectively and sufficient blood does not circulate to the lungs and body tissue.
    d. When the ventricles become hypertrophied due to viral or bacterial infection.

    Correct answer: C
    Rationale: Heart failure occurs when the heart muscle fails to pump effectively and sufficient blood does not circulate to the lungs and body tissues. The development of plaque may contribute to ineffective blood flow, but is not a primary cause of heart failure. Pulse pressure would increase, not decrease during heart failure. Hypertrophy may be a result of heart failure, but is not a primary cause.

2. List four types of angina.

    Stable angina
    Unstable angina
    Variant (Prinzmetal's angina)
    Refractory angina

3. Hypertension is usually defined as:

    a. Systolic blood pressure < 90 mmHg and diastolic blood pressure > 60 mm Hg
    b. Diastolic blood pressure > 90 mmHg and systolic blood pressure > 140 mm Hg
    c. Diastolic blood pressure < 60 mmHg and systolic blood pressure > 80 mm Hg
    d. Systolic blood pressure > 120 mmHg and diastolic blood pressure < 80 mm Hg

    Correct answer: B

4. Digoxin has the following action:

   a. Increases the ability of the heart to respond to adrenal hormones
   b. Strengthens atrial contractility and decreases pulmonary artery resistance
   c. Decreases atrial irritability and restores normal conduction
   d. Increases cardiac contracility without elevating the oxygen requirement of the myocardium

   Correct answer: D

5. The primary goal of andrenergic therapy for all forms of shock is to:

   a. Decrease the likelihood of myocardial infarction
   b. Increase blood flow to maintain adequate kidney function
   c. Increase blood flow through the coronary and cerebral vessels
   d. Stimulate the release of stress hormones to reduce peripheral perfusion

   Correct answer: C

6. Drugs that affect the cardiovascular system are often given to counteract the effects of shock. In the table below, draw a line from the description of the shock (left) to the correct type of shock (right).

Table 1

Description	Type of shock
Characterized by decreased cardiac output	Cardiogenic
Results from profound vasodilation and decreased peripheral resistance often resulting from gram-negative bacteria	Septic
Results from a decreased volume of circulating blood	Hypovolemic
Generally due to injury	Traumatic
Extensive vasodilation and decreased peripheral resistance often resulting from systemic allergic responses	Anaphylactic

Situation: S.M is a 64-year-old with heart failure who has been maintained on digoxin 0.125 mg, PO daily for a number of years without problems. He is now admitted to the hospital with bilateral ankle edema, weight gain of 12 pounds, dyspnea on exertion and fatigue. His admission ECG (electrocardiogram) showed atrial fibrillation. His digoxin level was 0.9 ng/ml. He was placed on the following medications:

- Digoxin 0.125 mg, PO daily
- Lasix 80 mg IVP now, then Lasix 40 mg, PO BID
- K-Dur 20 mEq, PO BID
- Amiodarone (Cordarone) 200 mg, PO daily
- Heparin 1000 units/hour, IV (after a loading dose of 5,000 units)

7. What is the primary nursing concern when Digoxin and Lasix are given simultaneously?

Lasix causes potassium depletion. Digitalis toxicity is more likely in the presence of hypokalemia.

8. What are the signs of digitalis toxicity?

Initial symptoms would include cardiac irregularities including varying degrees of heart block, gastrointestinal distress, confusion, drowsiness and visual disturbances. Life-threatening symptoms would include severe ventricular dysrhythmias, bradycardia and cardiac arrest.

9. Based on the above clinical scenario, what do you think are the clinical indications for administering heparin to this client?

The client is showing typical signs of left-sided heart failure. This may lead to venous statis in the extremities which can precipitate the development of thrombi.

The ECG showed atrial fibrillation which can also precipitate the development of thrombi.

10. What must the nurse consider about the dosage of either digoxin or amiodarone when they are being administered together?

Amiodarone can significantly increase the digoxin level. The digoxin dose should be monitored and possibly decreased by 50%.

Critical Thinking Exercise: CHAPTER 7

Drugs Affecting the Blood Answer Key

Note: *It is recommended that the following exercises be reviewed with a partner or in a small group to achieve maximum student interaction and to enhance critical thinking skills.*

Situation: M.S. is a 54-year-old man who began having chest pain during lunch while at work. On admission to the emergency department via ambulance one hour later, M.S. was pale, diaphoretic, and complained of shortness of breath. He was diagnosed with unstable angina to rule out myocardial infarction (MI). The client reported no previous episodes of chest pain or pressure. He has smoked two packs of cigarettes daily for 25 years. There is no family history of heart disease.

After evaluation of initial lab results, presenting symptoms, and ECG, the diagnosis of an extensive anterolateral MI was made. The client was considered a candidate for thrombolytic therapy; tissue plasminogen activator (t-PA) was started immediately, using front-loaded dosing technique. A nitroglycerin (NTG) drip (50 mg/250 mL D5W) was started at 1.5 mL/h (5 mcg/min). A heparin bolus of 8000 units given IVP, and a drip was hung at 1000 units/hour. Metoprolol tartrate 25 mg and an aspirin were given orally. The client was transferred to ICU.

After 1.5 hours of t-PA, his chest pain returned and blood pressure was 96/60. NTG was given sublingually with no relief, and no ECG changes were noted. M.S. was sent to the cardiac catheterization lab for an emergency cardiac catheterization and possible percutaneous transluminal coronary angioplasty (PTCA). Results showed 90% blockage of left anterior descending coronary artery, and a successful PTCA was performed. A total of 23,000 units of heparin was given IVP, and 500,00 units of urokinase was given intracoronary.

1. What are the pharmacologic actions of heparin?

    Heparin is an anticoagulant; it inhibits activated Factors IX, X, XI, and XII, which are involved in the conversion of prothrombin to thrombin, thereby reducing clot formation; and potentiates the effects of antithrombin III.

    Heparin prevents the conversion of fibrinogen to fibrin.

    Higher doses of heparin neutralize thrombus formation and extension of existing thrombi.

2. What are the indicators for use of heparin in the client after a myocardial infarction (MI)?

Heparin is used in the treatment of thrombus formation and to prevent future thrombus formation.

Heparin acts immediately after intravenous administration.

3. What is the effect of a thrombolytic agent on the MI client?

The overall goal of thrombolytic therapy isto reestablish blood flow and prevent tissue damage.

Thrombolytic agents:

Dissolve thrombi in coronary arteries thus preserving cardiac function

Stimulate conversion of plasminogen to plasmin, degrading fibrin present in clots because plasmin is a proteolytic enzyme that breaks down fibrin, the framework of a thrombus.

4. What made the client eligible to receive thrombolytics?

Ischemic chest pain of 30 minutes duration

Chest pain unresponsive to sublingual NTG (nitroglycerin)

Client less than 75 years of age

No conditions that may predispose him to hemorrhage

Critical Thinking Exercise: CHAPTER 8

Drugs Affecting the Respiratory System Answer Key

Note: *It is recommended that the following exercises be reviewed with a partner or in a small group to achieve maximum student interaction and to enhance critical thinking skills.*

1. With which condition are antihistamines generally considered safe? Provide rationale as to why.

   Antihistamines are generally contraindicated with narrow-angle glaucoma because most have anticholinergic side effects which may aggravate this condition and increase intraocular pressure. Antihistamines are indicated for conditions such as contact dermatitis and allergic rhinitis and may be taken by pregnant clients, and those with peptic ulcer disease and prostatic hypertrophy upon the advice of their primary care provider.

2. Discuss the difference between antitussives and expectorants. What are the indications for the use of each type of medication?

   Antitussives are drugs used to relieve cough by suppressing the cough center in the medulla to relieve tissue irritation of the bronchial mucosa caused by excessive coughing. Expectorants on the other hand, do not reduce irritation from coughing, but stimulate the flow of respiratory secretions, thinning mucus and making it easier to clear from the respiratory tract. Some experts question the effectiveness of expectorants.

3. Discuss the advantages and disadvantages of using inhaled corticosteroids.

   Inhaled corticosteroids suppress inflammation in the airways, which decreases mucus secretion, decreases edema in the mucosa of the airway, and helps repair damaged epithelium. Inhaled corticosteroids also increase the number and sensitivity of beta$_2$-adrenergic receptors, improving the response to beta$_2$-adrenergic bronchodilators. It was previously thought that serious systemic effects would not occur unless the inhaled forms are used in long-term, high-dose therapy. Recent studies have shown that even inhaled steroids at normal doses cause side effects, such as impaired growth in children.

Situation: S.S. is a 32-year-old woman with a long history of bronchial asthma. She is currently maintained on theophylline (Theo-Dur) 200 mg twice a day. She uses a fluticasone (Flonase) inhaler, one puff, twice a day. When respiratory wheezing increases, she uses an albuterol (Proventil) inhaler, two puffs every four hours, until her breathing improves.

4. What clinical manifestations would you expect to see in S.S. if her serum theophylline level was > 20 mcg/mL?

   A serum theophylline level greater than 20 mcg/mL indicates the client may experience toxicity. Onset may be sudden and the client may initially experience a sudden onset with arrhythmias and seizures as the first signs. The margin of safety for xanthines is narrow, especially in the young, elderly, and debilitated. Tremors occur with high serum levels of theophylline; the nurse should report this symptom to the prescribing practitioner for serum monitoring and possible dosing changes.

   Other assessment indicators include:
   - **Anorexia**
   - **Nausea**
   - **Vomiting**
   - **Headache**
   - **Anxiety**

5. Because albuterol (Proventil) is a $Beta_2$ agonist drug, you would expect to see what kind of a response related to adrenergic receptors?

   $Beta_2$-adrenergic receptors such as albuterol (Proventil) act on the smooth muscles of the bronchi and bronchioles. They stimulate increased production of cyclic adenosine monophosphate (cAMP), which induces relaxation of the smooth muscle, allows the airways to dilate and provides reduction of wheezing in the client.

   Given this information, the nurse would expect:
   - **More bronchodilation**
   - **Less cardiac effects**
   - **Less peripheral vasoconstriction**

After an acute attack of asthma during which S.S. was treated with aerosolized albuterol and systemic corticosteroids, her primary care provider is considering adding an additional medication she hopes will prevent future attacks.

6. What medications would you expect the primary care provider to consider?

    Most likely the medication that will be added is the xanthine bronchodilator, theophylline (Theo-Dur) because it can be administered orally and the client can continue taking the medication safely at home. Others include a leukotriene receptor antagonist, such as zafirlukast (Accolate).

Critical Thinking Exercise: CHAPTER 9

Drugs Affecting the Renal System Answer Key

Note: *It is recommended that the following exercises be reviewed with a partner or in a small group to achieve maximum student interaction and to enhance critical thinking skills.*

Situation: L.L. is a 72-year-old female who has had chronic CHF (congestive heart failure) for five years. She currently takes sustained-release diltiazem (Cardizem) 180 mg po qd for hypertension and digoxin (Lanoxin) 0.25 mg q a.m. to improve her cardiac function. She is admitted to the hospital after reporting increasing dyspnea and edema in her ankles and feet. On admission, she was started on oxygen per nasal cannula and intravenous fluids through a peripheral line. Your assessment reveals crackles in the lower lobes of both lungs. Her respiratory rate is 22, pulse 100, and BP 170/92.

1. A new order is written for furosemide (Lasix) 20 mg IV push now.

   a. What is the action of furosemide (Lasix)?

   It is a loop diuretic. It blocks the reabsorption of sodium and chloride in the loop of Henle, which results in decreased water reabsorption. This enhances diuresis.

   b. Describe two benefits of furosemide (Lasix) for this client.

   Pulmonary edema is reduced. Decreased blood volume lowers blood pressure, reducing the workload of the heart.

   Peripheral edema is reduced.

2. Identify at least two drug interactions among the drugs L. L. is taking.

   Diltiazem (Cardizem) and furosemide (Lasix) both lower blood pressure. Given together, the client is at increased risk of postural hypotension.

   Lasix promotes excretion of potassium; hypokalemia increases the risk of digoxin toxicity.

3. A blood sample is drawn to measure serum electrolytes.

   a. Which electrolytes are influenced most by furosemide (Lasix)?

      Sodium

      Chloride

      Potassium

   b. Explain why electrolytes must be closely monitored when clients are receiving loop diuretics and digoxin (Lanoxin).

      As noted above, significant potassium loss can occur with Lasix.

      Hypokalemia increases the risk of digoxin toxicity with potentially fatal dysrhythmias.

4. If L.L. is discharged on furosemide (Lasix), list three important client teaching points.

   Take in the morning to avoid nighttime voiding.

   Change positions slowly to prevent dizziness and loss of balance.

   Report weakness, confusion, gastrointestinal distress, or palpitations.

   Protect yourself from direct sunlight.

   Record weight daily.

5. L.L. is discharged home with prescriptions for diltiazem (Cardizem), digoxin (Lanoxin), and furosemide (Lasix). One month after discharge she tells the home health nurse she feels weak and nauseated. She also says she feels like her heart is skipping beats. The home health nurse should immediately suspect ______________.

   The home health nurse should immediately suspect hypokalemia.

Critical Thinking Exercise: CHAPTER 10

Drugs Affecting the Digestive System Answer Key

Note: *It is recommended that the following exercises be reviewed with a partner or in a small group to achieve maximum student interaction and to enhance critical thinking skills.*

Situation: J.L. is a 50-year-old man with ESRD (end-stage renal disease). He was hospitalized when his AV access clotted off. He had a renal transplant several years ago that he rejected. He has been dependent on hemodialysis since his rejection. J.L.'s past medical history includes hypertension, end-stage renal disease, history of ulcers, ventricular tachycardia and atrial fibrillation, chronic pancreatitis, anemia, Staphylococcus aureus sepsis, and steroid-induced diabetes mellitus. A Tenckhoff catheter was inserted during the current hospitalization and J.L. was placed on continuous cycling-assisted peritoneal dialysis (CCPD) with plans to discharge him on continuous ambulatory peritoneal dialysis (CAPD). His current medications are:

- Ferrous sulfate (Feosol) 325 mg PO bid
- Terazosin (Hytrin) 10 mg PO at HS
- Amiodarone (Cordarone) 200 mg PO QD
- Sucralfate (Carafate) 1g PO qid
- Epoetin alpha (Epogen) 6000 units SC 3x/wk
- Docusate sodium (Colace) 100 mg PO bid
- Calcitrol (Rocaltrol) 25 mcg, 2 tabs PO bid
- Calcium carbonate (Tums) 420 mg, 3 tabs with meals
- Nifedipine (Procardia XL) 120 mg PO bid at 10 a.m. and 10 p.m

1. What antacids are contraindicated in renal clients and why?

    Magnesium-based antacids are contraindicated for renal clients because of their poor excretion of magnesium.

2. Identify the reasons J.L. is taking docusate sodium (Colace).

    J.L. is hypertensive and has cardiomyopathy with a history of arrhythmias. Thus he is receiving docusate sodium to avoid straining with defection.

3. In regard to his other medications, when would you give him sucralfate (Carafate) and why?

   Schedule the sucralfate (Carafate) two hours after the other medications because it may bind to certain compounds in the gastrointestinal tract and inhibit their bioavailability.

4. How do you think popular opinion and the media influence the choice of over-the-counter antacids? Discuss some of the positive and negative implications involved.

   This question is opened-ended in order to cause the learner to refer back to the review module to reinforce their rationales.

5. What are some of the nursing implications of self-medication with over-the-counter antacids?

   This question is opened-ended in order to cause the learner to refer back to the review module to reinforce their rationales.

6. Fill in the letter of the drug you feel would be most appropriate for the condition listed to the right. There may be more than one correct answer. A list of drugs is located at the bottom of the page for reference.

Peptic ulcers:	A, B, G, J, K, N
Gastric reflux:	A, B, G
Constipation:	F, L, O
Diarrhea:	D, E, I
Nausea and vomiting:	C
Motion sickness:	H
Flatulence:	M
Stress ulcers:	A, B, J, K
GERD:	A, B, G

Drugs:

A. Aluminum hydroxide
B. Magnesium hydroxide
C. Dramamine
D. Lomotil
E. Psyllium
F. Biscodyl
G. Reglan
H. Antivert
I. Imodium
J. Zantac
K. Tagamet
L. Colace
M. Mylicon
N. Amoxicillin
O. Metamucil

Critical Thinking Exercise: CHAPTER 11

Drugs Affecting the Endocrine System Answer Key

Note: *It is recommended that the following exercises be reviewed with a partner or in a small group to achieve maximum student interaction and to enhance critical thinking skills.*

Situation: : S.L. is an 80-year-old woman with a history of hypertension and adult onset diabetes mellitus. She has just moved to the area and has come for an initial visit. S.L. has had hypertension for 20 years and diabetes for 10 years. Until eight months ago, the diabetes was treated with diet and an oral hypoglycemic agent. However, she began to lose weight, her thirst and urine output increased, and her blood sugar increased substantially, despite increasing doses of the hypoglycemic agent. She was then started on insulin. S.L. monitors her blood glucose at home twice a day. Five years ago, she had a left radical mastectomy performed for breast cancer. She now has metastasis to the bones. S.L.'s current medications are:

- Enalapril (Vasotec) 5 mg bid
- Hydrochlorothiazide and triamterene (Dyazide) 50 mg qd in a.m.
- Tamoxifen 20 mg bid
- NPH insulin 20 IU before breakfast, 5 IU before supper
- Humalog Insulin 5 IU before breakfast, 2 IU before supper
- Oxycodone (OxyContin) 10 mg q 12 hrs

1. Hydrochlorothiazide (HCTZ) is one of the drugs ordered for S.L.'s hypertension. Given she has diabetes, what teaching should be done for this client?

   Monitor carefully for hyperglycemia. Hyperglycemia is an adverse effect associated with hydrochlorothiazide. If hyperglycemia occurs, the primary care provider may have to alter the client's diet or adjust the insulin dose.

2. If S.L. takes her NPH insulin at 7 a.m., during what time period should the drug peak?

   1 p.m. and 7 p.m.

3. S.L. is complaining about severe hot flashes. She has a bottle of unused estrogen in her medi¬cine cabinet, and she says she is going to start taking it. How would you respond?

    1 p.m. and 7 p.m.

4. S.L.'s family knows to be alert to a possible hypoglycemic reaction around supper time related to her NPH insulin, but they are uncertain if they should anticipate a similar reaction to the Humalog insulin. What is the nurse's best response?

    Advise the risk of hypoglycemia is greatest 30-90 minutes after injection.

Discussion questions:

5. Discuss the role of the estrogen in the body.

    Estrogens are ovarian hormones that promote the development and maintenance of sexual characteristics in females, influence growth of female reproductive tissue and regulate and maintain the menstrual cycle. The presence estrogen has a major effect on bone mass because it blocking bone resorption. Estrogen elevates blood level of high- density lipoproteins and lower blood levels of low-density lipoproteins.

6. What kind of symptoms would the nurse expect to see in a client with hypothyroidism?

    Manifestations of hypothyroidism in adults include bradycardia, cold dry skin, brittle hair, low body temperature, fatigue, cold intolerance, flat affect, slowed cognition, and weight gain. Hypothyroidism is a chronic condition requiring lifelong hormone replacement therapy (HRT).

7. Discuss client teaching considerations the nurse should address with the client who has type 2 diabetes mellitus.

    The client should be advised to perform self blood glucose testing to monitor therapeutic benefit and to adhere to other regimens prescribed to control the disease, such as nutrition and exercise plan.

    The client should also be instructed to carry an emergency source of carbohydrate to treat hypoglycemia and carry emergency identification that provides identification to others that they are diabetic. Other teaching considerations include: allow insulin to warm to room temperature prior to injection to reduce local irritation; rotate injection sites to prevent irritation of tissues from repeated injections.

Critical Thinking Exercise: CHAPTER 12

Drugs Affecting Reproduction Answer Key

Note: *It is recommended that the following exercises be reviewed with a partner or in a small group to achieve maximum student interaction and to enhance critical thinking skills.*

Situation: A 19-year-old woman who recently married schedules an appointment for the first time in the women's clinic. She is here for a follow-up visit after her wedding to evaluate how she is doing on her newly prescribed birth control pills. She was prescribed a 6-month supply of Ortho-Novum prior to her wedding date. She is upset and describes the following: The first two months went well. Then, upon realizing she would have her period on her wedding night, she adjusted her dose to prematurely have her period "out of the way" of her wedding night. This was successful, but ever since then, she has had breakthrough bleeding all month long. She has also experienced severe leg cramping, and this last month she has had feelings of anxiety over a "racing heart." She "hates these pills," but doesn't want to get pregnant yet in her marriage. She verbalizes wanting to stop the pill until she and her husband can decide on an alternative form of birth control. You also discover in your history taking that she has just refilled a prescription for her Accutane because, after all this stress, her acne has returned.

1. What do you need to advise the client about her birth control options? What do you do about the Accutane and these birth control options?

   The first priority in this situation is the Accutane use without a plan for birth control. This presents an urgent problem that the young woman must understand. Accutane has been proven to cause birth defects in the first trimester that are typically fatal, including hydrocephaly and trisomies.

   The next issue is to encourage her to try a different dosage of the estrogen/progesterone mix birth control pills. Usually by adjusting the dosage of the estrogen/progesterone combination pills, the symptoms commonly described above will improve. If she wants to continue the use of Accutane, her only safe alternative form of birth control is a different brand of pill.

   If she is willing to discontinue the use of the Accutane, then she is free to try alternative, nonpharmacological forms of birth control such as foam and condoms, diaphragms and foams, etc. Be sure to instruct the client the chances of pregnancy are higher in these alternative choices if used independently; risk of pregnancy is further reduced if these forms of contraceptives are used simultaneously.

2. What are some of the uses for estrogen?

Estrogens are used in the treatment or prevention of an assortment of disorders, including: menopause, osteoporosis, menstrual disturbances, acne in females, lactation suppression. It is also used as in oral contraceptives and in prostate cancer treatment in men. If a client on estrogen therapy develops deep vein thrombosis (DVT) or cardiac complications, the estrogen therapy must be discontinued.

Matching Question:

3. Match each drug listed in the right column to its action listed in the left column.

Table 1

Drug	Therapeutic Action
Depo-Testosterone	Increases protein synthesis
Pitocin	Induces labor
Progesterone	Supresses ovulation
Nordette	Decreases endometriosis
Estrogen	Ovulation stimulant

Critical Thinking Exercise: CHAPTER 13

Drugs Affecting the Integumentary System Answer Key

Note: *It is recommended that the following exercises be reviewed with a partner or in a small group to achieve maximum student interaction and to enhance critical thinking skills.*

Situation: : A 17-year-old mother brings her 18-month-old son in the clinic for the second time this month for what she describes as "the bugs are back." Upon assessment, you find the youngster has a thick head of lice. You also notice nits on the blanket he is carrying and in the seams of his clothing. After reviewing his chart, you find he was diagnosed with head lice approximately two weeks prior and sent home with a bottle of Nix shampoo from your sample stock. Instructions were provided to the mother. You begin to question the mother of her understanding of the previous visit and how she used the shampoo. You find out she did shampoo the head of the youngster, but upon further questioning, you discover the young mother's roommate also has a 3- year-old who is a constant playmate; they even sleep together in the same bed. The physician makes a diagnosis of lice and orders Kwell be administered to all exposed family members, household members, and playmates.

1. What is your next course of action?

    The parents or responsible party for the playmate should be immediately notified so they can speak to the physician and provide appropriate consent for treatment.

    Rationale: The mother has parental consent privileges for her child, but cannot approve or authorize treatment for a child who is unrelated to her. Therefore, the provider may give another prescription or sample of the anti-parasitic Nix to the mother for her son. Provide enough for the mother, the roommate's child, and the roommate as well.

2. What directions should be given regarding pretreatment?

Inquire if the mother is pregnant or anyone in the household has allergic conditions. Inform the mother that, even with proper application, the medication may cause stinging, itching or rash. The medication should be used only as prescribed and the physician should be called immediately if any severe rashes, pain, seizures or hypersensitivity reactions occur following treatment. This information also needs to be shared with the mother of the three-year-old playmate.

Rationale: Antiparasitics are contraindicated in pregnant women. Young children or infants receiving this medicine need to be carefully monitored since adverse CNS conditions can occur.

Situation: You also discover upon closer examination of the child his scalp is reddened and he has areas of excoriations with pustules scattered randomly over the reddened areas. You suspect these may be infected areas because of the scratching. You confirm with your clinic's primary care provider that the child does have a secondary infection, probably impetigo.

---

3. What should be prescribed?

A Neosporin ointment applied locally, as well as an oral antibiotic, will be necessary to completely treat the impetigo. An antibiotic should be prescribed for the scalp infection. A 7-day course of Amoxicillin will be sufficient.

4. What other instructions would you want to provide for this mother?

After shampooing the hair of everyone in the household, wash all the sheets and pillowcases in hot, soapy water and then place in a hot dryer. All of the clothes that have been worn prior to the shampooing must also be washed before being worn again. The mother may also want to thoroughly vacuum the carpet and furniture. Washing all of the used towels and washcloths in hot, soapy water would also be recommended as would encouraging all family members to wash their hands after toileting.

Encourage the mother that this condition is easily treatable and that because her child has lice, it doesn't mean she is a bad mother. Help her to recognize that prevention through good hygiene is the most effective and least costly line of defense.

Matching Question:

5. Match the medication listed on the left to its appropriate therapeutic action on the right.

Table 1

Medication	Appropriate Therapeutic Action
Antiparasitics	Applied to living tissue in order to kill pathogens that may cause illness to the host
Bacteriostatic agents	Reduce the growth of organisms or prevent replication without killing the entire population
Soaps	A substance that breaks down particles to be washed away; not antibacterial by nature
Antiparasitics	Must be used with caution and with precise instructions for young children and the elderly due to the risk of CNS toxicity
Steroids	Can mask superinfections when used in conjunction with antibiotic creams or ointments
Cold water	The first line of treatment for burns
Emollients and protectants	Provides comfort either by their anti-inflammatory capabilities or by their lubricating properties
Prophylactic agents	Soothing and cooling; form a protective coating on the skin to keep out light, air and dust
Bactericidals	Kill bacterial organisms, except for viral, fungal or spore populations
Keratolytics	Soften and loosen the outer layer of skin; remove excess growth of the epidermis

Bibliography

Abrams, A. C., Goldsmith, T. L. (2003). *Clinical drug therapy: Rationales for nursing practice* (7th ed.). Philadelphia: Lippincott, Williams & Wilkins.

American Diabetes Association. *Tight diabetes control*. Retrieved February 15, 2005, from http://www.diabetes.org/type-1-diabetes/tight-control.jsp.

Carpenito-Moyet, L. J. (2003). *Handbook of nursing diagnosis* (10th ed.). Philadelphia: Lippincott, Williams & Wilkins.

Carpenito-Moyet, L. J. (2003). *Nursing diagnosis: Application to clinical practice*. (10th ed.). Philadelphia: Lippincott, Williams & Wilkins.

Craig, C., Stitzel, R. E. (2003). *Modern pharmacology with clinical applications* (6th ed.). Philadelphia: Lippincott, Williams & Wilkins.

Deglin, J. H., & Vallerand, A. H. (2004). *Davis's drug guide for nurses* (9th ed.). Philadelphia: F.A. Davis Company.

Dipiro, J. T., Talbert, R. L., Yee, G.C., Matzke, G. R., Wells, B.G., Posey, M. L. (2002). *Pharmacotherapy: A pathophysiologic approach* (5th ed.). New York: McGraw-Hill.

Evans, M. E., & Reiss, B. S., Broyles, B.E. (2001). *Pharmacological aspects of nursing care* (6th ed.). Stamford, CT: Thomson Delmar Learning.

Gahart, B. L., & Nazareno, A. R. (2004). *Intravenous medications 2005: A handbook for nurses and allied health professionals* (21st ed.). St. Louis, MO: Mosby.

GlaxoSmithKline. *Eskalith®/Eskalith CR®: Prescribing information*. Retrieved January 20, 2005, from http://www.gsk.com/products/prescriptionmedicines.jsp.

Haist, S. A., Robbins, J. B., Gomella, L. G. (2002). *Internal medicine on call* (3rd ed.). New York: McGraw-Hill/Appleton & Lange.

Hill, K., & Rolant, P.D. (2001). Mosby's rapid review series: *Nursing pharmacology* (2nd ed.). St. Louis, MO: Mosby.

Hodgson, B. B.(2004). *Saunders nursing drug handbook 2005*. Philadelphia: W. B. Saunders.

Institute for Safe Medication Practices. *Dangerous abbreviations and dose designations*. Retrieved January 21, 2005, from http://www.ismp.org/msaarticles/ specialissuetableprint.htm.

Institute for Safe Medication Practices. *ISMP's list of high alert medications*. Retrieved January 21, 2005, from http://www.ismp.org/MSAarticles/highalert.htm.

Joint Commission on Accreditation of Healthcare Organizations. Focus on five: Addicted to abbreviations? Break the habit! *Joint Commission Perspectives on Patient Safety* (January 2002) [newsletter]. Retrieved January 21, 2005, from http://www.jcrinc.com/subscribers/patientsafety.asp?durki=1080.

Joslin Diabetes Center. *Goals for blood glucose control*. Retrieved February 15, 2005, from http://www.joslin.harvard.edu/education/library/wbggoal.shtml.

Joslin Diabetes Center. *Questions and answers about Glucovance from Joslin Diabetes Center*. Retrieved January 21, 2005, from http://www.joslin.harvard.edu/education/library/glucovance.shtml

Karch, A. M. (2004). 2005 *Lippincott's nursing drug guide*. Philadelphia: Lippincott Williams & Wilkins.

Kee, J. L., & Hayes, E. R. (2002). *Pharmacology: A nursing process approach* (4th ed.). Philadelphia: W. B. Saunders.

Lacy, C. F., Armstrong, L. L., Goldman, M. P., & Lance, L. L. (2004). *Drug information handbook* (12th ed). Hudson, Ohio: Lexi-Comp, Inc.

Lehne, R. A. (2004). *Pharmacology for nursing care* (5th ed.). Philadelphia: W.B. Saunders Company.

Lewis, S. M., Heitkemper, M. M., & Dirsken, S. R. (2003). *Medical surgical nursing: Assessment and management of clinical problems* (6th ed.). St. Louis, MO: Mosby.

Lilley, L. L, & Aucker, R. S. (2001). *Pharmacology and the nursing process* (3rd ed.). St. Louis, MO: Mosby.

Linton, A.D., Matteson, M.A., & Maebius, N.K. (Eds.). (2000). *Introductory nursing care of adults*. Philadelphia: W.B. Saunders.

McEvoy, G. K. Miller, J., Litvak, K. *AHFS drug information* (2004). Bethesda, MD: American Society of Health System Pharmacists, Inc.

McKenry, L. M., & Salerno, E. (2002). *Mosby's pharmacology in nursing* (21st ed.). St. Louis, MO: Mosby.

Melander, S. D., Alexander C., Angel, S. W., Cooper, C., Egbert, P. A., Evinger, L. K., et al. (2004). *Review of critical care nursing: Case studies and applications* (3rd ed.). Philadelphia: W. B. Saunders Company.

National Diabetes Information Clearinghouse. (2001). *Medicines for people with diabetes*. Retrieved January 20, 2005, from http://diabetes.niddk.nih.gov/dm/pubs/medicines_ez/index.htm.

Nursing drug handbook. (2004) (25th ed.). Philadelphia: Lippincott, Williams & Wilkins

Pickar, G. D. (2003). *Dosage calculation* (7th ed.). Stamford, CT: Delmar Thomson Learning.

2005 Physicians' Desk Reference (2004) (59th ed.). Montvale, NJ: Thomson Healthcare.

Physicians' desk reference for nonprescription drugs and dietary supplements 2004 (25th ed.). Montvale, NJ: Thomson Healthcare.

Skidmore-Roth, L. (2004). *Mosby's 2005 nursing drug reference*. St. Louis, MO: Mosby.

Taylor, C., Lillis, C., LeMone, P., (2004). *Fundamentals of nursing: The art and science of care*. (5th ed.). Philadelphia: Lippincott, Williams & Wilkins.

Venes, D., Thomas, C. L., & Taber, C. W. (2004). *Taber's cyclopedic medical dictionary* (20th ed.). Philadelphia: F. A. Davis